Recent Results in Cancer Research 109

W. Hinkelbein G. Bruggmoser
R. Engelhardt M. Wannenmacher (Eds.)

Preclinical Hyperthermia

With 182 Figures and 40 Tables

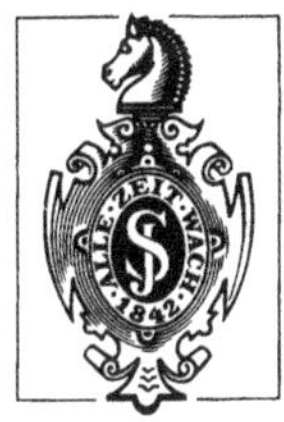

Springer-Verlag Berlin Heidelberg GmbH

Dr. Wolfgang Hinkelbein
Dipl. Phys. Gregor Bruggmoser
Prof. Dr. Rupert Engelhardt
Prof. Dr. Dr. Michael Wannenmacher

Abteilung Strahlentherapie (Med. Klinik)
Radiologische Klinik
Albert-Ludwigs-Universität
Hugstetter Straße 55, 7800 Freiburg, FRG

DOI 10.1007/978-3-642-83263-5

Library of Congress Cataloging-in-Publication Data
Preclinical hyperthermia / W. Hinkelbein ... [et al.] (eds.).
p. cm. - (Recent results in cancer research; 109)
Papers presented during an International Symposium on "Preclinical Hyperthermia and Combined Treatment Modalities in Normal Tissues and Tumors", held Dec. 5-6, 1986 in Freiburg, West Germany.
Includes bibliographies and index.

1. Cancer - Thermotherapy - Evaluation - Congresses. 2. Cancer - Adjuvant treatment - Evaluation - Congresses. I. Hinkelbein, W. (Wolfgang), 1948- . II. International Symposium on "Preclinical Hyperthermia and Combined Treatment Modalities in Normal Tissues and Tumors" (1986: Freiburg im Breisgau, Germany) III. Series.
[DNLM: 1. Combined Modality Therapy - congresses. 2. Hyperthermia, Induced - congresses. 3. Neoplasms - therapy - congresses.
W1 RE106P v. 109 / QZ 266 P923 1986]
RC261.R35 vol. 109 [RC271.T5] 616.99'4
s-dc19 [616.99'40632] DNLM/DLC 88-6464

Preface

The rate of local failure and the poor control of systemic disease constitute a big challenge for all physicians involved in cancer therapy. It is for this reason that we have to consider all treatment modalities which either can have toxic effects on tumors or are able to enhance the action of radio- and chemotherapy. Hyperthermia is a measure which can do both. Currently, hyperthermia is coming into clinical use in locoregional (superficial tumors and deep-seated tumors in the pelvis), whole-body (systemic disease), and local perfusion (mainly tumors of the extremities) applications. Heat treatment is regularly used in combination with either chemotherapy or irradiation, the optimism underlying such treatment being based on experimental data gained in recent years.

In this situation it is very useful that clinicians and scientists are discussing together preclinical hyperthermia with respect to its clinical relevance. The most interesting points are the importance of thermotolerance for the radiosensitizing effect of heat, the effects of combined treatment modalities on normal tissues and tumors, and the sequencing and timing of the therapeutic measures involved. Particular attention should be paid to the experiments with human tumor material.

The main purpose of this book is to protect the initial clinical trials with hyperthermia against avoidable errors and to help design ongoing clinical studies.

Freiburg, March 1988 M. Wannenmacher

Contents

*List of Contributors**

* The address of the principal author is given on the first page of each contribution.

[1] Page on which contribution begins.

Modification of Heat Action and Thermal Enhancement of Radio- and Chemotherapy

*Hyperthermic Toxicity and the Modulation of Heat Damage to Cell Protein Synthesis in HeLa Cells**

R. H. Burdon

Department of Bioscience and Biotechnology, Todd Centre, University of Strathclyde, Glasgow G4 ONR, Scotland

Introduction

The possibility that heat shock proteins (hsps) might be involved in the development of thermotolerance is suggested by a number of experimental approaches, including mutational analysis of hsp genes (Craig and Jacobson 1984) and kinetic analysis of hsp levels and thermotolerance development (Landry et al. 1982; Li and Werb 1982; Li and Mak 1985; Laszlo and Li 1985). Nevertheless, one finding of experiments aimed at determining the cytotoxic effects of hyperthermia on cultured mammalian cells was that tolerance to hyperthermic toxicity could be achieved by depletion of calcium ions from the culture medium (Lamarche et al. 1985). Moreover, addition of the protein synthesis inhibitor cycloheximide did not prevent the development of thermotolerance after hyperthermia (Hall 1983; Widerlitz et al. 1986). The fact that both calcium depletion and cycloheximide addition can block heat-induced hsp gene activation casts some doubt on the possible role of hsps in thermotolerance development.

In order to investigate this dilemma, and because cell killing is suggested to be related to the ability of cells to recover their cellular protein synthetic capacity (Schamhart et al. 1984), we have examined the effect of heat on cellular protein synthesis in relation to these observations.

Hyperthermia and Protein Synthesis Inhibition

An immediate effect of hyperthermic treatment of HeLa cell cultures is the inhibition of cellular protein synthesis (Fig. 1). Whilst rapid recovery is possible on return to 37° C, it nevertheless depends on the severity of the initial hyperthermic treatment. That the initial inhibitory effects may be due, amongst other things, to the damaging effects of oxygen-derived free radicals is suggested by the fact that pretreatment of the cells with 5 mM sodium azide or 50 mM mannitol decreased

* This work was partly supported by grants made available by the Cancer Research Campaign and the Scottish Home and Health Department.

Recent Results in Cancer Research, Vol. 109

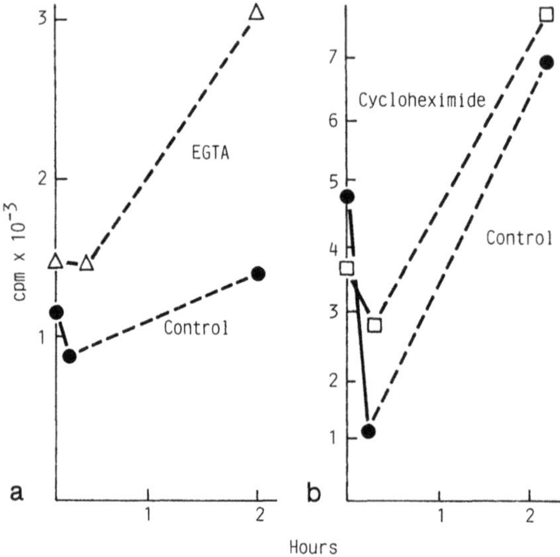

Fig. 1 a, b. Effects of EGTA and cycloheximide on the heat-induced inhibition of ^{35}S-methionine incorporation into HeLa cell protein. Triplicate HeLa cell cultures were grown as monolayers (0.5×10^6 cells per 2.5 cm diameter dish) for 24 h in Eagles MEM medium supplemented by 10% calf serum. In **a**, triplicate cultures were pretreated with 0.5 mM EGTA for 15 min at 37° before being subjected to 45° C for 10 min (△—△) and returned to 37° C for 2 h (△----△). Untreated control cells were subjected to 45° for 10 min (○—○) and then 37° C for 2 h (○----○). **b** is similar to **a**, but cells were pretreated with 20 µg/ml cycloheximide (□) or left as controls (●). The incorporation of ^{35}S-methionine into protein after the above treatments is measured over 30 min at 37° C. (See Burdon et al. 1987)

the extent of the initial heat-induced inhibition of protein synthesis (Burdon et al. 1987). Conversely, treatment with diethyldithiocarbamate (an inhibitor of superoxide dismutase and glutathione peroxidase) has a marked sensitizing effect (Burdon et al. 1987). Despite this suggested involvement of oxygen-derived radicals, we found that the ability of metronizadole to increase the inhibitory effect of heat was quite limited. This drug, which is known to sensitise hypoxic cells in radiotherapy (Willson 1977), increased the inhibitory effect of 45° C for 10 min by only 15%, and decreased subsequent recovery by only 20% at a concentration of 0.01% (w/v).

This general experimental approach was extended to include an examination of the effects of calcium ion depletion and cycloheximide addition. From Fig. 1 a it can be seen that EGTA pretreatment of HeLa cells dramatically reduced the inhibitory effects of heat and stimulated recovery of protein synthetic capacity. Cycloheximide treatment had similar although less pronounced effects (Fig. 1 b).

Table 1. Effect of hyperthermia and lipid peroxidation in HeLa cells[a]

Expt.	Treatment	nmol TBA reactive product per 10^{10} cells ± SD
1	37° C	327.6 ± 40.9
	45° C 60 min	450.5 ± 204.8
2	37° C	593.9 ± 16.4
	45° C	368.6 ± 24.5
	45° C 15 min, 37° 2 h	532.4 ± 8.2
	42° C 1 h	327.6 ± 8.2
	42° C 2 h	409.6 ± 28.6
3	37° C	716.8 ± 100.3
	45° C 10 min	552.9 ± 24.5
	45° C 10 min plus cycloheximide (20 µg/ml)	430.1 ± 16.3
	45° C 10 min plus EGTA (0.5 mM)	655.3 ± 32.7

[a] Triplicate monolayer cultures of HeLa cells were established with 10^7 cells in 20 ml medium, in a flat plastic culture vessel of 175 cm^2. The cells were allowed to grow to 2.5×10^7 (3 days) before exposure to the various experimental conditions described. After treatment, each monolayer culture was washed three times with 0.9% NaCl (w/v) and the cells scraped off into 2 ml 0.9% NaCl for malonaldehyde measurement. Trichloroacetic acid was added to a final concentration of 10% (w/v) and the suspension centrifuged at 2000 *g* for 5 min. 1 ml of the supernatant was removed and added to 1 ml 0.75% 2-thiobarbituric acid. Samples were heated at 90° C for 20 min and then spun at 10000 *g* for 10 min. The levels of thiobarbituric acid reactive products in each supernatant fraction were determined by measuring the difference between absorbances at 532 and 580 nm, and using malonaldehyde as standard. (See Gutteridge 1986; Walls et al. 1976)

Hyperthermia and Lipid Peroxidation

In view of the possibility of free radical involvement and because membranes have been claimed to be primary cellular targets for hyperthermic damage, the levels of lipid peroxidation in HeLa cells following hyperthermia have been examined. A significant increase in lipid peroxidation (Table 1) following prolonged hyperthermia was difficult to detect routinely by the TBA method (see Gutteridge 1986; Burdon et al. 1987). However, a problem with such prolonged hyperthermia is that a major portion of the cells in the culture will have become non-viable (approx. 80%). When shorter exposure times are examined, or less high temperatures, a decrease in TBA-reactive material is actually observed (see Table 1). This decrease is blocked by EGTA and accelerated by cycloheximide. It may well be that there is a significant, but low, steady state level of lipid hydroperoxide in the HeLa cell cultures. On brief heat treatment these peroxides might be broken down and so lessen the level of TBA-reactive material. Whether or not the breakdown products are subsequently damaging to the protein synthetic system will have to be examined.

Table 2. Effect of *t*-butylhydroperoxide on lipid peroxidation in HeLa cells[a]

Treatment	nmol TBA reactive product per 10^{10} cells ± SD
None	409.6 ± 20.5
50 μM *t*-butylhydroperoxide (3 h)	675.8 ± 40.9
50 μM *t*-butylhydroperoxide (3 h) plus cycloheximide (20 μg/ml)	430.1 ± 20.5
50 μM *t*-butylhydroperoxide (3 h) plus EGTA (0.5 mM)	552.9 ± 81.8

[a] The procedures adopted were as described for Table 1.

Calcium Ions, Cycloheximide and Lipid Peroxidation

Further experiments were carried out in light of the effects of EGTA and cycloheximide. Calcium ions have previously been reported to alter the rate of lipid peroxidation observed when liposomes, or erythrocyte membranes, are exposed to iron salts (see Halliwell and Gutteridge 1985). This may be through effects on the organisation of lipids in the membranes. The further experiments performed did, however, indicate that cycloheximide can influence events involving free radicals. For example, *t*-butylhydroperoxide treatment of HeLa cells increases levels of cellular lipid peroxidation (Table 2) as well as inhibiting cellular protein synthesis. What is important, however, is that both the increase in lipid peroxidation and the inhibition of protein synthesis brought about by *t*-butylhydroperoxide can be prevented by cycloheximide (Table 2, Fig. 2). EGTA was also protective but to a lesser degree (Table 2). Lipid peroxidation in this situation is likely to be initiated by a

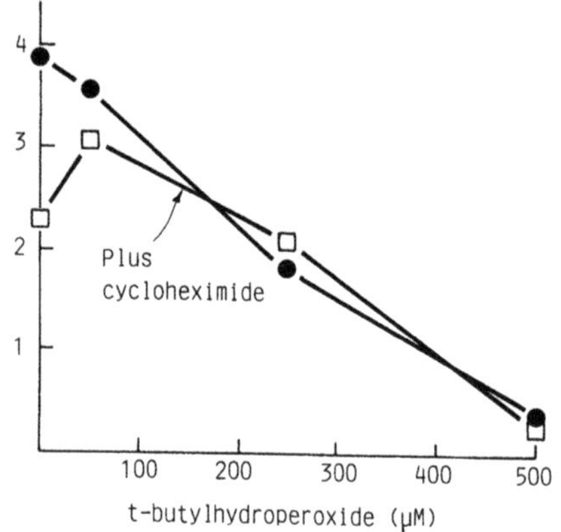

Fig. 2. Effects of *t*-butylhydroperoxide and cycloheximide on ^{35}S-methionine incorporation into HeLa cell protein. Triplicate HeLa cell cultures as in Fig. 1 were exposed for 60 min with varying concentrations of *t*-butylhydroperoxide in the presence (□) or absence (●) of 20 μg/ml cycloheximide. After such exposure the cultures were washed and then assayed for ability to incorporate ^{35}S-methionine into protein over 30 min at 37° C as in Fig. 1

radical species derived from the *t*-butylhydroperoxide, and the observation that cycloheximide can neutralise this process may have relevance to the situation following hyperthermia. In this latter situation explanations for the heat-induced increase in lipid peroxidation may be different and embrace changes in cellular membrane structures and altered compartmentation. Such changes may lead to abnormal reactions producing oxidative stress and subsequent lipid peroxidation that are not directly affected by cycloheximide. On the other hand potentially damaging radicals resulting from the heat-induced lipid peroxidation events may be neutralised, or scavenged in some way, by cycloheximide. Recent data indicate that cycloheximide will inhibit the heat-induced destabilisation of cellular RNA (Ralhan and Johnston 1986).

Recovery of Protein Synthetic Activity After Hyperthermia and Development of Tolerance in the System

As already mentioned, recovery of protein synthesis following hyperthermia is important, and whilst it can be stimulated by EGTA and cycloheximide, it can be blocked by low levels of actinomycin D sufficient to block ribosomal RNA synthesis. This, together with molecular hybridisation experiments, has led to the suggestion that heat-induced damage to components of the protein synthetic system might be rectified by the import of fresh components such as ribosomes from the nucleolus (Burdon 1987). Recovery of protein synthesis is also prevented if cellular levels of non-protein thiol are depressed, although not by inhibitors of superoxide dismutase (Burdon et al. 1987). However, it is known that intracellular levels of superoxide dismutase increase considerably after heat shock (Loven et al. 1985).

Following recovery from an initial hyperthermic exposure (45° C, 10 min), the protein synthetic system manifests an ephemeral (24-h) thermotolerance, inasmuch as a second exposure to hyperthermia within that time results in a lesser inhibitory effect followed by another recovery (Fig. 3). The ability to mount this second round of "recovery" is also prevented by low doses of actinomycin D (Fig. 3). Another reagent which will impair this manifestation of thermotolerance in the protein synthetic system is benzaldehyde (Fig. 4). Benzaldehyde, an antitumour agent, is already known to impair the development of cellular thermotolerance (Mizuno et al. 1984). The explanation for the effectiveness of benzaldehyde in this context is not clear. We find it neither blocks heat-induced hsp gene activation nor does it significantly increase levels of lipid peroxidation, although it is believed to modify the proteins of mammalian cell membranes (Miyakawa et al. 1979). As might be anticipated, however, the protective effects of cycloheximide and EGTA (see Fig. 1) continued to be manifest even when cells were exposed to a second period of hyperthermia.

Thus while hsps might be involved in the normal development of thermotolerance in the protein synthetic system following hyperthermia, possibly by stabilising the production of ribosomes (Burdon 1987), other routes to thermotolerance development are possible. Indeed, these need not necessarily involve hsp gene activation. For example, EGTA or cycloheximide may simply produce tolerance as a

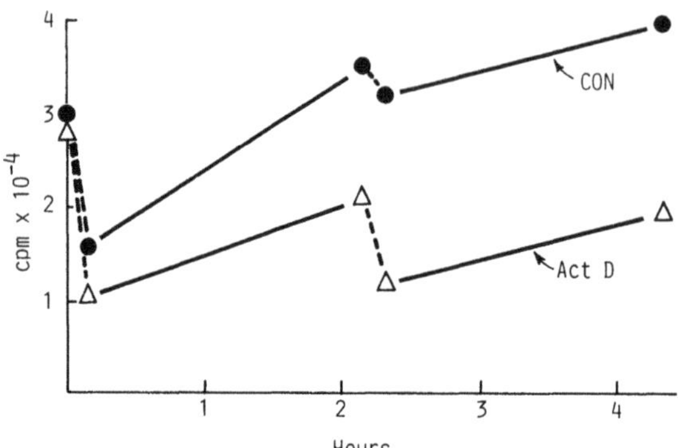

Fig. 3. The effect of low levels of actinomycin D *(Act D)* on the ability of HeLa cells to incorporate ^{35}S-methionine into protein following repeated hyperthermic tratments. Triplicate HeLa cell monolayer cultures were set up as described in Fig. 1. After 24 h, actinomycin D at 0.05 μg/ml was added to one set (△) whereas there were no addition to the set of control *(CON)* cultures (●). After 15 min, each set was subjected to 45° C for 10 min (-----), recovery for 2 h at 37° (—), a second 10-min treatment at 45° (-----) and a second 2-h period of recovery at 37° C (—). After the various treatments the cultures were washed three times with fresh medium and then their ability to incorporate ^{35}S-methionine at 37° C for 30 min was determined as in Fig. 1

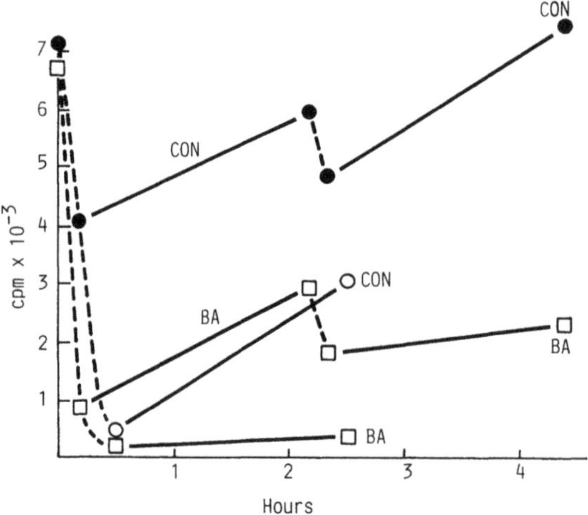

Fig. 4. The effect of benzaldehyde *(BA)* on the ability of HeLa cells to incorporate ^{35}S-methionine into protein following repeated hyperthermic treatments. The procedure adopted was exactly as described in Fig. 3 except that 0.3 mM benzaldehyde was used in place of actinomycin D. *CON*, control cultures

result of "quenching" of "limiting" the potential free radical mediated damage (Wolff et al. 1986). Whilst such a proposal stems from the use of "unnatural" agents, it may be a useful step to a mechanistic explanation of naturally induced thermotolerance. An alternative insight offered by the use of EGTA and cycloheximide is into the mechanisms underlying the activation of the hsp genes themselves. The observation that *both* reagents block hsp gene activation is significant, although cycloheximide only blocks hsp gene activation if added during the recovery period at 37° C, following the initial hyperthermic treatment. Addition during the initial hyperthermia has no effect (Slater et al. 1981), suggesting that if free radicals are involved in the induction mechanism then they are more likely to be derived *subsequent* to the initial heat-induced lipid peroxidation changes.

Summary

That some of the effects of hyperthermia on HeLa cell protein synthesis may involve free radical activity is suggested by experiments with free radical scavengers. A possible source of damaging free radicals induced by heat may lie in peroxidative events within lipid-containing membranes. These can be blocked by EGTA. Other experiments with *t*-butylhydroperoxide indicate that cycloheximide can also neutralise peroxidative effects. These effects are discussed in the light of observations that calcium depletion (or EGTA treatment) can induce thermotolerance and that cycloheximide does not prevent the development of thermotolerance.

References

Burdon RH (1987) Thermotolerance and the heat shock proteins. In: Bowler K (ed) Animals cells and temperature, symp 41, Society for Experimental Biology. 269-283

Burdon RH, Gill V, Rice-Evans C (1987) Oxidative stress and heat shock protein induction in human cells. Free Radical Res Commun 3: 129-139

Craig EA, Jacobson K (1984) Mutations of the heat inducible 70 kilodalton genes of yeast confer temperature sensitive growth. Cell 38: 841-849

Gutteridge JM (1986) Aspects to consider when detecting and measuring lipid peroxidation. Free Radical Res Commun 1: 173-184

Hall BG (1983) Yeast thermotolerance does not require protein synthesis. J Bacteriol 156: 1363-1365

Halliwell B, Gutteridge JM (1985) Free radicals in biology and medicine. Clarendon, Oxford

Lamarche S, Chretien P, Landry J (1985) Inhibition of the heat shock response and synthesis of glucose regulated proteins in Ca^{2+}-deprived rat hepatoma cells. Biochem Biophys Res Commun 131: 868-876

Landry J, Bernier D, Chretien P, Nichole LM, Tanguay RM, Marceau N (1982) Synthesis and degradation of heat shock proteins during development and decay of thermotolerance. Cancer Res 42: 2457-2461

Laszlo A, Li GC (1985) Heat-resistant variant of Chinese hamster fibroblasts altered in expression of heat shock protein. Proc Natl Acad Sci, USA 82: 8029-8033

Li GC, Werb Z (1982) Correlation between synthesis of heat shock proteins and development of thermotolerance in Chinese hamster fibroblasts. Proc Natl Acad Sci USA 79: 3218-3222

Li GC, Mak JY (1985) Induction of heat shock protein synthesis in murine tumours during the development of thermotolerance. Cancer Res 45: 3816-3827

Miyakana T, Zundel J-L, Sakaguchi K (1979) Selective inhibitory effect of benzaldehyde on the growth of SV40-transformed cells. Biochem Biophys Res Commun 87: 1024-1030

Mizuno S, Ishida A, Miwa N (1984) Enhancement of hyperthermic cytotoxicity and prevention of thermotolerance induction by benzaldehyde in SV-40 transformed cells In: Overgaard J (ed) Hyperthermic oncology, vol 1. Taylor and Francis, London, pp 99-102

Ralhan R, Johnston GS (1986) Destabilisation of cytoplasmic mouse mammary tumour RNA by heat shock: prevention by cycloheximide pretreatment. Biochem Biophys Res Commun 137: 1028-1034

Schamhart DHJ, van Walraven HS, Wiegant FAC, Linnemans WAM, van Rijn J, van den Berg J, van Wijk R (1984) Thermotolerance in cultured hepatoma cells: cell viability, cell morphology, protein synthesis and heat shock protein. Radiat Res 98: 82-95

Slater A, Cato ACB, Sillar GM, Kioussis J, Burdon RH (1981) The pattern of protein synthesis induced by heat shock of Hela cells. Eur J Biochem 117: 341-346

Walls R, Kumar KS, Hochstein P (1976) Aging of human erythrocytes. Arch Biochem Biophys 174: 463-468

Widerlitz RB, Magun BE, Gerner EW (1986) Effects of cycloheximide on thermotolerance expression, heat shock protein synthesis, and heat shock protein mRNA accumulation in rat fibroblasts. Mol Cell Biol 6: 1088-1094

Willson RL (1977) Metronidazole (Flagyl) in cancer radiotherapy: a historical introduction. In: Fingold SM, McFadzean JA, Roe FJC (eds) Metronidazole: proceedings, Montreal. Excerpta Medica, Amsterdam, p 185

Wolff SP, Graner A, Dean RT (1986) Free radicals, lipids, and protein degradation. Trends Biochem Sci 11: 27-31.

Membranes as Targets for Hyperthermic Cell Killing

A.W.T. Konings

Radiopathologisch Laboratorium, Rijksuniversiteit van Groningen, Bloemsingel 1,
9713 BZ Groningen, The Netherlands

Introduction

The purpose of this review is to describe briefly the latest findings concerning the possible role of cellular membranes as a primary target in hyperthermic cell killing. Mammalian cell membranes mainly consist of phospholipids, cholesterol, and proteins. The structure of lipids and proteins can be characterized by their equilibrium state and thermal fluctuations around it. The equilibrium state of membrane lipids is the bilayer with the lipid molecules oriented perpendicular to the bilayer plane. This equilibrium state is responsible for the function of a membrane as a permeability barrier. Exposure to temperatures above 37° C tends to cause phase separation of non-bilayer-forming lipids, manifest by appearance of three-dimensional aggregates of tubular micelles (inverted micelles). This may severely influence permeability. The equilibrium state of intrinsic membrane proteins in most cases is given by one or more bilayer-spanning α-helices. Positional fluctuations of whole proteins is essential for many membrane processes.

The lipids and proteins in a membrane are in dynamic equilibrium with each other. The physical state of the lipid component of the membrane may have significant effects on the properties of the proteins and as such modulate their conformation and activity. When the temperature is raised, the mobility of the phospholipid acyl chains and head group increases and a less ordered state is the result. The lipids of most biomembranes appear to exist mainly in the fluid state at normal physiological temperatures. Decreasing the temperature will ultimately rigidify the membranes. Below the "phase transition temperature" the molecules are arranged in an ordered quasicrystalline or gel state. It may also be that only parts of the membrane will rigidify after lowering the temperature, because for only some of the lipids is the transition temperature reached. This may lead to lipid phase separation accompanied by a clustering of proteins as depicted in Fig. 1.

From this introduction it may be clear that small temperature changes can drastically alter the structure of biomembranes and as a result of this, influence many membrane-related cellular functions. An illustration of heat-induced changes in the plasma membrane of a cell is given in Fig. 2.

Recent Results in Cancer Research, Vol. 109

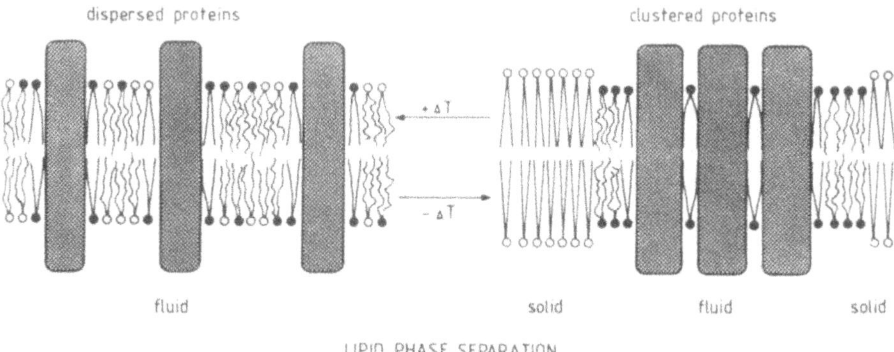

Fig. 1. Effect of temperature changes on the fluidity of phospholipids in a protein-containing bilayer. The *small circles* represent the polar headgroups of the phospholipids. The *tails on the circles* represent the fatty acyl chains; these may be in a fluid or rigid state, depending on the actual temperature and the type of lipid (transition temperature)

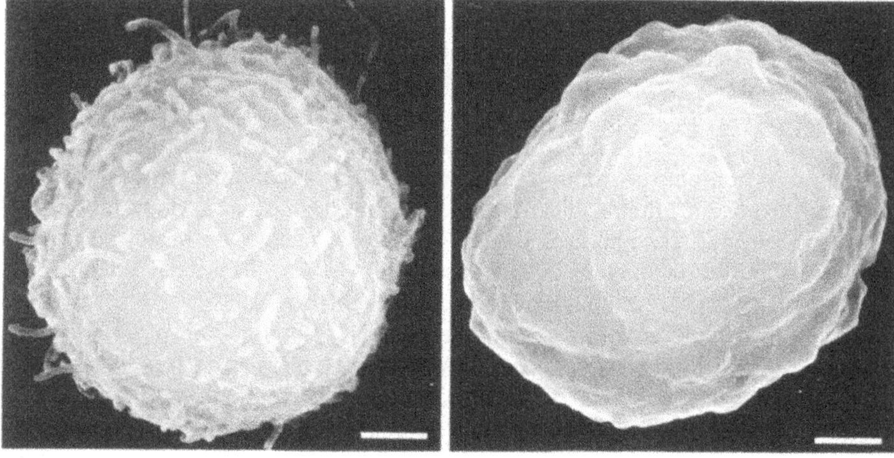

Fig. 2. Surface morphology of a control *(left)* and heated *(right)* mouse fibroblast LM cell from suspension cultures. Hyperthermia treatment was for 30 min at 43° C. Cell surface changes are characterized by a reduction in the number of microvilli and an increased bleb formation. Length scale on the micrograph: 1 μm. (Picture taken by C. E. Hulstaert, Medical Electronmicroscopy, Groningen)

Relation of Cellular Lipid Composition and Thermal Sensitivity

Cholesterol is an important lipid molecule of the plasma membrane of eukaryotic cells. This molecule has been shown to exert a variety of physical effects on a phospholipid bilayer, including permeability changes. This is probably the result of the ordering of phospholipid acyl chains by cholesterol, when these lipids are in the fluid state. As stated above, membrane functions may be controlled through

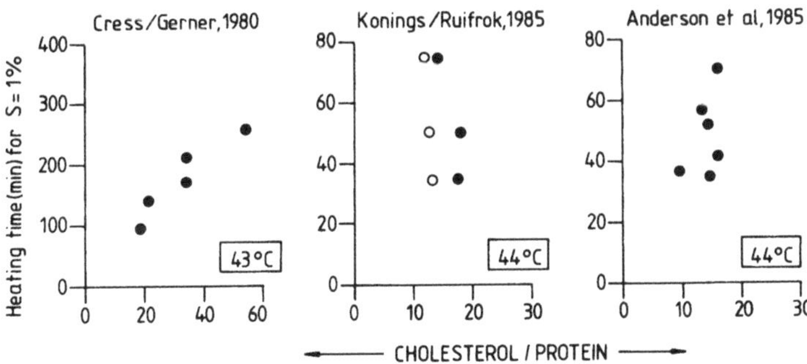

Fig. 3. Relation of heat sensitivity and cholesterol/protein ratio in different cell lines. Data are given as μg cholesterol per mg protein. The *open circles* represent data points of the different cells, cultured in the same medium. Although these cells contained less cholesterol, the heat sensitivity was not altered

alterations in lipid fluidity and lipid organization. As a result of this, protein conformational changes may occur which might become expressed in altered catalytic activities of membrane-bound enzymes. For instance the Ca^{2+} pump activity of sarcoplasmatic reticulum is modulated by membrane fluidity. Cholesterol decreases the energetic efficiency of Ca^{2+} pumping (Ca^{2+}/ATP ratio).

Raising the temperature of cells will result in more fluid membranes, especially because of the higher degree of disorder of the phospholipid acyl chains. It may be expected that cells with a higher cholesterol content will be more heat resistant because the more cholesterol is present in the membranes, the less increase in membrane fluidity might occur.

Different Cell Lines

The above-mentioned hypothesis was first tested by Cress and Gerner (1980), who measured the cholesterol content of five mammalian cell lines and reported a positive correlation between heat sensitivity at 43° C and cholesterol levels, when expressed on the basis of cellular protein. Comparable investigations have since been performed by other groups, but correlations similar to those reported by Cress and Gerner (1980) have never been confirmed. In Fig. 3 the results of Cress and Gerner are compared with those of two other groups. The cholesterol/protein ratios of the cells examined by Anderson et al. (1985) and by Konings and Ruifrok (1985) did not differ very much, while clear differences in heat sensitivity were seen. We (Konings and Ruifrok 1985) found that when the three cell lines used were adapted to a different nutrient medium, less cholesterol was present in the cells but the heat sensitivity did not alter. We believe that especially the latter experiments provide evidence that cholesterol is not a determining factor in heat sensitivity. This conclusion is supported by other reports in the literature. Yatvin et al. reported in 1983 that a change in membrane viscosity of P-388 and V-79 cells by cholesteryl hemisuccinate had no effect on heat sensitivity. Anderson et al.

(1984) found that in heat-resistant variants of B16 melanoma cells the cholesterol/protein ratio and cholesterol/phospholipid ratio decreased with increasing heat resistance. So this is just the opposite of what was expected. Raaphorst et al. (1985) could not observe a relationship between cholesterol as well as phospholipid content of cells with thermal sensitivity of normal and X-ray transformed C3H 10T½ mouse embryo cells.

State of Thermotolerance

If thermosensitivity of cells is determined by membrane lipid composition and membrane fluidity, one might expect that in these respects thermotolerant cells would be different from normal cells. Gerner et al. (1980) reported an increase in cholesterol content of CHO cells during the development of thermotolerance (TT) at 42° C. No such effects were evident in experiments reported by Gonzalez-Mendez et al. (1982), Anderson and Parker (1982), Konings and Ruifrok (1985), or Burns et al. (1986). Extensive investigations on thermotolerant mouse fibroblasts (Konings and Ruifrok 1985) have also revealed that no differences were apparent in phospholipid composition, fatty acid composition of the phospholipids, or membrane fluidity. Table 1 shows no effect of TT in relation to cholesterol and phospholipid content and Table 2 illustrates that membrane fluidity of normal and

Table 1. Content of cholesterol and phospholipids in normal and thermotolerant fibroblasts

Condition of cells	Cholesterol (μg/mg prot.)	Phospholipids (μg/mg prot.)	Ratio chol/PL
Normal	12±1	119± 8	0.10
Thermotolerant	13±1	118±10	0.11

Data are mean ±SD of ten independent experiments.

Table 2. Fluidity measurements in normal and thermotolerant fibroblasts

Condition of the cells	Polarization values (P) and order parameters (S)					
	Whole cells		Plasma membranes		Liposomes	
	P	S	P	S	P	S
Normal	0.240±0.011	0.69±0.01	0.238±0.004	0.66±0.02	0.200±0.007	0.69±0.02
Thermo-tolerant	0.238±0.013	0.69±0.02	0.242±0.005	0.68±0.02	0.200±0.007	0.69±0.02

The fluidity is measured with diphenylhexatriene (DPH) and expressed in polarization values *(P)* or with the ESR probe 5-nitroxystearate and expressed in order parameters *(S)*. The data for P are the mean±SD of eight independent experiments and for S, the mean±SD of three independent experiments. Thermotolerance was achieved by incubation of the cells for 8 min at 44° C followed by 5 h at 37° C.

thermotolerant cells was the same. Additionally, when the phospholipids were extracted from the cells and reconstituted into bilayers of liposomes, no difference in membrane fluidity could be detected. The fluidity measurements were performed with two completely different methods. The ESR probe 5-nitroxystearate was used and the fluorescent probe diphenylhexatriene (DPH). The two probes have different locations in the lipid bilayer. Due to its penetration deep into the bilayer, especially DPH is a sensitive detector of conformational fluctuations of the phospholipid chains. Lepock et al. (1981) also observed a lack of correlation between thermotolerance and membrane lipid fluidity, although their experiments were hampered by the fact that two-thirds of the cells had lost clonogenic ability.

Manipulation of Fatty Acid Composition

Cellular Heat Sensitivity

From the data discussed thus far one may conclude that cholesterol is not an important factor in the regulation of heat sensitivity. Changing the cholesterol content in cells did not alter the cell's vulnerability to a heat treatment (Konings and Ruifrok 1985).

Experiments with *Escherichia coli* by Overath et al. (1970) showed that linolenic acid (18:3) supplemented cells were incapable of growth at temperatures above 40° C whereas oleic acid (18:1) supplemented cells could grow at temperatures up to 45° C. So the cells with the more fluid membranes were more heat sensitive. Similar observations have been made by McElhaney (1974) using *Acholeplasma laidlawii.* These observations were in accordance with an early postulation by Heilbrunn (1924), that the physical state of cellular fats might be related to the extent of cell killing by heat. Yatvin (1977) was the first to produce cell survival curves of *E. coli* supplemented with 18:1 or 18:3. His findings were as expected and in line with the observations of Overath et al. (1970) 18:3 supplemented cells were more heat sensitive than the 18:1 supplemented cells. This differential heat sensitivity is illustrated in Fig. 4. The observations with bacterial cells were followed up and confirmed with L1210 cells and mouse fibroblasts (Guffy et al. 1982; Konings and Ruifrok 1985). Cultured L1210 murine leukemia cells were supplemented with either oleic acid (18:1) or docosahexanoic acid (22:6). A fatty acid concentration dependent heat sensitivity was found, as shown in Fig. 5. Comparable results were obtained by arachidonic acid (20:4) supplementation of the mouse fibroblasts. The enrichment in polyunsaturated fatty acyl (PUFA) chains of the phospholipids of these cells was quite extensive in all subcellular fractions (from about 8% in normal cells to about 40% in the modified cells). The change in PUFA content was accompanied by a change in fluidity in all fractions. This is illustrated in Table 3. Although the difference in fatty acid composition in the fibroblasts was dramatic, the difference in heat sensitivity (Fig. 8a) was small as compared to the data obtained with the L1210 cells.

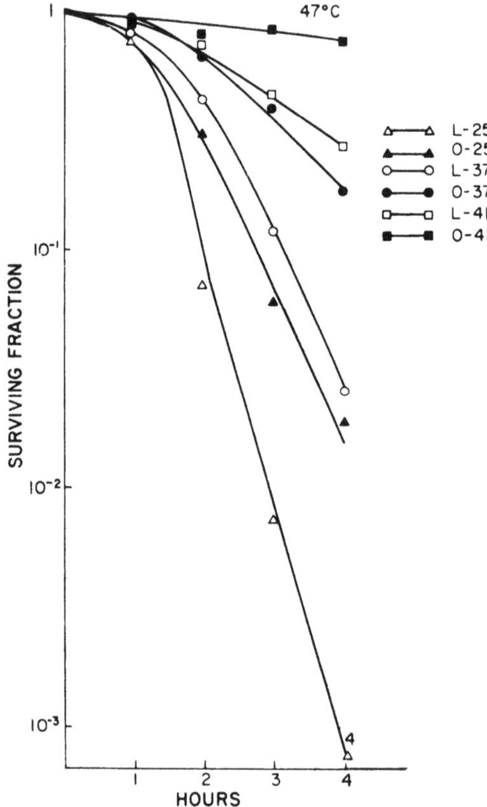

Fig. 4. Surviving fraction of linoleic *(L)* and oleic *(O)* acid substituted *E. coli* K1060 grown at 25°, 37°, or 41° C and heated at 47° C for times up to 4 h. (Yatvin 1977)

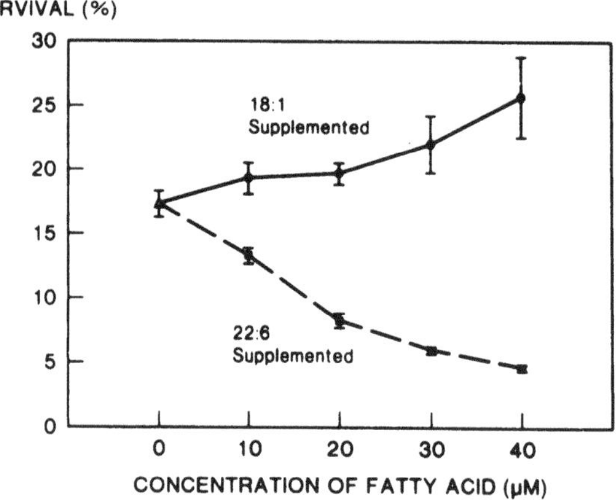

Fig. 5. Effect of concentration of supplemented fatty acid on thermosensitivity. L1210 cells were grown in media supplemented with either 22:6 or 18:1 at 0–40 μM and then heated at 42° C for 2 h. (Guffy et al. 1982)

Table 3. Polyunsaturated fatty acyl *(PUFA)* chains and degree of fluidity in subfractions of mouse fibroblasts

Cell fractions	Normal cells		Modified cells	
	% PUFA[a]	P[b]	% PUFA	P
Plasma membranes	6.2±0.8	0.247±0.006	44.3±6.8	0.223±0.005
Nuclear membranes	5.1±1.3	0.207±0.022	42.4±9.3	0.182±0.006
Mitochondria	5.5±1.1	0.200±0.007	37.9±8.1	0.184±0.010
Microsomes	9.0±2.4	0.242±0.005	41.7±9.7	0.202±0.008

[a] Polyunsaturated fatty acyl chains of the phospholipid fraction.
[b] The fluidity is measured as the degree of fluorescence polarization *(P)* of diphenylhexatriene (DPH). Data are given as means ± SD of four independent experiments.

State of Thermotolerance

It was of interest to examine whether cells with more fluid membranes (20:4 substituted cells) were still able to reach a normal state of thermotolerance. Therefore normal and PUFA-substituted mouse fibroblasts were heated for 8 min, at 44° C, a heat treatment which is not lethal to the cells but triggers the development of thermotolerance during incubation of the cells at 37° C. The cells with the more fluid membranes were still able to build up thermotolerance. This is shown in Fig. 6. The extent of the acquired thermotolerance of the PUFA cells was comparable to the acquisition of thermotolerance seen in normal cells (Konings 1985). At the level of 10% survival, cellular heat resistance is increased by a factor of about 2.3 for both the normal cells and the PUFA cells. Recently Burns et al. (1986) came to the same conclusion using L1210 leukemia cells.

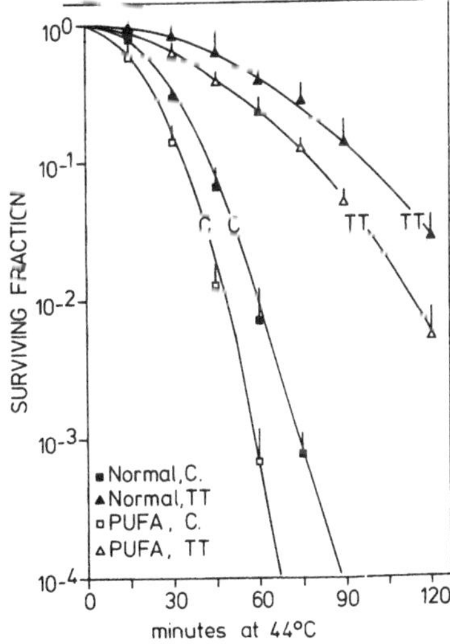

Fig. 6. Development of thermotolerance *(TT)* in normal and PUFA cells. Thermotolerance was obtained by incubation of the cells for 8 min at 44° C, followed by 5 h at 37° C. (Konings 1985)

Membrane-Active Agents

Many so-called membrane-active agents modify hyperthermic cell killing, a phenomenon often cited as evidence that the plasma membrane is the first choice as a cellular target in heat sensitivity. Although this is a rather convincing argument, one should always keep in mind that most of the agents used may penetrate the cell's interior and affect other cellular structures besides the plasma membrane. Amphotericin B interacts with cholesterol and is reported to be a hyperthermic sensitizer (Hahn et al. 1977). Short chain alcohols such as ethanol disrupt hydrophobic regions of membranes and sensitize cells to heat (Li and Hahn 1978), as in the case with some anesthetics (Yatvin 1977; Yau 1979). Addition of polyamines (Gerner et al. 1980) and DEAE-dextran (Molinski et al. 1984) markedly potentiates hyperthermic cell killing. Both these latter compounds are thought to interact with negatively charged residues on the cell surface, but especially polyamines may affect many intracellular processes.

Local anesthetics and especially procaine are popular membrane-active drugs often used in hyperthermia research protocols. Recent studies point to direct anesthetic - lipid interactions (Chan and Wang 1984). Local anesthetics may increase membrane fluidity in model lipid systems (Papahadjopoulos et al. 1970) and increase the lateral mobility of membrane proteins of lymphocytes (Woda et al. 1980).

Substituting cellular membranes with PUFA, resulting in an increased membrane fluidity, as well as treatment of cells with the local anesthetic procaine, sensitizes the cells for hyperthermic treatments. If the action of procaine is simply due to a fluidization of the lipid part of the membrane one might expect the cytotoxic and heat-sensitizing properties of procaine to be different in normal and PUFA substituted cells. This seems not to be the case, as is illustrated in Fig. 7. Addition of 10 mM procaine just prior to heating of the cells further sensitized the cells. The extent of sensitization by procaine of the PUFA cells was comparable to that found for normal cells. The enhanced thermosensitivity was expressed on the level of the shoulder (Dq) as well as on the level of the slope (Do) of the survival curves (Konings 1985).

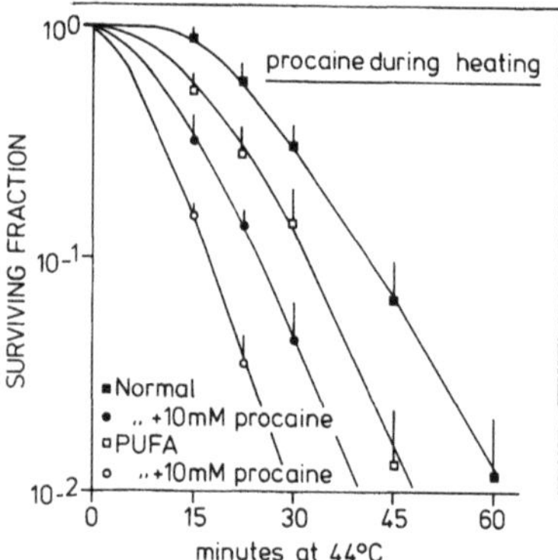

Fig. 7. Effect of PUFA supplementation during cell growth on cell survival after hyperthermia with and without 10 mM procaine. Procaine was present only during the heat treatment. (Konings 1985)

Further indications that procaine does not act via membrane lipid fluidity comes from experiments in which it is shown that procaine inhibits (or delays) thermotolerant development (Konings 1985), a phenomenon not seen by PUFA substitution (Fig. 6).

Membranes Versus DNA as Targets for Killing by Heat and Radiation

Membrane modification by lipid substitution may affect heat sensitivity, as discussed above. Such cellular alterations do not influence radiation-induced reproductive cell death (Wolters and Konings 1982), as is shown in Table 4. Substituting 5′-bromodeoxyuridine (BrdUrd) for thymidine in DNA sensitizes cells for radiation killing while no effect was found on heat sensitivity.

Apart from the substitution experiments, there is abundant further evidence that mechanisms leading to hyperthermic cell killing are different from those leading to cell killing by ionizing radiation. The influence of sulfhydryl compounds is different for heat sensitivity and radiosensitivity (Kapp and Hahn 1979), and the effect of pH changes is not the same (Freeman et al. 1981) when the two modalities are compared. The variation in radiosensitivity of different mutants and cell variants does not correspond with heat sensitivity (Reddy et al. 1981; Raaphorst et al. 1985).

When heat and radiation treatments are combined it seems that heat potentiates those molecular events in the cell that lead to radiation killing and not the other way around. While K+ loss from mouse fibroblasts could be shown even after moderate heat doses (Ruifrok et al. 1985), high dose radiation treatment did not result in K+ loss. The combination treatment did not enhance K+ loss above the level resulting from the hyperthermia treatment alone (Ruifrok et al. 1985). Separate modes of action in thermal radiosensitization and direct thermal death are also suggested from the results of experiments by Mivechi and Hofer (1983), where drugs were used to modify the effects. In a recent publication by Kampinga et al. (1986) three different cell lines with different heat sensitivities were compared for

Table 4. Molecular substitution in different cellular targets; effect on radiation and heat sensitivity[a]

Cellular target	Substituent	Sensitization of	
		Radiat. eff.	Heat eff.
Membranes	PUFA[b]	No[d]	Yes[e]
DNA	BrdUrd[c]	Yes[f]	No[f]

[a] Survival of mammalian cells was measured as clonogenic ability after radiation or hyperthermia.
[b] Polyunsaturated fatty acyl *(PUFA)* chains in phospholipid.
[c] 5′-bromodeoxyuridine *(BrdUrd)*, a thymidine analogue.
[d] Wolters and Konings (1982); George et al. (1983).
[e] Guffy et al. (1982); Konings and Ruifrok (1985).
[f] Raaphorst et al. (1984).

heat radiosensitizing characteristics. No correlation could be established between the two properties in the different cell lines.

It is assumed that repair of radiation-induced DNA damage is the mechanism underlying heat radiosensitization. While for heat killing membrane damage may be the critical event, for heat radiosensitization, heat-induced intracellular changes related to the DNA repair system will probably be critical. Together with heat-induced membrane damage an enhanced protein binding in nuclei isolated from heated cells has been observed (Roti Roti and Winward 1978; Tomasovic et al. 1978; Kampinga et al. 1985). Based on recovery experiments (post heat incubations) of normal and thermotolerant cells, it is postulated (Kampinga et al. 1987) that the rate of protein removal after the heat treatments is indicative of the extent of cell survival after hyperthermia. The observed enhanced binding of nuclear protein may possibly be a cause of heat radiosensitization. Restricted DNA accessibility for repair enzymes, because of the enhanced protein binding, may be the reason for the observed inhibition of repair of radiation-induced DNA damage.

Membrane Proteins as Target Molecules

Although the finding that lipid substitution of membranes points to this cell organelle as the important target for heat killing, it does not necessarily mean that the lipid molecules as such are the entities in cells that regulate thermosensitivity. There are at least two important observations that militate against a role of endogenous lipids as determinants of heat sensitivity:

1. Thermotolerant cells have the same lipid composition and membrane fluidity as normal cells.
2. In mouse fibroblasts extensive changes in PUFA content and membrane fluidity lead to only small increases in heat sensitivity.

The first item has been discussed earlier; the second is illustrated in Fig. 8. The results as shown in this figure stress the probability that via lipid fluidization, the endogenous important membrane components are critically altered. The most probable candidates as critical target molecules are the proteins of the membrane.

Heat-induced conformational changes of hyaluronate groups containing proteins (glycocalyx) are probably responsible for the observed changes in cell surface charge after hyperthermia (Sato et al. 1981). Heat-induced alternations in binding of hormone or antibody ligands to membrane receptors correlate with heat sensitivity measured in terms of cell survival (Stevenson et al. 1981). A comparable response was observed for insulin receptor binding (Calderwood and Hahn 1983) and for hyperthermia effects on binding of epidermal growth factor (Magun et al. 1981). Measurements of intrinsic protein fluorescence and of the protein fluorophore to transparanaric acid energy transfer demonstrate the existence of an irreversible transition in protein structure above 40° C, both in mitochondrial and in plasma membranes (Lepock et al. 1983). The latter authors hypothesize that the alterations in the structure of the proteins above 40° C could cause many of the observed changes in the plasma membrane and may be involved in hyperthermic cell killing.

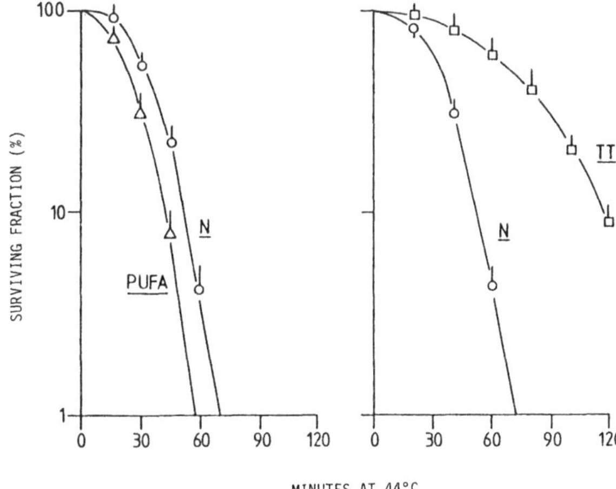

Fig. 8. Effect of increased membrane fluidity by PUFA substitution *(left)* as well as effect of heat-induced thermotolerance *(right)* on heat sensitivity in mouse fibroblasts. *PUFA*, polyunsaturated fatty acid substituted cells; *N*, normal cells; *TT*, thermotolerant cells

The next step in hyperthermia-related membrane research will be the identification of critical membrane proteins (e.g., enzymes, carrier systems) which may be the key molecules in the membrane responsible for the supposed role of this cellular organelle as a primary target in hyperthermic cell killing.

References

Anderson RL, Parker R (1982) Analysis of membrane lipid composition of mammalian cells during the development of thermotolerance. Int J Radiat Biol 42: 57-69

Anderson RL, Tao T-W, Hahn GM (1984) Cholesterol: phospholipid ratios decrease in heat resistant variants of B16 melanoma cells. In: Overgaard J (ed) Hyperthermic oncology Taylor and Francis, London, pp 123-126

Anderson RL, Lunec J, Cresswell SR (1985) Cholesterol content and heat sensitivity of nine mammalian cell lines. Int J Hyperthermia 1: 337-347

Burns CP, Lambert BJ, Haugstad BN, Guffy MM (1986) Influence of rate of heating on thermosensitivity of L1210 leukemia: membrane lipids and Mr 70,000 heat shock protein. Cancer Res 46: 1882-1887

Calderwood SK, Hahn GM (1983) Thermal sensitivity and resistance of insulin-receptor binding. Biochim Biophys Acta 756: 1-8

Chan DS, Wang HH (1984) Local anesthetics can interact electrostatistically with membrane proteins. Biochim Biophys Acta 77: 55-64

Cress AE, Gerner EW (1980) Cholesterol levels inversely reflect the thermal sensitivity of mammalian cells in culture. Nature 283: 677-679

Freeman ML, Boone MLM, Ensley BA, Gillette EL (1981) The influence of environmental pH on the interaction and repair of heat and radiation damage. Int J Radiat Oncol Biol Phys 7: 761-764

George AM, Lunec J, Cramp WA (1983) Effect of membrane fatty acid changes on the radiation sensitivity of human lymphoid cells. Int J Radiat Biol 43: 363-378

Gerner EW, Cress AE, Stickney DG, Holmes DK, Culver PS (1980) Factors regulating membrane permeability after thermal resistance. Ann NY Acad Sci 335: 215-233

Gonzalez-Mendez R, Minton KW, Hahn GM (1982) Lack of correlation between membrane lipid composition and thermotolerance in Chinese hamster ovary cells. Biochim Biophys Acta 692: 168-170

Guffy MM, Rosenberger JA, Simon I, Burns CP (1982) Effect of cellular fatty acid alteration on hyperthermic sensitivity in cultured L1210 murine leukemia cells. Cancer Res 42: 3625-3630

Hahn GM, Li GC, Shiu E (1977) Interaction of amphotericin B and 43° hyperthermia. Cancer Res 37: 761-764

Heilbrunn LV (1924) The colloid chemistry of protoplasm. IV. The heat coagulation of protoplasm. Am J Physiol 69: 190-199

Kampinga HH, Jorritsma JBM, Konings AWT (1985) Heat-induced alterations in DNA polymerase activity of HeLa cells and isolated nuclei. Relation to cell survival. Int J Radiat Biol 47: 29-40

Kampinga HH, Jorritsma JBM, Burgman P, Konings AWT (1986) Differences in heat-induced cell killing as determined in three mammalian cell lines do not correspond with the extent of heat radiosensitization. Int J Radiat Biol 50: 675-684

Kampinga HH, Luppes JG, Konings AWT (1987) Heat-induced nuclear protein binding and its relation to thermal cytotoxicity. Int J Hyperthermia 3: 459-465

Kapp DS, Hahn GM (1979) Thermosensitization by sulfhydryl compounds of exponentially growing Chinese hamster cells. Cancer Res 39: 4639-4645

Konings AWT (1985) Development of thermotolerance in mouse fibroblast LM cells with modified membranes and after procaine treatment. Cancer Res 45: 2016-2019

Konings AWT, Ruifrok ACC (1985) Role of membrane lipids and membrane fluidity in thermosensitivity and thermotolerance of mammalian cells. Radiat Res 102: 86-98

Lepock JR, Massicotte-Nolan P, Rule GS, Kruuv J (1981) Lack of a correlation between hyperthermic cell killing, thermotolerance, and membrane lipid fluidity. Radiat Res 87: 300-313

Lepock JR, Cheng K-H, Al-Qysi H, Kruuv J (1983) Thermotropic lipid and protein transitions in Chinese hamster lung cell membranes: relationship to hyperthermic cell killing. Can J Biochem Cell Biol 61: 421-427

Li GC, Hahn GM (1978) Ethanol-induced tolerance to heat and adriamycin. Nature 274: 699-701

Magun BE, Fennie CW (1981) Effects of hyperthermia on binding, internalization, and degradation of epidermal growth factor. Radiat Res 86: 133-146

McElhaney RN (1974) The effect of alterations in the physical state of the membrane lipids on the ability of *Acholeplasma laidlawii* B to grow at various temperatures. J Mol Biol 84: 145-147

Mivechi NF, Hofer RG (1983) Evidence for separate modes of action in thermal radiosensitization and direct thermal cell death. Cancer 51: 38-43

Molinski M, Calderwood SK, Stevenson MA, Hahn GM (1984) The polycation diethylaminoethyl dextran potentiates thermal cell killing. Int J Radiat Biol 46: 587-596

Overath P, Schairer HU, Stoffel W (1970) Correlation of in vivo and in vitro phase transitions of membrane lipids in *Escherichia coli*. Proc Natl Acad Sci USA 67: 606-612

Papahadjopoulos D, Jacobson K, Poste G, Shepherd G (1970) Effects of local anesthetics on membrane properties. I. Change in fluidity of phospholipid bilayers. Biochim Biophys Acta 211: 467-477

Raaphorst GP, Vadasz JA, Azzam EI (1984) Thermal sensitivity and radiosensitization in V79 cells after BrdUrd or IdUrd incorporation. Radiat Res 98: 167-175

Raaphorst GP, Vadasz JA, Azzam EI, Sargent MD, Borsa J, Einspenner M (1985) Comparison of heat and/or radiation sensitivity and membrane composition of seven X-ray-transformed C3H 10T½ cell lines and normal C3H 10T½ cells. Cancer Res 45: 5452-5456

Reddy NMS, Rao BS, Madhvanath U (1981) Comparison of sensitivity of rad mutants of diploid yeast to heat and gamma radiation: cellular target for heat inactivation. Int J Radiat Biol 40: 235-243
Roti Roti JL, Winward RT (1978) The effects of hyperthermia on the protein-to-DNA ratio of isolated HeLa cells chromatin. Radiat Res 74: 159-169
Ruifrok ACC, Kanon B, Konings AWT (1985) Correlation between cellular survival and potassium loss in mouse fibroblasts after hyperthermia alone and after a combined treatment with X rays. Radiat Res 101: 326-331
Sato C, Nakayama J, Kojima K, Nishimoto Y, Nakamura W (1981) Effects of hyperthermia on cell surface charge and cell survival in mastocytoma cells. Cancer Res 41: 4107-4110
Stevenson MA, Minton KW, Hahn GM (1981) Survival and concanavalin-A-induced capping in CHO fibroblasts after exposure to hyperthermia, ethanol, and X-irradiation. Radiat Res 86: 467-478
Tomasovic SP, Turner GN, Dewey WC (1978) Effect of hyperthermia on nonhistone proteins isolated with DNA. Radiat Res 73: 535-552
Woda BA, Yguerabide J, Feldman JD (1980) The effect of local anaesthetics on the lateral mobility of lymphocyte membrane proteins. Exp Cell Res 126: 327-331
Wolters H, Konings AWT (1982) Radiation effects on membranes. III. The effect of X irradiation on survival of mammalian cells substituted by polyunsaturated fatty acids. Radiat Res 92: 474-482
Yatvin MB (1977) The inflluence of membrane lipid composition and procaine on hyperthermic death of cells. Int J Radiat Biol 32: 513-521
Yatvin MB, Vorpahl JW, Gould MN, Lyte M (1983) The effects of membrane modification and hyperthermia on the survival of P-388 and V-79 cells. Eur J Cancer 19: 1247-1253
Yau TM (1979) Procaine-mediated modification of membranes and the response to X-irradiation and hyperthermia in mammalian cells. Radiat Res 80: 523-541

*Sulfhydryl Compounds as Thermosensitizers**

R. D. Issels

Gesellschaft für Strahlen- und Umweltforschung (GSF), Institut für Hämatologie, Medizinische Klinik III, Klinikum Großhadern, Ludwig-Maximilians-Universität, Marchioninistraße 15, 8000 München 70, FRG

Introduction

The cytotoxic effects of a number of widely used chemotherapeutic agents have been reported to be enhanced by heat (Hahn 1979; Hahn and Li 1982). The exact mechanism of this enhancement is not fully understood and might differ with the various compounds. Thermosensitization by sulfhydryl compounds in vitro has been observed by Kapp and Hahn (1979). We have previously reported that the thermosensitizing effect at 44° C and 43° C of sulfhydryl compounds like cysteamine can be modified by catalase (Issels et al. 1984). The enhancement of thiol cytotoxicity by hyperthermia was found to be due to the generation of activated oxygen species during the autoxidation of such compounds (Biaglow et al. 1984). The aim of this report was to evaluate the effects of cysteamine on heat survival curves at lower temperatures (42.5° C and 41.8° C). At these temperatures, the induction and development of thermotolerance have been shown to occur during the time of heating. We addressed the following questions: (a) to which extent the generation of activated oxygen species by cysteamine might be involved in the interaction between heat and cysteamine treatment at these temperatures; (b) the influence of cell density, and (c) the comparison of cysteamine with the thiol compound aminopropylamino-ethylthiophosphate (WR2721).

Material and Methods

Cell Cultures

Chinese hamster ovary (CHO) cells were grown in McCoys's Medium 5A supplemented with 10% (v/v) calf and 5% (v/v) fetal calf serum, penicillin (0.05 g/liter), streptomycin (0.05 g/liter), and neomycin sulfate (0.1 g/liter). Cells were main-

* This work was supported by grants SFB 324/Is-B3 from the Deutsche Forschungsgemeinschaft. Part of the work was presented at the 11th Annual Meeting of the American Association for Cancer Research (AACR), Los Angeles, CA, 1986.

Recent Results in Cancer Research, Vol. 109

tained in exponential growth at 37° C in a 5% CO_2 atmosphere. Under such conditions, the population doubling time of exponential-phase cells was approximately 13-15 h, and colony-forming efficiency was 80%-90%.

Heat Drug Exposure

At Low Cell Density. Twenty-four hours prior to drug exposure at the different temperatures, exponentially growing cells were trypsinized (0.25% for 2 min) and counted, and dilutions of known cell numbers were inoculated in four to six replicate T-25 flasks (Lux, Lab Tec, USA) containing 4.5 ml of fresh medium (total volume). The flasks were placed in a 37° C incubator containing 5% CO_2 and air until treatment. For combined drug and heat treatments, thiols were added directly to the warm medium (pH 7.4). The flasks were placed horizontally in a circulating water bath (W45/EB, Haake AG, Berlin, West Germany) at the indicated temperatures (±0.05° C). Temperature equilibration of the medium in the flasks at the cell surface with the water bath temperature occurred in approximately 2.5 min. The medium pH ranged from 7.2 to 7.6 throughout the experiments. Control heat treatment survival curves were obtained each time cells were exposed to combined drug and heat treatments.

At High Cell Density. Essentially the same experimental protocol was used as described above except that CHO cells were plated 24 h prior to heat and drug treatment at high cell density ($\simeq 10^6$ cells/flask) in two replicate T-25 flasks containing 4.5 ml of fresh medium. After treatment, the cells were trypsinized (0.25% for 2 min) and counted, and dilutions of known cell numbers were inoculated in four to six replicate T-25 flasks for colony formation.

Clonogenic Cell Survival

After treatment the cells were incubated for 8-14 days for colony development. Following incubation, the colonies were rinsed with 0.9% NaCl solution, fixed, and stained with 20% ethanol containing 0.8% ammonium oxalate and 2% crystal violet. The surviving fraction was calculated after correction for cellular multiplicity (approximately 1.9), which was determined at the time of the drug and/or heat treatment. The multiplicity-corrected surviving fraction data, when plotted on log (surviving fraction) versus linear (dose) paper, yielded survival curves of which the slopes were fitted to straight lines by linear regression.

Chemicals

Cysteamine hydrochloride (β-mercaptoethylamine) was obtained from Sigma Chemical Co. and stored at 5° C in a dessicator. Stock solutions of cysteamine were freshly prepared as described by Kapp and Hahn (1979). Aminopropylamino-ethylthiophosphate (WR2721) was a gift of L. Gerweck, Boston, Mass. Catalase from bovine liver (17600 units/mg) and alkaline phosphatase (1000 units/ml) were obtained from Sigma.

Results

Heat Survival of CHO Cells Exposed to Cysteamine at 42.5° C and 41.8° C at Low Cell Density (10^2-10^4 Cells/Flask

The survival curves of CHO cells after continuous incubation (0-500 min) at 42.5°C or 41.8° C alone (control) show the typical development of thermotolerance during the time of heat treatment (see Fig. 1). The cytotoxic effects of heat for periods in excess of 3 or 4 h were markedly reduced at both temperatures. With addition of cysteamine (0.4 mM) to heat treatment at 42.5° C or 41.8° C, no such development of thermotolerance could be observed. The clonogenic surviving fraction of cells heated under these conditions was log-linearly reduced. The modifications by cysteamine of the effects of heat were even more pronounced at the lower temperature (41.8° C). Addition of catalase (50 μg/ml) could block the removal of the shoulder region, but not the inhibition of thermotolerance development by cysteamine at these temperatures. In control experiments, the addition of catalase alone did not modify the heat response of CHO cells at either temperature (data not shown).

Heat Survival of CHO Cells Exposed to Cysteamine at 41.8° C at High Cell Density ($\simeq 10^6$ Cells/Flask)

In order to study the influence of cell density upon the pronounced effect of cysteamine at 41.8° C, the same type of experiments (n = 3) were performed, except that cells were trypsinized after heat and drug treatment. As shown in Fig. 2, no inhibition of the development of thermotolerance could be observed for cells treated with cysteamine (0.4 mM) at 41.8° C under these experimental conditions. The addition of catalase (50 μg/ml) also showed no effect.

Heat Survival of CHO Cells Exposed to WR2721 at 41.8° C at High Cell Density ($\simeq 10^6$ Cells/Flask)

For comparison with the results obtained in cysteamine-treated cells at high cell density, we also used WR2721 under the same experimental conditions. The thiophosphate WR2721 can be hydrolyzed to its free thiol derivative WR1065 by the addition of alkaline phosphatase (20 U/ml) to the medium. In contrast to WR2721 (0.4 mM) alone, the free thiol derivative (WR2721 + AP) blocked the development of thermotolerance in CHO cells at 41.8° C (see Fig. 3). It should be noted that WR2721 + alkaline phosphatase at this high cell density showed no significant effect at 37° C (data not shown).

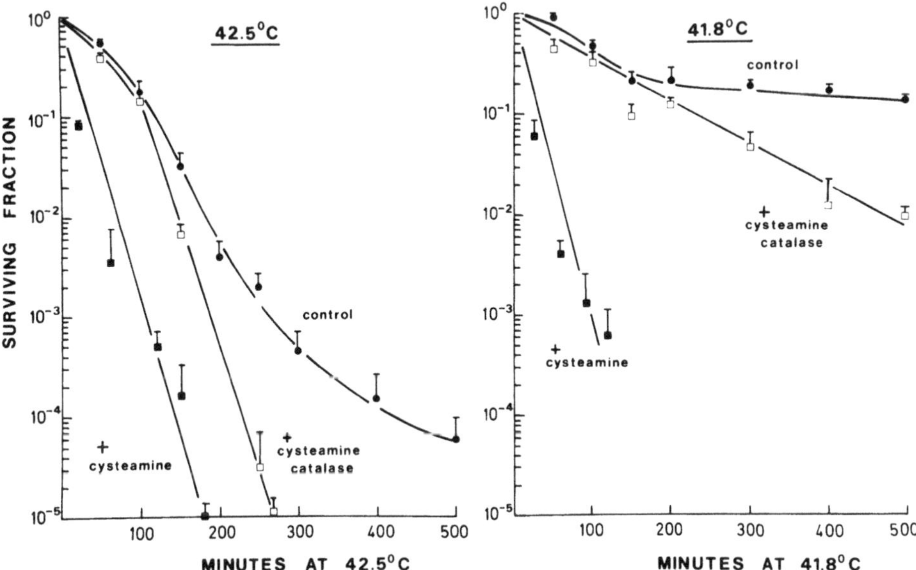

Fig. 1. Clonogenic cell survival of CHO cells exposed to 0.4 mM cysteamine at 42.5° C or 41.8° C for different periods (min). ■, cysteamine plus heat treatment; □, cysteamine plus heat treatment in the presence of 50 μg/ml catalase; ●, control: heat alone. The cell density at the time of heat and drug treatment was 10^2–10^4 cells/flask (for details see Material and Methods). *Bars*, SD

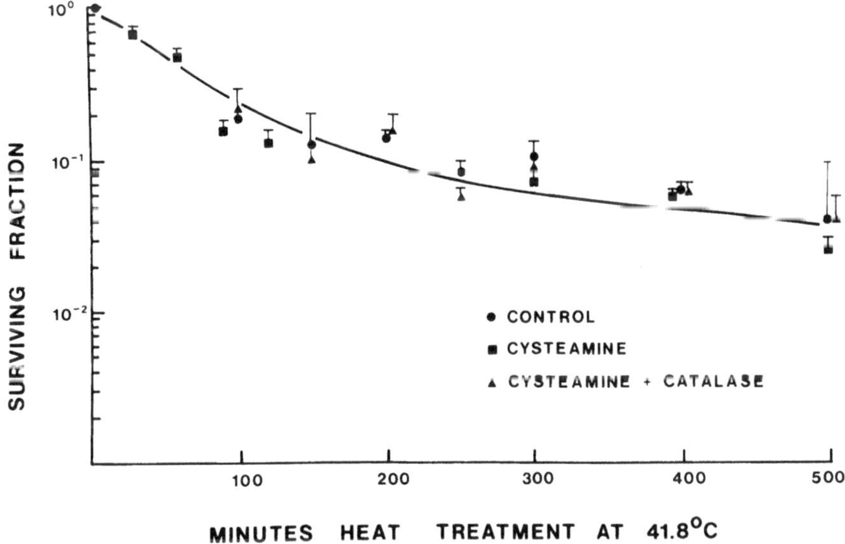

Fig. 2. Clonogenic cell survival of CHO cells exposed to 0.4 mM cysteamine at 41.8° C for different periods (min). ■, cysteamine plus heat treatment; ▲, cysteamine plus heat treatment in the presence of 50 μg/ml catalase; ●, control: heat alone. The cell density at the time of heat and drug treatment was $\simeq 10^6$ cells/flask (for details see Material and Methods). *Bars*, SD

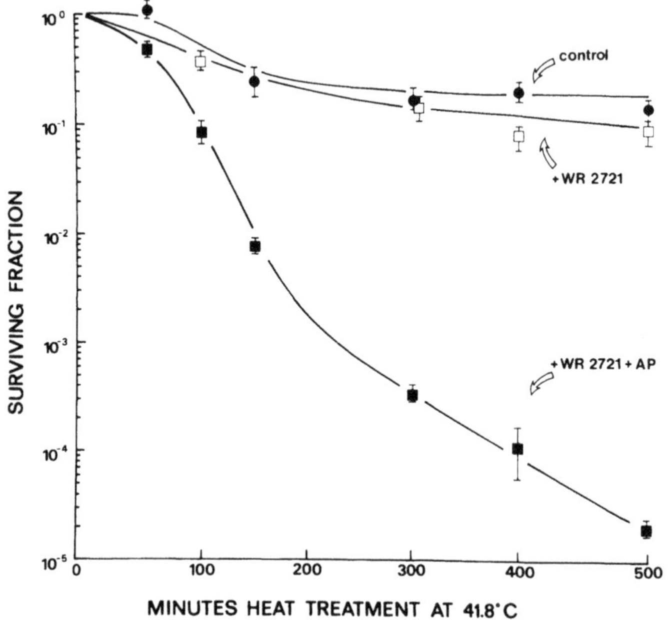

Fig. 3. Clonogenic cell survival of CHO cells exposed to 0.4 mM WR2721 at 41.8° C for different periods (min). ■, WR2721 plus heat treatment in the presence of 20 U/ml alkaline phosphatase; □, WR2721 plus heat treatment; ●, control: heat alone. The cell density at the time of heat and drug treatment was $\simeq 10^6$ cells/flask (for details see Material and Methods). *Bars*, SD

Discussion

Thermosensitization of CHO cells by sulfhydryl compounds like cysteamine (Kapp and Hahn 1979; Issels et al. 1984) based on the generation of activated oxygen species during autoxidation (Biaglow et al. 1984) seems to be essentially dependent upon the temperature used in the experiments. At temperatures above 42.5° C, the removal of the shoulder of survival curves was most likely explained by interaction with hyperthermic repair processes. The previous data suggested that the production of H_2O_2 is the first reaction step in the mechanism of thermosensitization by cysteamine at 44° C and 43° C. In the present study during incubation of CHO cells at 42.5° C and 41.8° C combined with cysteamine, the development of thermotolerance normally induced in these cells could not be observed. Since the effect of cysteamine at lower temperatures could not be blocked by the addition of catalase, mechanisms other than the production of H_2O_2 by thiols may be involved. The temperature-dependent increase of glutathione in CHO cells by thiols (Issels et al. 1985) might be of critical importance. Why the effect of cysteamine is completely dependent on cell density remains unclear in this study. However, at high cell density the free thiol derivative of WR2721 seems to inhibit the development of thermotolerance in CHO cells. More recently, we were able to demonstrate that WR2721, like other thiols, promotes cystine uptake in CHO cells and increases the content of glutathione (Issels et al. 1986). Further studies are in progress to investigate whether perturbation of the glutathione status of cells during combined heat and thiol treatment is related to the observed thermosensitizing effects of such compounds.

References

Biaglow IE, Issels RD, Gerweck LG, Varnes ME, Jacobsen B, Mitchell JB, Russo A (1984) Factors influencing the oxidation of cysteamine and other thiols: implications for hyperthermic sensitization and radiation protection. Radiat Res 100: 298-312

Hahn GM (1979) Potential for therapy of drugs and hyperthermia. Cancer Res 39: 2264-2268

Hahn GM, Li GC (1982) The interactions of hyperthermia and drugs: treatments and probes. Natl Cancer Inst Monogr 61: 457-460

Issels RD, Biaglow JE, Epstein L, Gerweck LE (1984) Enhancement of cysteamine cytotoxicity by hyperthermia and its modification by catalase and superoxide dismutase in Chinese hamster ovary cells. Cancer Res 44: 3911-3915

Issels RD, Bourier S, Biaglow JE, Gerweck LE, Wilmanns W (1985) Temperature-dependent influence of thiols upon glutathione levels in Chinese hamster ovary cells at cytotoxic concentrations. Cancer Res 45: 6219-6224

Issels RD, Nagele AH, Boening B, Bourier S, Wilmanns W (1986) Promotion of cystine uptake in Chinese hamster ovary cells by WR2721 and related aminothiols (abstr). 34th Annual meeting of Radiation Research Society, Las Vegas, (Fi-1) p 142

Kapp DS, Hahn G (1979) Thermosensitization by sulfhydryl compounds of exponentially growing Chinese hamster cells. Cancer Res 39: 4630-4635

Therapeutic Benefit from Combined Heat and Radiation

S. A. Hill and J. Denekamp

Cancer Research Campaign, Gray Laboratory, Mount Vernon Hospital,
Northwood, Middlesex HA6 2RN, Great Britain

Introduction

The response of both tumours and normal tissues to heat, X-rays or a combination of the two is complex. Both agents can act directly by causing cell death or the loss of proliferative capacity. In addition, both agents can act indirectly, by damaging the vasculature and thereby leading to ischaemic cell death as blood vessels collapse or are occluded by thrombi (Fig. 1). When the two agents are combined there may be a synergism, antagonism or sensitisation of the action of either agent by the other. The response to both agents can be modulated by physiological changes, particularly by oxygenation or acidity changes that may follow from alterations of the patterns of blood flow. If heat and X-rays are to be used clinically in a way that will be safe and will give the maximum therapeutic advantage, it is important to be able to understand and separate these different elements in the response. It is possible to go some way towards this by studying the time course of the response of tumours and normal tissues to each agent separately and to the combination.

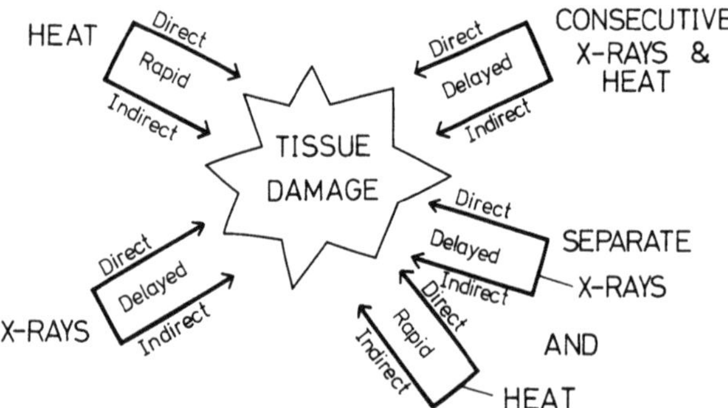

Fig. 1. Summary of actions of heat and X-rays, applied either alone or in combination

Recent Results in Cancer Research, Vol. 109

Time Course of Injury

The time course of response to X-rays differs markedly from one tissue to another. Tissue or tumour damage is not manifest until the total cell population is depleted. This occurs within days in some tissues (e.g. intestine, buccal mucosa) but is delayed for months, or even years, in others (e.g. kidney, lung, brain). This pattern of response can be rationalised in terms of the proliferation kinetics of each tissue. Irradiated cells can continue to function indefinitely after moderate radiation doses (e.g. 10–30 Gy). However, their ability to divide indefinitely is impaired after quite low doses (a few gray) because of damage to the chromosomes. This damage is only expressed at mitosis and is generally detected as the inability to segregate the chromosomes properly and to produce a viable clone of offspring. In tissues with a high rate of cell turnover the damage is expressed at a mitosis soon after irradiation, whereas in those with a very slow turnover the damage may remain latent for weeks or months, until division is attempted and then fails. This turnover generally correlates with the natural lifetime of the differentiated cells in the tissue, since natural loss and replacement are finely balanced. A knowledge of the cell proliferation pattern in a tissue allows one to predict the time at which radiation injury will occur.

By contrast, damage inflicted by heat is expressed rapidly and is not related to mitotic events. Cells die within hours, and tissue or tumour damage is usually evident within a day or two. Since heat disrupts all components of the cell (DNA, RNA, protein, membranes), by contrast with the specific damage to DNA from X-rays, there is less opportunity for normal cell functions to continue whilst concealing a latent genetic defect.

The contrast between the time of apparent tissue injury from heat and X-rays has previously been demonstrated for skin and for intestine (Law et al. 1978; Hume et al. 1979). We have recently investigated this for a late responding tissue, the kidney. Localised renal irradiation leads to progressive renal failure at 3–6 months after irradiation. This can be detected in terms of an inability to excrete radiolabelled EDTA (an inulin substitute), or as failure to concentrate the

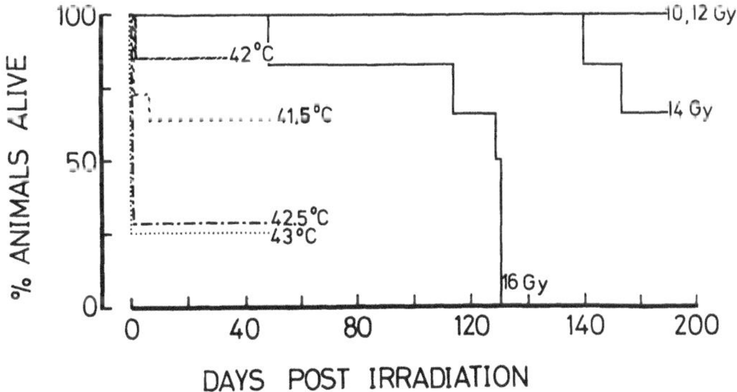

Fig. 2. Patterns of death as a function of time after localised treatment of the mouse kidney with single doses of either hyperthermia (30 min) or X-rays

urine (and hence excessive urine production) (Williams and Denekamp 1983). Figure 2 shows that extreme renal failure leads to most deaths at 100–130 days after 16 Gy, and even later deaths after 14 Gy. Lower doses (10–12 Gy) do not lead to total renal insufficiency even after 200 days. By contrast, mice treated with localised hyperthermia die within a day or two of treatment after doses of 41.5° –43° C for 30 min. Table 1 summarises these data for several normal tissues. Similarly, with tumours, shrinkage occurs within a few days after heating, whereas it is much slower after X-irradiation.

The studies on rapidly proliferating tissues have shown that when heat and X-rays are used in close sequence a radiosensitising effect is observed. The same pattern of damage occurs after the combined treatment as after X-rays alone, but the X-ray dose needed to cause a particular effect is reduced. For example, in skin 30 Gy X-rays alone are as effective as 20 Gy combined with 1 h exposure in a waterbath at 42.5° C, i.e. a thermal enhancement ratio, TER, of 1.5 (Law et al. 1978). It appears that radiosensitisation enhances the effect observed with X-rays, without modifying its time course. This is most likely to result from treatments given in close sequence. It is for this reason that an interval of 3–4 h may give a safety margin, especially for late reacting tissues, which ultimately may lead to life-threatening side-effects (Stewart and Denekamp 1978; Hill and Denekamp 1979). Even though current combined modalities may not show any enhanced normal tissue morbidity, it is important to be aware that such enhancement should be expected if deep tissues are heated in combination with a full tolerance dose of radiotherapy. In such a case, small sensitisation factors of only 1.05 or 1.1 could be disastrous and could lead to increased damage many months or years after treatment, even though much larger factors (TER 1.3–1.5) will not be detectable if the radiotherapy regime is 30%–50% below a tolerance dose. Damage caused by the *cytotoxic* effects of heat, by contrast, will be apparent soon after the treatment.

Table 1. Differences in time course of radiation-induced and heat-induced injury

Tissue	Time of expression of peak injury in response to			Reference
	Heat (days)	X-rays (days)	Heat + X-rays (days)	
Intestinal mucosa	<1 day	3–4	3–4	Hume et al. 1979
Skin: ear	1–5	25–30	25–30	Law et al. 1978
Skin: tail	1–2	20	20	Hume and Myers 1984
Kidney	1–2	100–200	Not known	Present results
Tumours:				
CA NT	2–5	15–30	15–30	Hill, unpublished
CA MT	3–6	10–20	10–20	
SA F	2–5	7–14	7–14	

Vascular Effects

The differential effect of heat on tumours seems to be mediated, at least in part, by a greater sensitivity of the vasculature in tumours (Song 1984; Reinhold et al. 1985). Vascular shutdown has been observed, both by direct visualisation and by tracer isotope studies, to occur after 30-40 min heating at temperatures of 41.5°-43° C. At this thermal dose vasodilation is the characteristic response of normal tissues. A vascular collapse can be induced in normal tissues also, but it generally requires temperatures in excess of 46°-47° C. This greater thermal sensitivity of tumour vessels may result from an increased tendency of the blood in them to coagulate, or a greater sensitivity of the endothelium. Heat-induced changes in deformability of erythrocytes have been documented, and these may occur more readily in low oxygen tensions or in regions of higher acidity (von Ardenne and Krüger 1980). An alternative and plausible hypothesis is that proliferating endothelium in the fragile neovasculature of tumours is more thermosensitive than quiescent differentiated endothelium in the well structured vessels of normal tissues (Denekamp 1981). Some support for this comes from the in vitro studies of Fajardo et al. (1985). They showed that endothelial cells are more thermosensitive than fibroblasts in vitro, and that this thermosensitivity is further enhanced if the cultures are treated with endothelial cell growth factor.

Endothelial Proliferation

The endothelial cells in tumours have been shown to proliferate very much faster than those in normal tissues (Fig. 3). A median value for the labelling index (per-

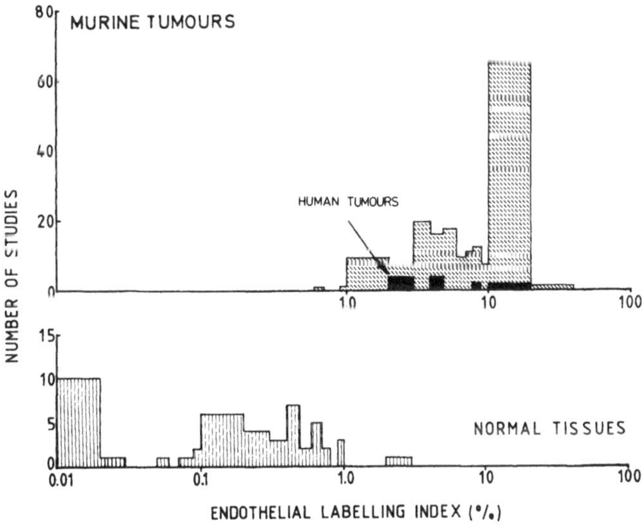

Fig. 3. Histograms showing the uptake of tritiated thymidine into the endothelial cells lining the blood vessels of murine tumours and normal tissues. (Data from Denekamp 1984)

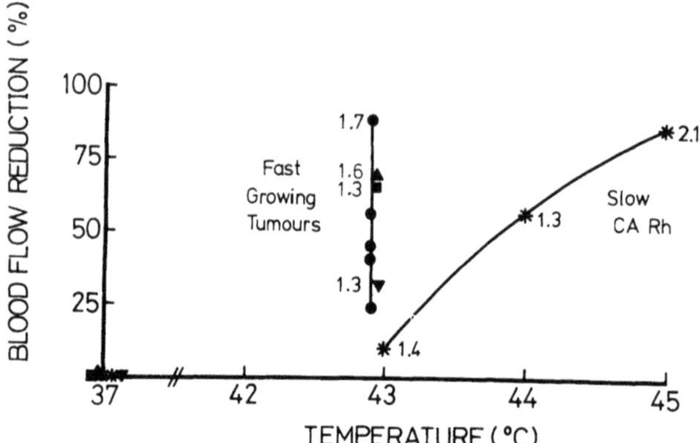

Fig. 4. Reduction in ^{86}RbCl extraction per gram of tumour 24 h after a 1-h treatment at the indicated waterbath temperature (Stewart and Begg 1983 and this study). TER values are listed for each tumour type (from Denekamp et al. 1980 and this study). ●, SA FA; ▲, CA MT; ■, CA NT; ▼, SA F; *, CA RH

centage of cells actively synthesising DNA) of rodent tumours is 9%, whereas that for normal vessels is 0.2%. Human tumour endothelial values are slightly lower, but the cells are still proliferating much faster than any normal adult endothelium. It would be desirable to know what the relationship is between thermal sensitivity and proliferation rate, so that the temperature at which a vascular response could be expected in human tumours would be known. Insufficient data exist to establish this relationship at present. However, blood flow data are available for several rodent tumours at the Gray Laboratory, as summarised in Fig. 4.

A significant reduction in relative blood flow (^{86}Rb extraction) was seen in four rapidly growing tumours (T_D 1–4 days) 1 day after immersion for 1 h at 42.8° C. In all these tumours an enhanced growth delay was seen if this thermal dose was added to a single dose of X-rays. Their endothelial labelling indices are not known. The fifth tumour, CA RH, is much more slowly growing (T_D 10–14 days) and has an endothelial labelling index close to that of human tumours. No enhanced growth delay had been seen at this temperature. In a further experiment, hardly any reduction in blood flow was seen after immersion for 1 h at 43.0° C although a significantly increased growth delay was seen at high radiation doses. After higher temperatures a thermally induced contribution to growth delay coincided with a massive decrease in blood flow (Fig. 4). Further studies are in progress to elucidate the relationship between endothelial turnover, vascular shutdown and induced tumour damage.

Thermally induced vascular collapse may lead to an avalanche of tumour cell death, if it is long-lasting. Temporary or partial vascular collapse may lead to an increase in the hypoxic fraction, with subsequent recovery to a reoxygenated status. Since hypoxic cells are very radioresistant, the timing of a subsequent dose of radiation would obviously need to be adjusted according to the kinetics of blood flow alterations.

Metastatic Spread

There has been some concern about whether vascular damage caused by moderate heat doses may lead to a greater shedding of tumour cells into the circulation, with a consequent increase in distant metastases. This may lead to an increased incidence (Dewhirst et al. 1985) or even to an atypical distribution of metastases (Lord et al. 1981). We have previously shown, for seven different rodent tumours, that the metastatic incidence was not significantly increased when a single dose of heat preceded, accompanied or followed a large single dose of X-rays (Hill and Denekamp 1982). However, in clinical use heat will be combined with smaller, less tumouricidal X-ray doses. We therefore designed the experiment illustrated in Table 2. Tumours were treated with a curative dose of radiation either when they reached 4.5 mm mean diameter, or 1 or 3 days later. The smaller the tumour size at the time of treatment, the lower the incidence of metastases (23%-60%). Other groups were treated at 4.5 mm with 5-Gy X-rays alone, or with 5 Gy followed by various heating regimes. These involved immersion for 30 min in saline and exposure to localised RF to achieve uniform temperatures of 39°, 41° and 43° C. By deliberately varying the RF power and circulating saline temperature, a non-uniform heating of 39° C at the surface and 43° C at depth was achieved. Either 1 or 3 days later treated tumours were given a curative dose of X-rays. Radiation alone (5 Gy) increased the metastatic incidence relative to those simply given a single curative treatment (controls). This was not further enhanced by the addition of mild or non-uniform hyperthermia. It was, however, significantly *reduced* by the addition of uniform heating for 30 min to 43° C. Data are not yet available for corresponding doses of heat alone, but further studies are in progress. These data indicate that inadequate treatment of a tumour, whether by X-rays alone or a combined local modality, may increase the risk of metastatic spread, presumably by disrupting the vasculature. This can be abolished by the addition of an effective and uniform heat dose, or by immediately using a large curative X-ray dose.

Table 2. Incidence of metastases after localised tumour treatment[a]

Test treatment	40 Gy + miso[b] (curative treatment) given at		
	4.5 mm	+1 day	+3 day
Control	23%	35%	60%
Inadequate treatments			
5 Gy	-	70%	88%
5 Gy + 39° C/30 min	-	55%	75%
5 Gy + 41° C/30 min	-	44%	100%
5 Gy + 39°-43° C/30 min	-	58%	100%
Effective treatments			
5 Gy + 43° C/30 min		35%	30%

[a] These data are preliminary, being derived from 10-16 animals in each group.

[b] 0.5 mg/g misonidazole injected 30 min before irradiation.

Conclusion

Before heat can be used as an adjunct to radiotherapy more information is needed about the relative contributions of direct cytotoxicity, indirect effects mediated by vascular collapse, and the independent or synergistic modes of action of the two modalities. The difference in time of expression of radiation and heat injury allows some of these factors to be unravelled. The vascular shutdown occurs at different temperatures in different tumours, and occurs at higher temperatures in normal tissues. There may be a correlation between thermal sensitivity and the rate of proliferation of the endothelial cells. Incomplete damage to the vasculature, whether caused by radiation or heat, may allow dissemination of a local tumour, whereas more effective treatments can prevent it.

References

Denekamp J (1981) Summary of Thermobiology Session II. Natl Cancer Inst Monograph 60: 311-314

Denekamp J (1984) Vasculature as a target for tumour therapy. In: Hammersen (ed) Angiogenesis. Karger, Basel, pp 28-38 (Progress in applied microcirculation, vol 4)

Denekamp J, Hill SA, Stewart FA (1980) Combined heat and X-ray treatment of experimental tumours. Henry Ford Hosp Med J 29: 45-51

Dewhirst MW, Sim DA, Forsyth K, Grochowski KJ, Wilson S, Bicknell E (1985) Local control and distant metastases in primary canine malignant melanomas treated with hyperthermia and/or radiotherapy. Int J Hyperthermia 1: 219-234

Fajardo LF, Schreiber AB, Kelly NI, Hahn GM (1985) Thermal sensitivity of endothelial cells. Radiat Res 103: 276-285

Hill SA, Denekamp J (1979) The response of six mouse tumours to combined heat and X-rays: implications for therapy. Br J Radiol 52: 209-218

Hill SA, Denekamp J (1982) Does local tumour heating in mice influence metastatic spread? Br J Radiol 55: 444-451

Hume SP, Myers R (1984) An unexpected effect of hyperthermia on the expression of X-ray damage in mouse skin. Radiat Res 97: 186-199

Hume SP, Marigold JCL, Field SB (1979) The effect of local hyperthermia on the small intestine of the mouse. Br J Radiol 52: 657-662

Law LP, Ahier RG, Field SB (1978) The response of the mouse ear to heat applied alone or combined with X-rays. Br J Radiol 51: 132-138

Lord PF, Kapp DS, Morrow D (1981) Increased skeletal metastases of spontaneous canine osteosarcoma after fractionated systemic hyperthermia and local X-irradiation. Cancer Res 41: 4331-4334

Reinhold HS, Wikey-Hooley JL, van den Berg AP, van den Berg-Blok A (1985) Environmental factors, blood flow and microcirculation. In: Overgaard J (ed) Hyperthermic oncology 1984, vol 2. Taylor and Francis, London, pp 41-52

Song CW (1984) Effect of local hyperthermia on blood flow and microenvironment. A review. Cancer Res 44: 4721s-4730s

Stewart FA, Denekamp J (1978) The therapeutic advantage of combined heat and X-rays on a mouse fibrosarcoma. Br J Radiol 51: 307-316

Stewart FA, Begg AC (1983) Blood flow changes in transplanted mouse tumours and skin after mild hyperthermia. Br J Radiol 56: 477-482

von Ardenne M, Krüger W (1980) The use of hyperthermia within the frame of cancer multistep therapy. Ann NY Acad Sci 335: 356-361

Williams MV, Denekamp J (1983) Sequential functional testing of radiation-induced renal damage in the mouse. Radiat Res 94: 305-317

*Correlation Between Polymerase β Activity and Thermal Radiosensitization in Chinese Hamster Ovary Cells**

E. Dikomey and H. Jung

Institut für Biophysik und Strahlenbiologie, Universität Hamburg, Martinistraße 52, 2000 Hamburg 20, FRG

Introduction

The efficacy of sparsely ionizing radiation in killing cells is enhanced when irradiation is combined with heat. The mechanisms of this so-called thermal radiosensitization are not yet completely understood, but there are several indications that the enhanced radiosensitivity is a consequence of impaired repair of radiation-induced damage in heated cells. Among the enzymes involved in the repair of DNA lesions, polymerase β is of particular importance since it performs the major portion of the repair synthesis. With respect to both our understanding of the molecular processes of DNA repair and the application of heat as an adjuvant to radiotherapy, it is of great interest to study whether the enhancement of radiation effects in heated cells is caused by reduced polymerase β activity.

Effect of Heat on Radiosensitivity

Figure 1 shows some survival curves of Chinese hamster ovary (CHO) cells determined by the colony forming assay. When compared with exposure to X-rays at 0° C alone (Fig. 1, t = 0), not only do heat treatments at 43° C for 30 or 60 min result in a reduced survival after the heat treatment alone but, in addition, the radiosensitivity of the surviving cells is clearly enhanced. The increase in radiosensitivity was quantified by the thermal enhancement ratio (TER) determined at a survival level of 10%; that is $TER = D(X)_{10\%}/D(H,X)_{10\%}$, where $D(X)_{10\%}$ and $D(H,X)_{10\%}$ are the doses required to reduce survival to 10% by X-irradiation alone or by the combination with heat, respectively, the survival of nonirradiated cells being normalized to 100%. The sensitization ratios for cells heated at 43° C for 30 or 60 min were $TER = 1.33 \pm 0.02$ and $TER = 1.84 \pm 0.07$, respectively. In general, the TER is found to increase with increasing duration and temperature of the heat

* This study was supported by Bundesministerium für Forschung und Technologie (01 VF 8516).

Recent Results in Cancer Research, Vol. 109

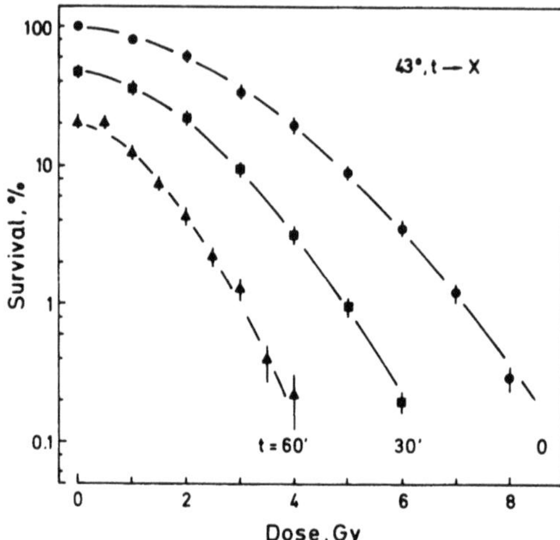

Fig. 1. Thermal radiosensitization in CHO cells. Cells were heated at 43° C for the times indicated before being exposed at 0° C to graded doses of X-rays

treatment (Ben Hur et al. 1974; Holahan et al. 1984; Robinson and Wizenberg 1974) and is most pronounced when both modalities are given simultaneously (Sapareto et al. 1978).

The cellular heat sensitivity can be reduced by preceding heat treatment; this phenomenon is termed thermotolerance (for review see Henle and Dethlefsen 1978). In CHO cells, thermotolerance was induced by acute pretreatment at 43° C for 45 min and was found to be maximally developed after a time interval of 16 h at 37° C (Dikomey et al. 1984). When CHO cells were irradiated at the time of maximal thermotolerance, their radiosensitivity was not significantly different from the sensitivity of normal cells (Fig. 2, TER = 1.04 ± 0.05). However, thermotolerance was found to modify the effect of a combined treatment. In thermotolerant cells, survival after exposure at 43° C for 60 min was higher than in normal cells and, in addition, the thermal radiosensitization in the surviving cells was reduced. A ratio of TER = 1.36 ± 0.02 was obtained for thermotolerant cells, as compared to TER = 1.84 ± 0.07 for normal cells. A similar decrease in TER was also observed when the CHO cells were made thermotolerant by chronic pretreatment at 40° C for 16 h. For other cell lines, the induction of thermotolerance is generally reported to result in a decrease in thermal radiosensitization (Hartson-Eaton et al. 1984; Haveman 1983; Holahan et al. 1984, 1986; Jorritsma et al. 1986).

Pretreatment at a higher temperature followed by a lower temperature (step-down heating) leads to a pronounced increase in the cellular heat sensitivity (Dikomey et al. 1984; Jung 1982, 1986). This phenomenon is termed thermosensitization. Heating at 40° C for 5 h only slightly reduced survival of CHO cells and did not affect radiosensitivity (Fig. 3, closed squares). On the other hand, when cells were made thermosensitive by pretreatment at 43° C for 30 min, which alone reduced survival to about 50%, further heating at 40° C for 5 h resulted in a drastic decrease in survival. However, the thermal enhancement obtained after the pretreatment alone (TER = 1.38 ± 0.02; Fig. 3, open circles) was not enhanced further when the pretreatment at 43° C was followed by incubation at 40° C for 5 h (TER = 1.40 ± 0.01, Fig. 3, closed circles). These results show that the radiosensitiv-

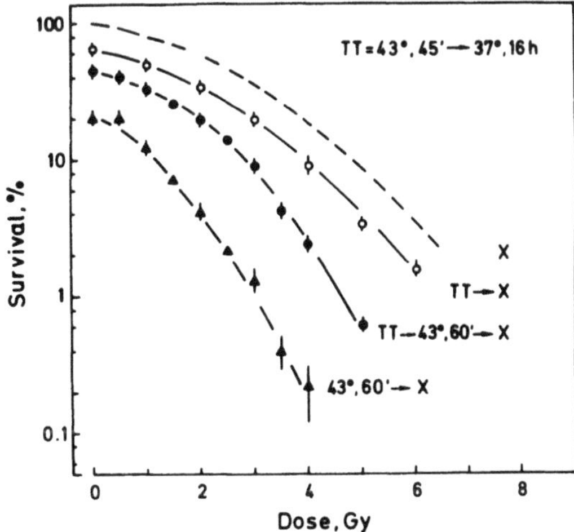

Fig. 2. Thermal radiosensitization in thermotolerant CHO cells. Normal cells and cells made thermotolerant by pretreatment *(TT)* were exposed either to graded doses of X-rays alone or to a combination of a second heat treatment at 43° C for 60 min immediately followed by irradiation

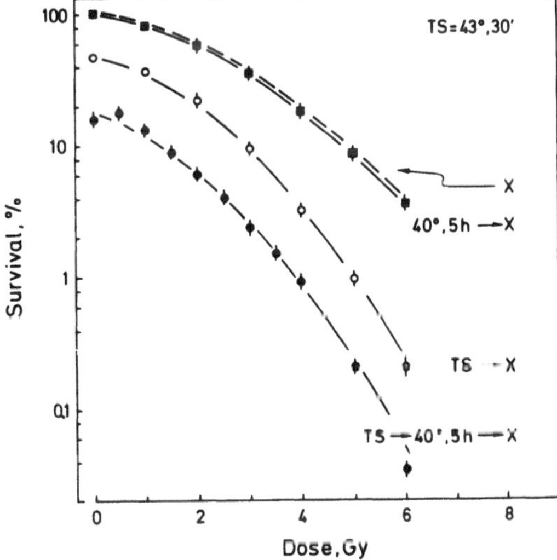

Fig. 3. Thermal radiosensitization in thermosensitive CHO cells. Normal cells and cells made thermosensitive by pretreatment *(TS)* were exposed either to graded doses of X-rays alone or to a combination of a second heat treatment at 40° C for 5 h immediately followed by irradiation

ity of CHO cells is not affected by thermosensitization although this leads to an increase in cellular heat sensitivity. Similar observations were made for HeLa and EAT cells (Jorritsma et al. 1986). Thus, in step-down heated cells the surviving fraction after heat alone does not correlate with the TER measured when heat is followed by X-irradiation.

Effect of Heat on Polymerase β Activity

Polymerase β activity was measured by the incorporation of tritium-labeled TTP in activated calf thymus DNA. Cells were homogenized and then mixed with activated calf thymus DNA and the four nucleotide triphosphates. Since the activity of polymerase α was completely depressed by addition of the specific inhibitor aphidicolin, the amount of DNA-incorporated ^{3}H-TTP is a measure of the polymerase β activity (Dikomey et al. 1987).

Heating of CHO cells at 43° C leads to a reduction in polymerase β activity (Fig. 4). During the first 30 min the polymerase β activity decreased very rapidly, followed by a decrease at a lower rate. For CHO cells, biphasic response curves are obtained for all temperatures ranging from 40° to 46° C (Dikomey et al. 1987); this has also been observed for HeLa and EAT cells (Jorritsma et al. 1986).

We studied the effect of thermotolerance on the heat sensitivity of polymerase β in CHO cells. Thermotolerance was induced by acute pretreatment at 43° C for 45 min followed by incubation at 37° C for 16 h; this resulted in three- and fourfold decreases in the initial and the final sensitivity of polymerase β at 43° C, respectively (Fig. 4, open circles). A reduction in the heat sensitivity of polymerase β at 43° C was also observed when CHO cells were made thermotolerant by chronic pretreatment at 40° C for 16 h (Dikomey et al. 1987). In CHO cells, the induction of thermotolerance always resulted in reduced heat sensitivity of polymerase β

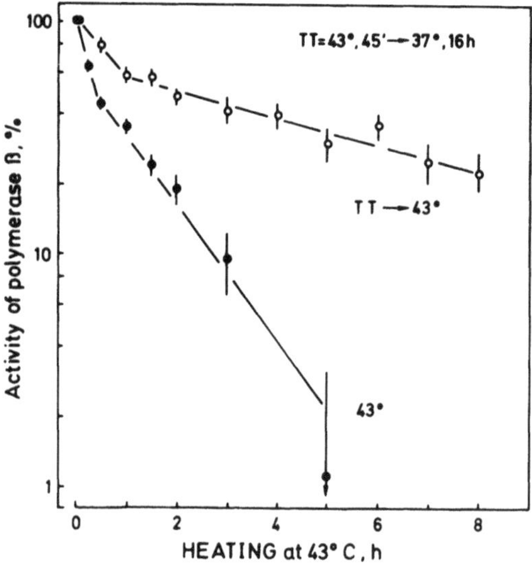

Fig. 4. Reduction in polymerase β activity after heating at 43° C of normal CHO cells and cells made thermotolerant by pretreatment *(TT)*

(Denman et al. 1982; Dewey and Esch 1982; Dikomey et al. 1987), whereas in HeLa and EAT cells heat sensitivity of polymerase β was found not to be altered by thermotolerance induction (Jorritsma et al. 1986; Kampinga et al. 1985).

The effect of step-down heating on heat sensitivity of polymerase β is shown in Fig. 5. CHO cells were exposed to 43° C for 30 min before being incubated at 40° C. Pretreatment alone reduced the enzyme activity to 43%. But in pretreated cells the enzyme sensitivity at 40° C was not significantly different from the sensitivity in normal cells. Thus, the heat sensitivity of polymerase β was not altered when CHO cells were made thermosensitive. The same result has been reported for HeLa and EAT cells (Jorritsma et al. 1986).

In Fig. 6, the TER values obtained from the survival curves shown in Figs. 1-3 and from other experiments are plotted versus the polymerase β activity measured

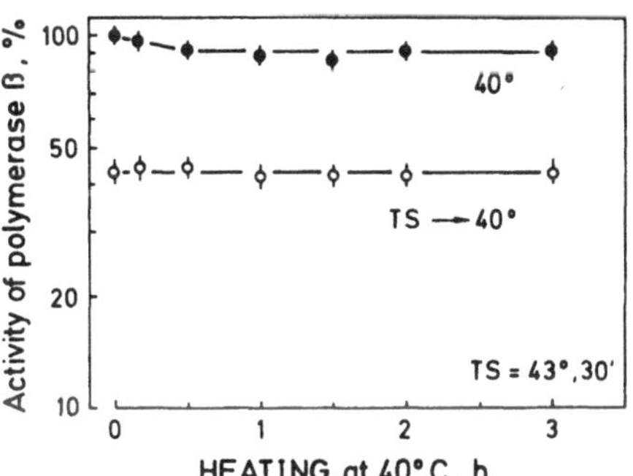

Fig. 5. Reduction in polymerase β activity at 40° C in normal CHO cells and in cells made thermosensitive by pretreatment *(TS)*

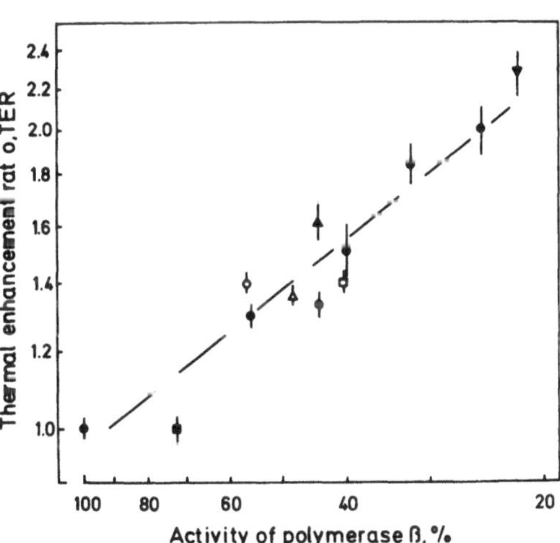

Fig. 6. Correlation between polymerase β activity and the thermal enhancement ratio, *TER*, in CHO cells after identical heat treatments. Cells were exposed to single (■, 42°; ●, 43°; ▲, 44°; ▼, 45°) or combined heat treatments (△: 43°, 45 min→37°, 16 h→43°, 60 min; ○: 40°, 16 h→43°, 60 min; □: 43°, 30 min→40°, 5 h) and then either analyzed for the polymerase β activity or exposed to graded doses of X-rays to determine the radiosensitivity and thus the thermal enhancement ratio

after single and multiple heat treatments. It becomes obvious that the radiosensitivity of preheated CHO cells is higher the lower the polymerase β activity is at the beginning of irradiation. A heat treatment leading to a reduction in polymerase β activity is always found to enhance the radiosensitivity when heat is combined with X-rays. And, in contrast, a heat treatment which does not result in a further decrease in the enzyme activity (such as the sequence 43° C→40° C) does not cause a further increase in radiosensitivity. For CHO cells, a similar correlation between polymerase β activity and radiosensitivity was observed by Mivechi and Dewey (1985). A treatment with glycerol resulted in a reduced effect of heat on polymerase β activity and also led to a decrease in thermal radiosensitization. In addition, the authors showed that the activity of polymerase β recovered with time after heat treatment with the same kinetics as were found for the decrease in the thermal radiosensitization. A good correlation between reduction in polymerase β activity and increase in radiosensitivity after single and combined heat treatments has also been observed for HeLa cells, whereas there is only a moderate correlation for EAT cells (Jorritsma et al. 1986).

These results indicate that, at least for CHO and HeLa cells, the increase in radiosensitivity observed when X-rays are combined with heat may be causally related to the reduction in polymerase β activity by the preceding heat treatments. The mechanism of this thermal enhancement might be that the reduction in the enzyme activity in heated cells, which is due to a competitive inhibition (Dikomey et al. 1987), leads to a reduced rate of repair of radiation-induced damage as measured for the DNA strand break repair in heated cells (Dikomey 1982; Jorritsma and Konings 1983; Mills and Meyn 1983). As a consequence of a depressed repair the possibility of misrepair should be enhanced, leading to an increased yield of chromosomal aberrations (Dewey et al. 1978) and thus causing increased radiosensitivity as is generally observed in heated cells.

Summary

The enhancement of the radiosensitivity of CHO cells was determined for various single and multiple heat treatments followed by X-irradiation at 0° C to prevent repair during exposure. Furthermore, the reduction in the activity of DNA polymerase β was determined after the same heat treatments. The thermal enhancement ratios for cell killing, calculated on the 10% survival level for the various experimental conditions, showed a clear-cut correlation with the activity of DNA polymerase β measured by the end of the various heat treatments. These results indicate that the thermal radiosensitization observed in many biological systems might be associated with the transient loss of polymerase β activity.

References

Ben Hur E, Elkind MM, Bronk BV (1974) Thermally enhanced radioresponse of cultured Chinese hamster cells: inhibition of repair of sublethal damage and enhancement of lethal damage. Radiat Res 58: 38-51

Denman DL, Spiro IJ, Dewey WC (1982) Effects of hyperthermia on DNA polymerases α and β: relationship to thermal cell killing and radiosensitization. In: Dethlefsen LA (ed) Proceedings of the 3rd international symposium: cancer therapy by hyperthermia, drugs and radiation. Natl Cancer Inst Monogr 61: 37-39

Dewey WC, Esch JL (1982) Transient thermal tolerance: cell killing and polymerase activities. Radiat Res 92: 611-614

Dewey WC, Sapareto SS, Betten DA (1978) Hyperthermic radiosensitization of synchronous Chinese hamster cells: relationship between lethality and chromosomal aberrations. Radiat Res 76: 48-59

Dikomey E (1982) Effect of hyperthermia at 42 and 45° C on repair of radiation-induced DNA strand breaks in CHO cells. Int J Radiat Biol 41: 603-614

Dikomey E, Eickhoff J, Jung H (1984) Thermotolerance and thermosensitization in CHO and in RIH cells: a comparative study. Int J Radiat Biol 46: 181-192

Dikomey E, Becker W, Wielckens K (1987) Reduction of DNA polymerase β activity of CHO cells by single and combined heat treatments. Int J Radiat Biol 52: 775-785

Hartson-Eaton M, Malcolm AW, Hahn GM (1984) Radiosensitivity and thermosensitization of thermotolerant Chinese hamster cells and RIF-1 tumors. Radiat Res 99: 175-184

Haveman J (1983) Influence of a prior heat treatment on the enhancement by hyperthermia of X-ray-induced inactivation of cultured mammalian cells. Int J Radiat Biol 43: 267-280

Henle KJ, Dethlefsen LA (1978) Heat fractionation and thermotolerance: a review. Cancer Res 38: 1843-1851

Holahan EV, Highfield DP, Holahan PK, Dewey WC (1984) Hyperthermic killing and hyperthermic radiosensitization in Chinese hamster ovary cells: effects of pH and thermal tolerance. Radiat Res 97: 108-131

Holahan PK, Wong RSL, Thompson LL, Dewey WC (1986) Hyperthermic radiosensitization of thermotolerant Chinese hamster ovary cells. Radiat Res 107: 332-343

Jorritsma JBM, Konings AWT (1983) Inhibition of repair of radiation-induced strand breaks by hyperthermia, and its relationship to cell survival after hyperthermia alone. Int J Radiat Biol 43: 506-516

Jorritsma JBM, Burgman P, Kampinga HH, Konings AWT (1986) DNA polymerase activity in heat killing and hyperthermic radiosensitization of mammalian cells as observed after fractionated heat treatments. Radiat Res 105: 307-319

Jung H (1982) Interaction of thermotolerance and thermosensitization induced in CHO cells by combined hyperthermic treatments at 40 and 43° C. Radiat Res 91: 433-446

Jung H (1986) A generalized concept for cell killing by heat. Radiat Res 106: 56-72

Kampinga HH, Jorritsma JBM, Konings AWT (1985) Heat-induced alterations in DNA polymerase activity of HeLa cells and of isolated nuclei: relation to cell killing. Int J Radiat Biol 47: 29-40

Mills MD, Meyn RE (1983) Hyperthermic potentiation of unrejoined DNA strand breaks following irradiation. Radiat Res 95: 327-338

Mivechi NF, Dewey WC (1985) DNA polymerase α and β activities during the cell cycle and their role in heat radiosensitization in Chinese hamster ovary cells. Radiat Res 103: 337-350

Robinson JE, Wizenberg MJ (1974) Thermal sensitivity and the effect of elevated temperatures on the radiation sensitivity of Chinese hamster cells. Acta Radiol Ther Phys Biol 13: 241-248

Sapareto SA, Hopwood LE, Dewey WC (1978) Combined effects of X-irradiation and hyperthermia on CHO cells for various temperatures and orders of application. Radiat Res 73: 221-233

Effect of Heat and Combined Treatments on Normal Tissues

The Problem of Defining Thermal Dose

M. P. Law and S. B. Field

MRC Cyclotron Unit, Hammersmith Hospital, Du Cane Road,
London W12 OHS, Great Britain

Introduction

The rationale for using hyperthermia to treat malignant disease is based on experimental studies which suggest that tumours may be more susceptible to thermal injury than normal tissues (Field and Bleehen 1979). In particular, solid tumours may have an inadequate vascular supply so that many tumour cells may be in an environment (low nutrient and oxygen supply, low pH) which increases thermal sensitivity. Another consequence of a low blood flow is that removal of heat from a locally heated tumour may be poor so that it reaches higher temperatures than adjacent normal tissues.

Hyperthermia also enhances biological responses to both ionising radiations and chemotherapeutic agents. The factors which increase tumour susceptibility to direct thermal damage, however, are unlikely to increase thermal enhancement of damage caused by other modalities. Indeed, animal studies show that thermal enhancement of radiation damage to tumour and normal tissue is similar for a given degree of hyperthermia (Field et al. 1980; Overgaard 1982). Only if tumour reaches a higher temperature than normal tissue will a therapeutic gain be achieved for the simultaneous application of heat and irradiation (Fig. 1).

A therapeutic gain after combined therapy may be achievable in the absence of a marked temperature difference between tumour and normal tissue if the two modalities are separated in time. This has been demonstrated in both experimental (Fig. 1) and clinical studies (Overgaard 1981) when heat is given 3-4 h after the radiation. In this case the interactive effect of heat and radiation will have decayed and any therapeutic advantage will probably result from a greater susceptibility of acidic tumour cells to heat.

Preclinical studies of hyperthermia should consider the various factors which affect the relative responses of tumour and normal tissues. There is thus a need for systematic investigation of physiological responses of various cells and tissues, including those in man, and studies of underlying mechanisms which may suggest ways of optimising treatment. In order to quantitate such studies, a satisfactory method of expressing thermal does is required. A rigid definition of "thermal dose", however, has not been accepted.

Recent Results in Cancer Research, Vol. 109

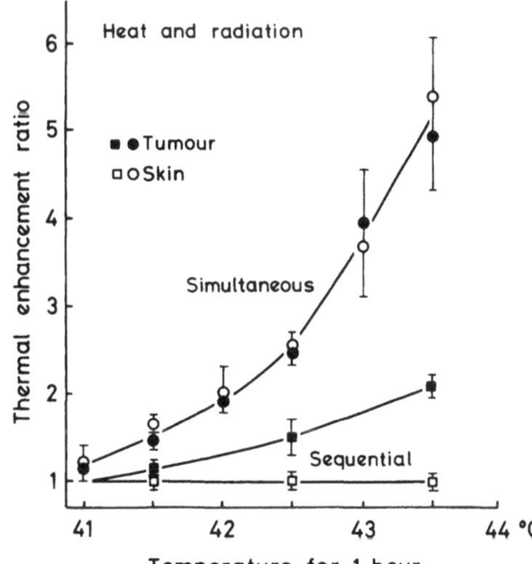

Fig. 1. Thermal enhancement ratio after simultaneous or sequential treatment at various temperatures. In the sequential treatment heat was given 4 h after radiation. Results for a murine mammary carcinoma and its surrounding skin are compared. (Overgaard 1980, 1984)

The Concept of Thermal Dose

Dose is used to provide a means of predicting a biological response following administration of a medicine or something analogous to a medicine and to provide a means of communication regarding the effects of a given amount of a medicine or something analogous to medicine. A dose unit, therefore, must be a well defined and measurable physical quantity. The biological response must be related to the dose in a meaningful and quantitative manner. Proper means of intercomparison should be possible.

Radiotherapists have become accustomed to using energy deposited to describe the dose of radiation as this relates clearly to the resulting biological effect. Absorbed energy, however, cannot be used satisfactorily to predict the biological response to hyperthermia, as illustrated by Hahn (1982). If a thermally insulated culture dish initially at 37° C is heated quickly to 43° C no cells are killed. If the system is kept at 43° C with no energy allowed to enter or leave, cell killing will begin as a result of the cells being at the elevated temperature. The effect of heat depends on the temperature and duration of heating, not on the energy required to produce the temperature rise. Thus for a fixed temperature, time is a reasonable measure of thermal dose.

The problem of using time at a given temperature is that treatments are given at different temperatures and the temperature is probably not constant. One solution is to use some means of relating a given treatment to an equivalent time at a reference temperature. Although different cells and tissues have different sensitivities to heat, there is a general relationship between temperature and time to cause a given response, as described by Dewey et al. (1977). This relationship is given by:

$$t_2 = t_1 \, A(T_1 - T_2)$$

where t is the heating time, T is the temperature and A is a factor which depends on the temperature range (Sapareto and Dewey 1984). Mean values for A, ob-

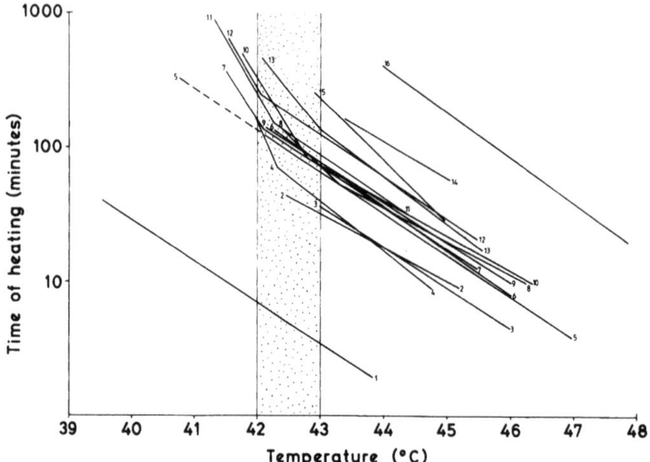

Fig. 2. Relationship between time of heating and temperature for a chosen level of damage in a range of normal tissues and tumours in situ. Each line represents a different biological system. (Field and Morris 1983)

tained by reviewing data for both normal tissues and tumours, are 2 for temperatures above about 42.5° C and 6 for those below 42.5° C (Fig. 2; Field and Morris 1983). Sapareto and Dewey (1984) proposed that 43° C should be used as a reference temperature and that all treatment be described as equivalent minutes of heating at 43° C. They showed that survival of Chinese hamster ovary cells heated at different temperatures for different times fitted a single curve when plotted as a function of equivalent minutes at 43° C, although data below the inflection temperature deviated somewhat from the single line.

Potential Problems with the Concept of Thermal Dose

A number of difficulties are involved in the definition of thermal dose outlined above:

1. The "inflection temperature", the temperature at which the relationship between time and temperature changes, has been determined only in a limited number of tissues, and these results together with those for cells in vitro suggest that the inflection temperature may vary between 42° and 43° C.
2. Although the factor of 2 for temperatures above 42.5° C is well established, there is considerable uncertainty about the value in the lower temperature range. Computer simulation to allow for different values of transition temperature and slope of the iso-effect curve in the low temperature region, however, have been carried out by Hand (reported by Field 1987). It was shown that the choice of parameters could have an important effect on the "thermal dose" especially at low temperatures below the transition.
3. In clinical practice there are considerable fluctuations in temperature during any one treatment which might lead to changes in thermal sensitivity due to the

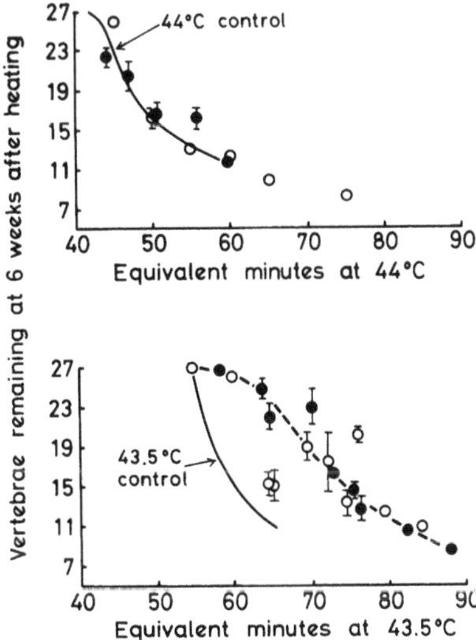

Fig. 3. Application of the relationship between heating time and temperature to define a thermal dose. Simulation of a treatment at varying temperatures was achieved by immersing tails of baby rats alternately in water baths of different temperatures. Heating was either for equal times at the two temperatures (●) or for times required to cause equal effects (○). *(Above)* Results of six cycles of heating at 43° C and 45° C matched to 44° C according to the "heat dose" formula, showing an accurate prediction. *(Below)* Results of three cycles of heating at 42° C and 45° C similarly matched to 43.5° C showing an effect of thermotolerance, i.e. an increase in time of 20%. (Field and Morris 1984)

development of thermotolerance or "step-down" sensitisation. A recent study using the baby rat tail, aimed at simulating clinical conditions, shows that variation in thermal sensitivity resulting from variations in temperature during treatment may be small. The measured biological effects were in good agreement with those expected for a given equivalent time calculated using the formula (Fig. 3). The maximum difference between observed and expected heating times was 20%, equivalent to an error in temperature of 0.3° C (Field and Morris 1984). Such a discrepancy is small compared with other uncertainties in a typical hyperthermia treatment. Extreme changes, however, such as half of the treatment at 45° C followed by the other half at 41° C, would certainly result in step-down sensitisation and invalidate the use of the formula.

4. The time-temperature relationship may change during fractionated treatment. Evidence from cells in vitro and skin in mouse shows that the induction of thermotolerance does not alter the slope of the iso-effect curves relating heating time and temperature although it does increase the inflection temperature and decrease thermal sensitivity (Bauer and Henle 1979; Law 1979).
5. The time-temperature relationship for the interaction between heat and radiation is similar to that for heat alone although the inflection temperature is at the lower temperature of about 41.5° C (Hume and Marigold 1985).
6. The time-temperature relationships for the interaction between heat and chemotherapeutic agents are not known.

The formula, however, provides a practical method of comparing hyperthermal treatments under conditions likely to occur in normal clinical practice and its use is the best approach available at present.

Fractionation and the Role of Thermotolerance

The formula put forward for the definition of thermal dose does not account for changes in biological sensitivity which depends on a number of factors. These factors include individual susceptibility, temperature distribution within a tissue, overall treatment time, various modifying factors and previous treatment. Similar factors influence the response to radiation and drugs but the radiotherapist and chemotherapist have learnt by experience how to modify their treatment schedules to give the optimum response. An additional problem for treatment planning in hyperthermia is introduced by the possibility of the development of thermotolerance during fractionated treatment.

It is well established that transient thermotolerance develops in normal tissues and tumours after an acute treatment at temperatures of 42.5 °C or greater (Law 1987). For a given tissue, the degree of thermotolerance is greater and is expressed later as the severity of the initial heat treatment is increased (Law et al. 1979; Overgaard 1984; Field and Morris 1985). Despite different capacities to develop thermotolerance there is a general relationship between heating time and temperature required for its induction. This relationship is similar to that for direct thermal injury (Law 1981; Nielsen and Overgaard 1982; Field and Morris 1985).

The limited number of studies of fractionated hyperthermia indicate that, for a given cell line or tissue, there is a maximum thermotolerance which cannot be exceeded (Henle et al. 1979; Law et al. 1984; Overgaard and Nielsen 1984; Nielsen and Overgaard 1985). In addition, the maximum thermotolerance induced by a given fractionation regime depends on the size of each fraction rather than on the number of fractions. It is the same as that after a single heat treatment of the same size as each fraction (Law et al. 1984).

The development of maximal thermotolerance depends on the interval between fractions (Overgaard and Nielsen 1984; Nielsen and Overgaard 1985; Law 1985). This is illustrated for the mouse ear in Fig. 4, which illustrates the response to two heat treatments. The results can be divided into several groups:

1. If the second fraction is given when thermotolerance after the first is developing, the development of thermotolerance is delayed but reaches the same maximum value as that observed after a single treatment and then decays.
2. If the second treatment is given when thermotolerance after the first is maximal, the maximal degree of thermotolerance is maintained for a period of time before decaying.
3. If the second treatment is given when thermotolerance is decaying there is a further increase to maximal thermotolerance again followed by decay.

The degree of thermotolerance at any given time during a fractionated hyperthermia treatment, therefore, will depend on the tissue and protocol being used. If short interfraction intervals are used, thermotolerance may build up to the maxi-

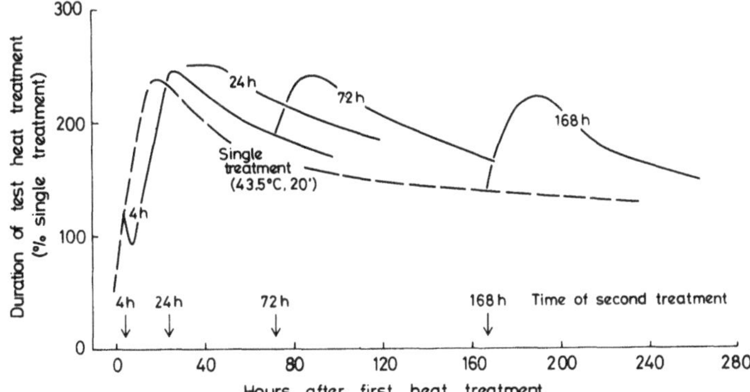

Fig. 4. Thermotolerance induced in the mouse ear after two fractions of heat. Thermotolerance was expressed as the duration of a test treatment at 43.5° C required to cause thermal damage in 50% of the ears. Values greater than 100% indicate thermotolerance. *Broken line*, thermotolerance after a single treatment of 20 min at 43.5° C; *solid lines*, thermotolerance after two treatments of 20 min at 43.5° C separated by 4, 24, 72 or 168 h. (Law 1987)

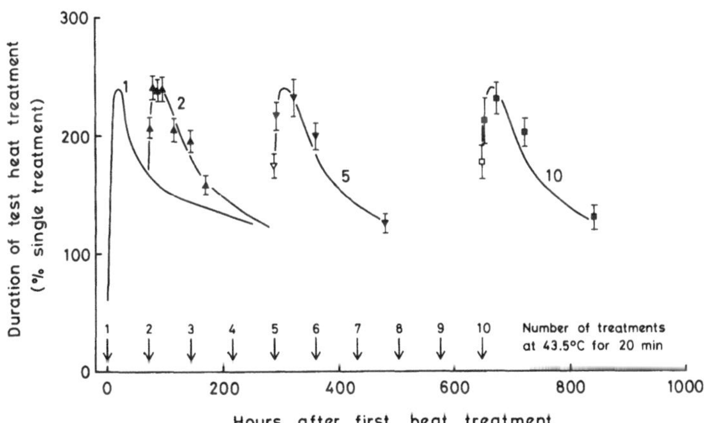

Fig. 5. Thermotolerance induced in the mouse ear by treatments of 20 min at 43.5° C given at 72-h intervals. Thermotolerance was assessed as in Fig. 4. The *solid line* indicates results for one treatment. ▲, two treatments; ▽, four treatments; ▼, five treatments; □, nine treatments; ■, ten treatments. (Law et al. 1987)

mum during the early fractions. If fractions are repeated when thermotolerance is maximal, this maximum will be maintained throughout treatment. If fractions are repeated at longer intervals there will be increases and decreases in thermotolerance throughout treatment, as shown in Fig. 5.

Animal studies show that thermotolerance in tumours is similar to that in normal tissues. Whether or not there will be differences in the responses to fractionated treatment which can be exploited in cancer therapy is not known. At present, the accepted approach is to allow sufficient time between each fraction for thermotolerance to decay. Clearly, more information about response of tumours and normal tissues to fractionated hyperthermia is required for the optimisation of clinical treatment.

Conclusions

1. Tumours are likely to be more susceptible to direct thermal damage than normal tissues. However, when heat is given simultaneously with radiation or chemotherapy to enhance response, a therapeutic advantage appears to be obtained only if tumour tissue reaches a temperature which is significantly higher than that in surrounding normal tissue. A therapeutic advantage may be obtained in the absence of a temperature differential, however, if heat is given a few hours after radiation. In the latter case, there will be no enhancement of normal tissue response but heat is likely to kill acidic tumour cells.
2. A method of defining thermal dose is required for comparison of experimental and clinical results. In a theoretical situation with temperature fixed and constant, duration of heating is a satisfactory method of describing thermal dose. In the real situation, when temperature is not fixed and is variable, a biologically equivalent dose must be used. The use of the biological iso-effect relationships to define a thermal dose equivalent appears to be acceptable for heat treatments in the normal clinical range. There may be differences in the iso-effect relationship when using heat in combination with other modalities.
3. Thermal dose is defined for a single treatment only. When considering fractionated treatment the development of thermotolerance is of particular importance. Present data indicate that the maximal thermotolerance which develops during or after fractionated hyperthermia is equal to that observed after a single fraction. The time course of thermotolerance depends on the interval between fractions.
4. The concept of "thermal dose" based on time-temperature relationships is useful for planning treatments and comparing responses of patients. It must not, however, substitute for the basic clinical data, which should be retained.

References

Bauer KD, Henle KJ (1979) Arrhenius analysis of heat survival curves from normal and thermotolerant CHO cells. Radiat Res 78: 251-263

Dewey WC, Hopwood LE, Sapareto SA, Gerweck LE (1977) Cellular responses to combinations of hyperthermia and radiation. Radiology 123: 463-474

Field SB (1987) Biological effects of hyperthermia. In: Field SB, Franconi C (eds) Physics and technology of hyperthermia. Nijhoff, The Hague

Field SB, Bleehen NM (1979) Hyperthermia in the treatment of cancer. Cancer Treat Rev 6: 63-94

Field SB, Morris CC (1983) The relationship between heating time and temperature: its relevance to clinical hyperthermia. Radiother Oncol 1: 179-186

Field SB, Morris CC (1984) Application of the relationship between heating time and temperature for use as a measure of thermal dose. In: Overgaard J (ed) Hyperthermic oncology 1984, vol 1. Taylor and Francis, London, pp 183-186

Field SB, Morris CC (1985) Experimental studies of thermotolerance in vivo. I. The baby rat tail model. Int J Hyperthermia 1: 235-246

Field SB, Hume SP, Law MP (1980) The response of tissues to heat alone or in combination with radiation. In: Okada S, Imamura M, Terashima T, Yamaguchi H (eds) Proceedings, 6th international congress of radiation research, 13-19 May 1979. Japanese Association for Radiation Research, Tokyo (ISSN 0538-6586)

Hahn GM (1982) Hyperthermia and cancer. Plenum, New York

Henle KJ, Bitner AF, Dethlefsen LA (1979) Induction of thermotolerance by multiple heat fractions in Chinese hamster ovary cells. Cancer Res 39: 2486-2491

Hume SP, Marigold JCL (1985) Time-temperature relationships for hyperthermal radiosensitisation in mouse intestine: influence of thermotolerance. Radiother Oncol 3: 165-171

Law MP (1979) Induced thermal resistance in the mouse ear: the relationship between heating time and temperature. Int J Radiat Biol 35: 481-485

Law MP (1981) The induction of thermal resistance in the ear of the mouse by heating at temperatures ranging from 41.5-45.5° C. Radiat Res 85: 126-134

Law MP (1985) Thermotolerance induced in the mouse ear by fractionated hyperthermia depends on the interval between fractions. Strahlentherapie 161: 541 (Abstr)

Law MP (1987) The response of normal tissues to hyperthermia. In: Urano M (ed) Hyperthermia and oncology, vol 1. VNU Scientific, The Netherlands

Law MP, Coultas PG, Field SB (1979) Induced thermal resistance in the mouse ear. Br J Radiol 52: 308-314

Law MP, Ahier RG, Somaia S, Field SB (1984) The induction of thermotolerance in the ear of the mouse by fractionated hyperthermia. Int J Radiat Oncol Biol Phys 10: 865-873

Law MP, Ahier RG, Somaia S (1987) Thermotolerance induced by fractionated hyperthermia: dependence on the interval between fractions. Int J Hyperthermia 3: 433-439

Nielsen OS, Overgaard J (1982) Importance of preheating temperature and time for the induction of thermotolerance in a solid tumour in vivo. Br J Cancer 46: 894-903

Nielsen OS, Overgaard J (1985) Studies on fractionated hyperthermia in L1A2 tumour cells in vitro: response to multiple equal heat fractions. Int J Hyperthermia 1: 193-203

Overgaard J (1980) Simultaneous and sequential hyperthermia and radiation treatment of an experimental tumor and its surrounding normal tissues in vivo. Int J Radiat Oncol Biol Phys 6: 1507-1517

Overgaard J (1981) Fractionated radiation and hyperthermia: experimental and clinical studies. Cancer 48: 1116-1123

Overgaard J (1982) Influence of sequence and interval on the biological response to combined hyperthermia and radiation. Natl Cancer Inst Monogr 61: 325-332

Overgaard J (1984) Hyperthermia and radiation. Biological rationale and clinical experience. Proceedings, Varian's 4th European clinac users meeting, 25-26 May 1984, Malta

Overgaard J, Nielsen OS (1984) Influence of thermotolerance on the effect of multifractionated hyperthermia in a C3H mammary carcinoma in vivo. In: Overgaard J (ed) Hyperthermic oncology 1984, vol 1. Taylor and Francis, London, pp 211-214

Sapareto SA, Dewey WC (1984) Thermal dose determination in cancer therapy. Int J Radiat Oncol Biol Phys 10: 787-806

*Effect of Hyperthermia on Human Natural Killer Cells**

M. Onsrud

Kvinneklinikken, Regionsykehuset, 7000 Trondheim, Norway

Introduction

Natural killer (NK) cells, a subset of lymphocytes, have the ability preferentially to kill virus-infected cells and certain tumor cells in vitro (Herberman et al. 1979). NK cells have been proposed to represent a first level defense mechanism against tumor development and tumor spread in vivo (Herberman 1981; Pollack and Hallenbeck 1982). A correlation between defective NK activity and an increased incidence of malignant disease both in man and in mice supports this concept (Haliotis et al. 1980; Talmadge et al. 1980).

Natural killer cell activity can be modified in vitro by interferon, prostaglandins, and metabolic inhibitors (Saksela et al. 1979; Brunda et al. 1980). Fever is common both in infections and in neoplastic diseases. Whether the elevated temperature influences the prognosis of the disease in a favorable or an unfavorable way is unclear. Local or general hyperthermia (40°-43° C) has been applied in the treatment of cancer, most often in combination with radiotherapy. A constraint is placed on the clinical use of hyperthermia by the uncertainty over whether it affects in vivo tumor defense mechanisms. In some animal tumor systems heating seems to increase the frequency of distant metastases (Yerushalmi 1976; Schecter et al. 1978), whereas in other systems a decreased frequency has been reported (Shen et al. 1985). Azocar et al. (1982) found that human NK activity was depressed after incubation of lymphocytes at 39°-40° C for more than 4 h.

The studies presented here were undertaken to determine the thermal sensitivity of human NK cells under conditions relevant for hyperthermic therapy. The findings are correlated to lymphocyte viability, expression of surface markers, and ability to proliferate in vitro.

* This study was supported by the Norwegian Cancer Society.

Recent Results in Cancer Research, Vol. 109

Materials and Methods

Peripheral blood mononuclear cells were separated from defibrinated blood of healthy donors, and monocytes removed by the adherence technique. Nonadherent blood lymphocytes (PBL) suspended in RPMI 1640 Medium with 10% fetal bovine serum were used in the studies. Rosetting techniques were used to determine the T cell fraction and the fraction of cells bearing receptors for the Fc part of IgG (which is a marker for the NK cell fraction).

Hyperthermic treatment was performed in water baths held at temperatures of 37°, 40°, 41°, and 42° ±0.2° C. Tubes containing less than 3 ml of PBL suspensions were immersed for periods up to 3 h.

Cells of the erythroid leukemia cell line K562 labeled with ^{51}Cr were used as targets in the NK cell assay as previously described (Onsrud and Thorsby 1981). The proliferative capacity of PBL was determined by stimulation with phytohemagglutinin (PHA) for 3 days, and by mixed lymphocyte culture (MLC) for 6 days, and the results are given as ^{3}H-thymidine incorporation. Cell-mediated lympholysis (CML) of MLC-activated cells was determined against PHA-induced lymphoblasts of the MLC-stimulator cells.

Effects of Hyperthermia on NK Cell Activity

Lymphocyte suspensions kept in hyperthermic water baths for up to 3 h showed a decrease in subsequent NK activity which depended on the temperature and on the period of immersion. The results of one typical experiment are shown in Table 1. Effector cells kept at 37° C for similar periods normally showed unchanged activity. In some experiments exposure to 40° C for 1 h slightly potentiated the activity. For a given temperature the decrease in activity was related to the period of treatment in a semilogarithmic fashion (Fig. 1). A dramatic increase in thermal sensitivity was seen when the temperature was raised from 41° C to 42° C. Lymphocytes kept at 42° C for 1 h showed less than 10% of the cytotoxicity expressed by cells kept at 37° C for the same period of time. The supernatant of effector lymphocytes kept at 42° C for 3 h had no effect on the NK activity displayed by unheated lymphocytes (data not shown).

Table 1. Effect of hyperthermia on lymphocyte natural killer (NK) activity

Temperature	Period of treatment (h)			
	0	1	2	3
37° C	26[a]	28	29	28
40° C		29	28	22
41° C		23	20	14
42° C		3	1	0

[a] % cytotoxicity in a 3-h ^{51}Cr-release assay with K562 cells, effector/target = 10/1.

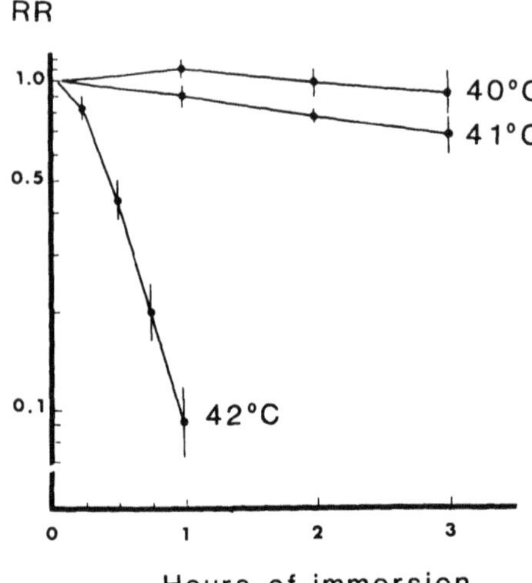

Fig. 1. The effect of hyperthermia on the NK activity of blood lymphocytes. Tubes of lymphocytes suspensions were immersed in water baths for various periods of time, and the cytotoxicity against K562 target cells was then determined in a 3-h ^{51}Cr-release assay at an effector: target ratio of 10:1. Relative response *(RR)* denotes the NK activity of heat-treated lymphocytes relative to the NK activity of lymphocytes kept at 37° C. Means ± SE of five experiments

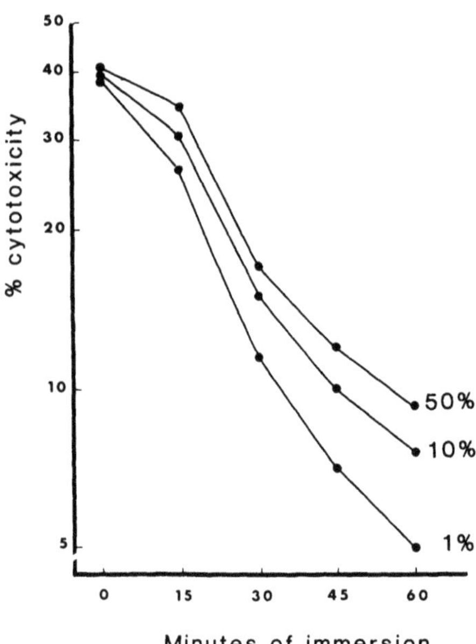

Fig. 2. The influence of serum concentration on the thermal sensitivity of NK cells. Lymphocytes from one donor were suspended in medium containing 1%, 10%, or 50% fetal bovine serum during treatment at 42° C for 3 h

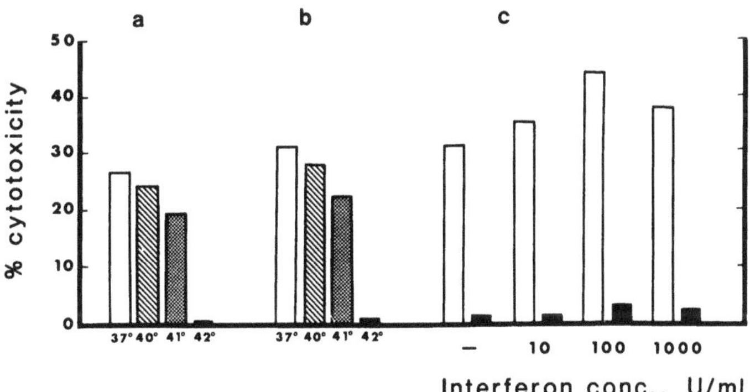

Fig. 3 a–c. Lack of repair of heat-induced damage to NK cells. Lymphocytes were kept at 37°, 40°, 41°, and 42° C for 3 h, and the NK activity was determined **a** immediately afterwards, **b** after further overnight incubation at 37° C, and **c** after overnight incubation with various concentrations of purified leukocyte interferon (Cantell and Hirvonen 1978). Mean values of four experiments

The thermal sensitivity curves were influenced by the serum concentration of the medium: High concentrations of fetal bovine serum provided a certain degree of protection against heat-induced cell damage (Fig. 2).

Various experiments were performed to see whether the heat-induced NK deficiency was reparable. Heat-treated lymphocytes were still hypo- or unresponsive when the NK assay period was extended from 3 h to 18 h (data not shown). When the heated cells were incubated at 37° C overnight before being tested in a 3-h NK assay, the response profile was the same as when they were tested directly after heating (Fig. 3 a, b). Overnight treatment with various concentrations of interferon potentiated the NK activity of the effector cells exposed to 37° C, whereas no effect was seen on the cells exposed to 42° C for 3 h (Fig. 3 c).

Table 2. Differential effect of hyperthermia on NK activity and on proliferation in MLC

Temperature (3 h)	NK activity[a]	Proliferation in MLC[b]	
		Responder capacity	Stimulator capacity
37° C	26.7±4.6	4.47±0.14	3.77±0.57
40° C	21.6±4.1	4.39±0.20	3.92±0.67
41° C	18.0±3.7	4.51±0.12	3.73±0.45
42° C	0.7±0.4	4.40±0.15	3.69±0.76

[a] % cytotoxicity against K562 target cells.

[b] Log_{10} cpm ^{3}H-thymidine in 6 days MLC. Mean±SE of four experiments.

Difference in Thermal Sensitivity of NK Cells and T Cells

T-lymphocyte proliferation as estimated from the ^{3}H-thymidine incorporation of MLC was not significantly affected by pretreatment of the MLC-responder cells for 3 h at 42° C (Table 2). Similarly, heating did not significantly change the MLC-stimulating capacity of the lymphocytes.

The cytotoxicity expressed in the CML assay with PHA lymphoblasts as targets was less sensitive to hyperthermia than was the NK activity of fresh lymphocytes from the same cell donor (Table 3).

The PHA responsiveness of lymphocytes pretreated at 42° C for 3 h was slightly lowered when determined after 3 days of culture (Fig. 4a). This depression can be explained by a delay in the proliferation kinetics of the heated cells (Fig. 4b).

Table 3. Differential effect of hyperthermia on NK activity and on cell-mediated lympholysis *(CML)*

Effector cell type	Minutes at 42° C			
	0	15	30	45
Fresh NK cells	40[a]	37	15	10
MLC-activated cells (CML)	35[b]	36	36	27

[a] % cytotoxicity against K562 targets in a 3-h assay, effector/target = 10/1.

[b] % cytotoxicity against PHA lymphoblasts in a 6-h assay, effector/target = 50/1.

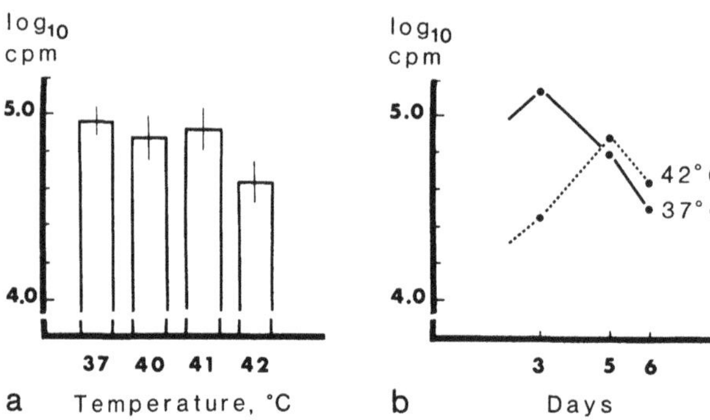

Fig. 4a, b. The effect of hyperthermia on PHA-induced lymphoproliferation. Lymphocytes were kept at various temperatures for 3 h before being stimulated by PHA. The responses are given as the logarithmic value of counts per minute *(cpm)*. **a** Harvesting on day 3 of culture, mean ± SE of five experiments. **b** Harvesting performed on various days

Table 4. Effect of hyperthermia on lymphocyte viability and expression of surface markers. Results after overnight incubation are shown in parentheses

Temperature (3 h)	Viability[a] (%)	Fc_γ-receptor[b] (%)	E-rosettes[c] (%)
37° C	100 (98±1)	15±4 (9±2)	61±5 (53±5)
40° C	99±1 (97±1)	10±3 (6±1)	57±9 (55±3)
41° C	98±1 (93±2)	9±2 (5±1)	47±3 (51±4)
42° C	95±1 (81±5)	4±1 (4±1)	34±3 (48±2)

[a] Determined by trypan blue exclusion.
[b] % of cells bearing receptors for IgG.
[c] % of cells forming rosettes with sheep erythrocytes. Mean±SE of five experiments.

Effects of Hyperthermia on Viability and Expression of Surface Markers

After exposure to 42° C for 3 h no significant depression of lymphocyte viability was seen (Table 4). After further overnight incubation at 37° C the viability, as determined by trypan blue exclusion, was still above 80%. Both the number of cells expressing Fc-receptors and the number of cells showing E-rosettes were significantly reduced after heat exposure. When reexamined after overnight incubation at 37° C the number of Fc-receptor bearing lymphocytes was still low, whereas the number of cells with T cell characteristics was normalized.

Discussion

The results presented here show that NK cells, in contrast to cells proliferating in MLC and PHA assays, are highly sensitive to heating at 42° C. The NK deficiency appears not to be reparable. The damage exerted on T cells seems to be more easily repaired.

The discrepancy between the changes in NK activity and in lymphocyte viability could indicate that the heat damages some structures necessary for the lytic event without killing the effector cells. The NK cells, however, account for less than 15% of circulating lymphocytes. The results could therefore be compatible with a preferential killing of NK cells by the hyperthermia. The permanent depression of NK activity and Fc-receptor expression favor this view. Furthermore, interferon, which potentiates NK activity by recruiting pre-NK cells, could not restore the cytotoxicity. This indicates that also NK precursors are thermosensitive. Heat appears to have a direct effect on the NK effector cells, as the supernatant of heated cells had no suppressive effect on the NK activity of unheated effector cells.

Little is known about the thermal sensitivity of other immunocompetent cells. Hopwood et al. (1984) found that heating of human lymphocytes at 42° C for 4 h decreased the PHA response and the proliferation in MLC by 25%. They also showed that the cytotoxic T cells in CML were more heat sensitive than the T cells proliferating in MLC. This study shows that the cytotoxic cells in CML are less heat sensitive than the fresh NK cells (Table 3).

The difference in thermal sensitivity of various lymphoid subpopulations may depend on differentiation and activation. While small T-lymphocytes are considered to be resting cells, the NK cells seem to have undergone some in vivo activation (Herberman et al. 1979). Certain differentiation products could be particularly heat sensitive. Interestingly, the Fc-receptor for IgG which is expressed on NK cells seems to be a marker for differentiation rather than a marker of a particular lymphoid cell subpopulation (Pichler and Broder 1981). Some serum factors may be of importance for the stability of such thermosensitive surface structures (Fig. 2).

The preferential effect of heating on NK cells may have practical consequences and provide the means for separating unwanted NK cells from T cells, i.e., in the cloning of specific antigen-reactive cells. Whether in vivo hyperthermia (or fever) has a similar differential effect is unknown. It is too early to draw any conclusions as to the impact of hyperthermic therapy on the cancer defense mechanisms.

References

Azocar J, Yunis EJ, Essex M (1982) Sensitivity of human natural killer cells to hyperthermia. Lancet I: 16-17

Brunda MJ, Herberman RB, Holden HT (1980) Inhibition of murine natural killer cell activity by prostaglandins. J Immunol 124: 2682-2687

Cantell K, Hirvonen S (1978) Large scale production in human leucocyte interferon containing 10^8 units per ml. J Gen Virol 39: 541-543

Haliotis T, Roder J, Klein M, Ortaldo J, Fauci AS, Herberman RB (1980) Chediak-Higashi gene in humans. I. Impairment of natural killer function. J Exp Med 151: 1039-1048

Herberman RB (1981) Significance of natural killer cells in cancer research. Human Lymph Diff 1: 63-76

Herberman RB, Djeu JY, Kay D, Ortaldo JR, Riccardi C, Bonnard GD, Holden GT, Fagnani R, Santoni A, Puccetti P (1979) Natural killer cells: characteristics and regulation of activity. Immunol Rev 44: 43-70

Hopwood LE, Zeevi A, Doquesnoy R (1984) Response of human peripheral lymphocytes to hyperthermia (meeting abstr). 32nd Annual meeting of the Radiation Research Society, 25-29 March 1984, Orlando, Florida, p 51

Onsrud M, Thorsby E (1981) Influence of in vivo hydrocortisone on some human blood lymphocyte subpopulations. I. Effect on natural killer cell activity. Scand J Immunol 13: 573-579

Pichler WJ, Broder S (1981) In vitro functions of human T cells expressing Fc-IgG or Fc-IgM receptors. Immunol Rev 56: 163-197

Pollack SB, Hallenbeck LA (1982) In vivo reduction of NK activity with anti-NK 1 serum: direct evaluation of NK cells in tumor clearance. Int J Cancer 29: 203-207

Saksela E, Timonen T, Cantell K (1979) Human natural killer cell activity is augmented by interferon via recruitment of "pre-NK" cells. Scand J Immunol 10: 257-266

Schechter M, Stowe SM, Moroson H (1978) Effects of hyperthermia on primary and metastatic tumor growth and host immune response in rats. Cancer Res 38: 498-502

Shen RN, Shidnia H, Brahmi Z, Hornback NB (1985) Decreased lung metastases and higher natural killer cell activity by whole-body hyperthermia in Lewis lung carcinoma and B16 melanoma (meeting abstr). International Clinical Hyperthermia Society meeting, 21-26 April 1985, Charleston, South Carolina

Talmadge JE, Meyers KM, Prieur DY, Starkey JR (1980) Role of NK cells in tumor growth and metastasis in beige mice. Nature 284: 622-624

Yerushalmi A (1976) Influence on metastatic spread of whole body or local tumor hyperthermia. Eur J Cancer 12: 455-463

*Effect of Hyperthermia at 40.5° C and Cytostatic Drugs on Human Bone Marrow Progenitor Cells**

H. A. Neumann and R. Engelhardt**

St. Josef Hospital, Medizinische Klinik, Ruhr-Universität, Gudrunstraße 56, 4630 Bochum, FRG

Introduction

Hyperthermia in clinical treatment is mostly used locally, either alone or in combination with radio- or chemotherapy. In the treatment of local tumors, this modality is of proven therapeutic benefit (Cavaliere et al. 1982; Dewhirst et al. 1983). A small group of clinicians, however, have tried to apply whole body hyperthermia. Their therapeutic aim is the thermal enhancement of cytostatic drug effects in the treatment of disseminated malignancies (Pettigrew et al. 1974; Barlogie et al. 1979; Bull et al. 1979; Parks et al. 1979; Neumann et al. 1982). In using this modality, it is of critical importance to know whether hyperthermia can damage normal bone marrow and, if enhancement of cytostatic drug effects is indeed achieved, whether the action might be not only on the tumor cells but also on the bone marrow cells. It was therefore the aim of our study to establish whether hyperthermia can enhance the cytotoxicity of several cytostatic drugs on normal human bone marrow cells. For the clinical application of whole body hyperthermia the temperatures and the treatment times must be restricted to a tolerable level. We therefore used a temperature of 40.5° C for 2 h.

Material and Methods

Bone Marrow Cultures

Bone marrow cells were obtained from normal volunteers by aspiration from the iliac crest into a heparinized syringe. Mononuclear cells of a density less than 1.077 g/ml were separated by density centrifugation in Ficoll-Paque (Farmacia Fine Chemicals). One hundred thousand washed cells were plated in the presence of 30% fetal calf serum, 5% phytohemagglutinin-leukocyte-conditioned medium (PHA-LCM); methylcellulose at a concentration of 0.9% (w/v) was used as vis-

* Dedicated to Professor Dr. med Dr. h. c. G. W. Löhr on his 65th birthday

** The authors thank Mrs. Marlies Braun for excellent technical assistance.

Recent Results in Cancer Research, Vol. 109

cous support. Incubation was performed in an incubator at 7.5% CO_2 in a moist atmosphere. After 10-12 days colonies could be evaluated under an inverted microscope. The incubation of the control dishes was performed at 37° C (Fauser and Messner 1978).

Preparation of PHA-LCM

PHA-LCM was prepared according to Aye (1977). Briefly, 1×10^6 peripheral leukocytes were incubated with 1% human serum albumin (Sigma chemicals), Iscoves modified Dulbeccos medium, and 1% phytohemagglutinin. After 4 days of culture the supernatant was harvested.

Hyperthermic Incubation

At the initiation of the cultures the dishes were placed in an incubator at 40.5° C. The temperature was monitored with an electronic thermosensor (ETW Waldkirch) in the methylcellulose of a sham culture containing the same amount of methylcellulose as the dishes containing the cell suspensions. After hyperthermic treatment, the cultures were placed in an incubator at 37° C and remained there for the rest of the incubation time. In order to simulate conditions that are compatible with clinical conditions, we chose a slow temperature increase and a slow temperature decrease, as shown in Figs. 1 and 2.

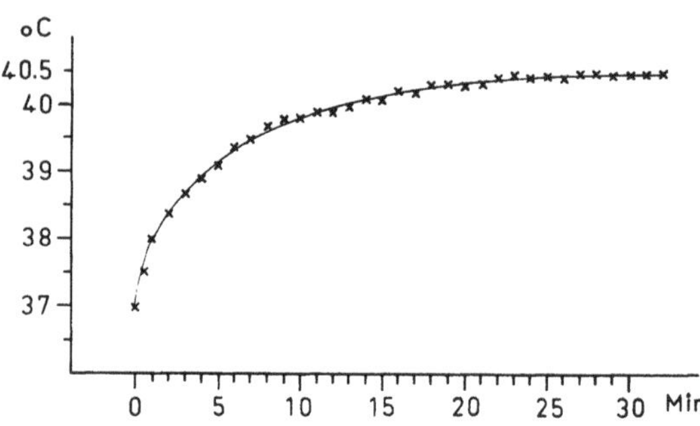

Fig. 1. Course of temperature increase in methylcellulose

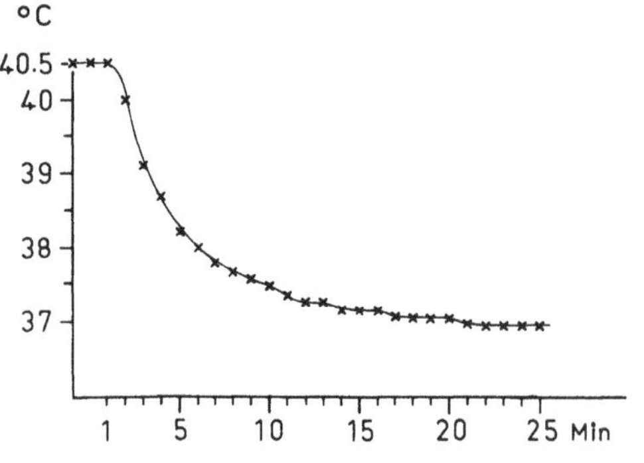

Fig. 2. Decline in the temperature after hyperthermic treatment when the culture dishes were placed in an incubator at 37° C

Drugs

The following drugs were tested: doxorubicin (Farmitalia), vincristine (Lilly), vinblastine (Lilly), cis-platin (Bristol), actinomycin D (MSD), etoposide (Bristol), bleomycin (Mack), peplomycin (Mack), and melphalan (Welcome). The drugs were dissolved with aqua bidest. Melphalan was dissolved with ethanol; further dilutions were performed with aqua bidest. The effect of the drugs was expressed as percent reduction in colony formation as a function of drug concentration. Drug exposure war performed continuously. For the assessment of a dose-respone curve at least seven or eight bone marrow samples from different donors were used.

Results

Bone marrow progenitor cells were plated in a methylcellulose assay. Plating efficiency ranged between 60 and 100 cells per 1×10^5 cells plated. There was no significant difference between colony formation obtained at 37° C incubation and after 2 h treatment at 40.5° C. At 37° C plating efficiency for CFU-C was 88 ± 17, at 40.5° C 77 ± 21. The effect of several cytostatic drugs on the colony forming capacity of human bone marrow progenitor cells (CFU-C) was assessed at 37° C and after a hyperthermic pulse at 40.5° C for 2 h. The dose-response curves are shown in Figs. 3–11. They showed homogeneous shapes independent of the donor. For each

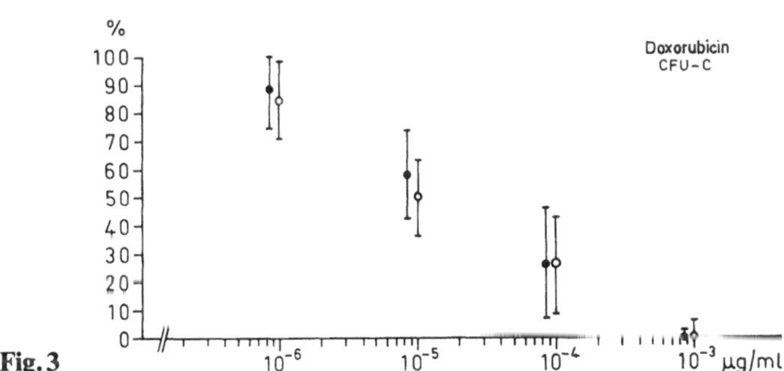

Fig. 3

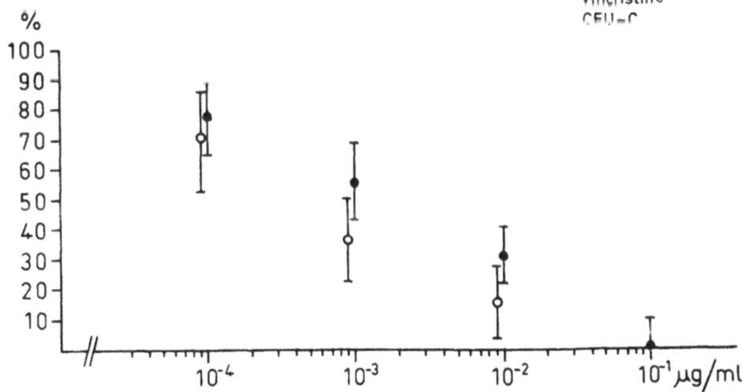

Fig. 4

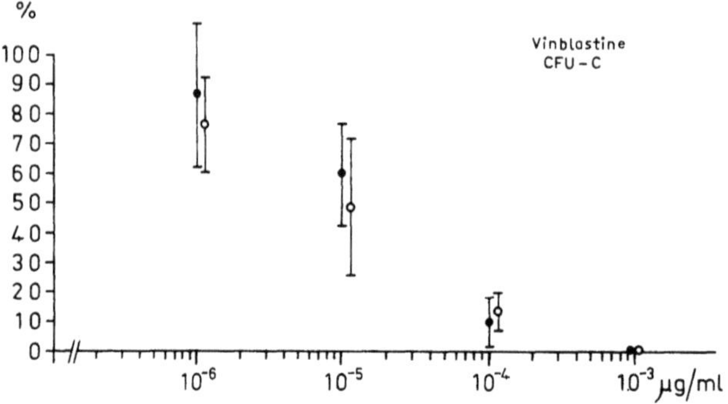

Fig. 5

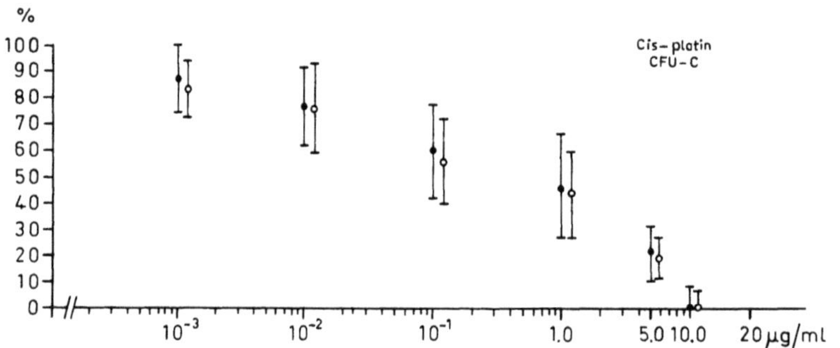

Fig. 6

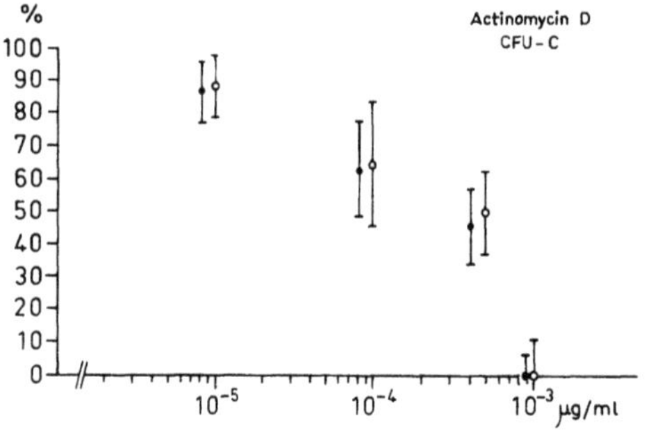

Fig. 7

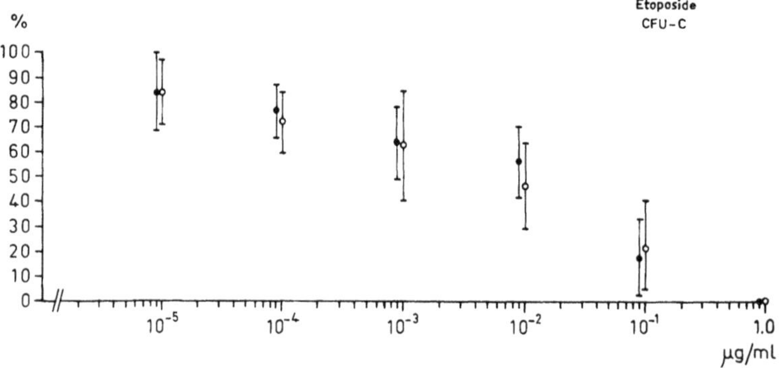

Fig. 8

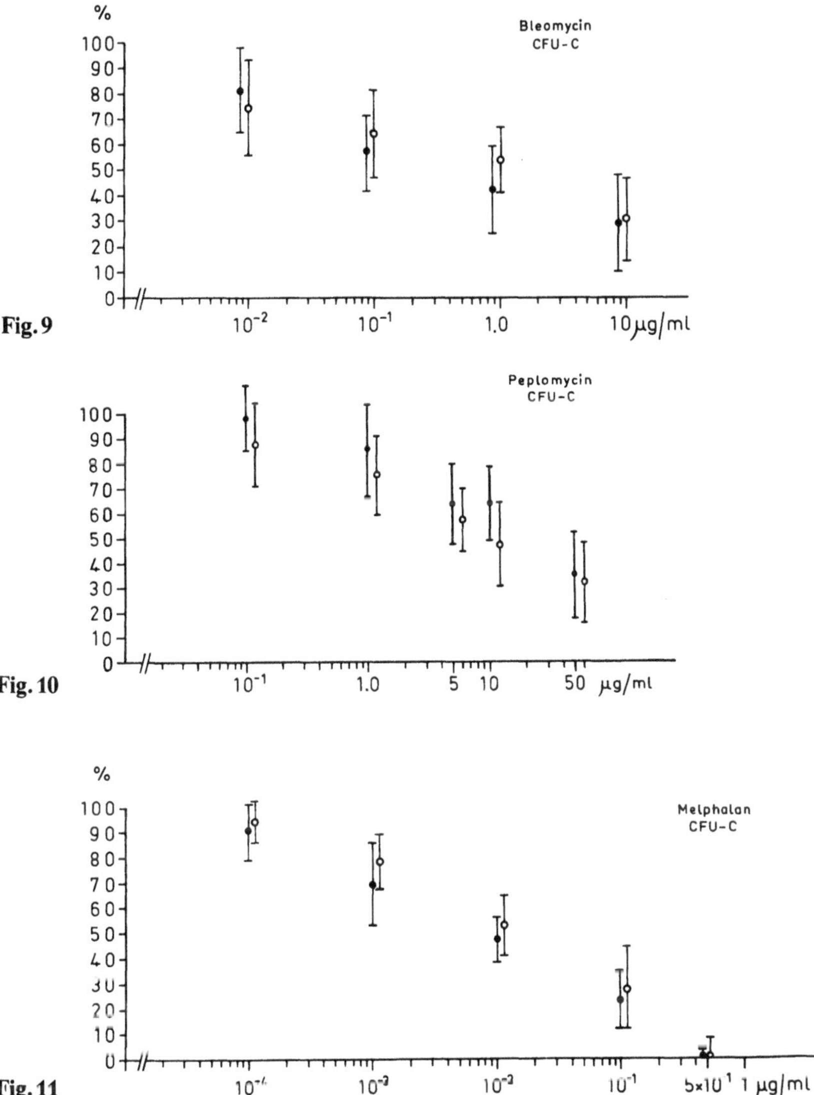

Figs. 3-11 *(pp. 59-61).* Dose-response curves of CFU-C under cytostatic treatment. The drugs are indicated in the charts. The *closed circles* indicate normothermic incubation, and the *open circles* hyperthermic incubation. Each dose response curve was established using at least seven different bone marrow samples. The drug effect is expressed as percent reduction in colony formation as a function of drug concentration

drug a typical dose-dependent reduction in colony formation was observed. With one exception (vincristine) there was no significant difference between dose-response curves at 37° C and those at 40.5° C for 2 h.

The incubation with vincristine showed colony formation up to a concentration of 10^{-1} μg/ml at 37° C, whereas at this concentration under hyperthermia no colony formation was observed. At lower concentrations of vincristine, no significant differences were observed between normo- and hyperthermic exposure.

Discussion

For the clinical application of whole body hyperthermia with the aim of enhancing drug cytotoxicity on malignant tumors, it is of great importance to investigate potential enhancement of cytotoxicity on normal tissue. In this case enhancement by hyperthermia would only result in an effect like that produced by a higher dose. The application of whole body hyperthermia can only lead to therapeutic benefit when thermal enhancement has a selective effect on tumor cells.

Elkon and co-workers (1981) have investigated the effect of hyperthermia on the pluripotent hematopoietic stem cell (CFU-S) in the mouse using the spleen cell colony assay described by Till and McCulloch (1961). Hyperthermic exposure was applied at temperatures ranging from 41.5° to 45.5° for 30 min. At 41.5° C no thermic damage was observed in the CFU-S. Bromer et al. (1982) have tested hyperthermic effects on human granulocytic progenitor cells (CFU-C). At a temperature of 41° C and short exposure, no reduction in colony formation was observed. After 12 h hyperthermic treatment, colony formation was reduced significantly. These observations are compatible with our results showing no difference between colony formation under normothermic and hyperthermic conditions. In combination with BCNU, O'Donell and co-workers (1979) were able to demonstrate enhancement of bone marrow toxicity at 41.8° C in the murine system.

In our studies we have used a rather low hyperthermic temperature. In these temperature ranges it is of interest whether some drugs thought to show linear thermal enhancement in tumor cell lines [e.g., melphalan and cis-platin (Hahn 1983)] might show the same kind of reactions when incubated with bone marrow cells. Under our conditions this was not the case. Vincristine has been described as a drug which shows no thermal enhancement at low temperatures (Halm, 1982) when tested in tumor cell lines. In our experiments at a dose of 10^{-1} μg/ml thermal enhancement was observed. Vincristine is a drug whose clinical use is not limited by bone marrow toxicity, and insofar the drug concentrations employed in our experiments do not reflect concentrations that are achievable in vitro. At concentrations lower than 10^{-1} μg/ml no difference between normothermic and hyperthermic incubation was seen. Equally the application of bleomycin and peplomycin is not limited by potential bone marrow toxicity. The dose-response curves for such drugs can only be used to prove that under the employed conditions no thermal enhancement of the drug effect is observed on normal bone marrow. Certainly, these observations cannot be extrapolated for higher temperatures. In conclusion, thermal enhancement of cytostatic drugs on the bone marrow might not be expected at 40.5° C for 2 h.

References

Aye MT, Niho Y, Till JE, McCulloch EA (1977) Studies of leukemic cell populations in culture. Blood 44: 205-214

Balogie B, Corry PM, Yip E, Lippmann I, Johnston DA, Khalil K, Tenczynski TF, Reilly E, Lawson R, Dosik G, Rigor B, Hankenson R, Freireich EJ (1979) Total-body hyperthermia with and without chemotherapy for advanced neoplasms. Cancer Res 39: 1481-1489

Bromer RH, Mitchell JB, Soares N (1982) Response of human hematopoietic precursor cells (CFU-C) to hyperthermia and radiation. Cancer Res 42: 1261-1265

Bull JM, Lees DE, Schutte WH, Wang Pang J, Smith R, Bynum G, Atkinson ER, Gottdiener JS, Gralnik HR, Shawker TH, de Vita VT (1979) Whole body hyperthermia: a phase I trial of a potential adjuvant to chemotherapy. Ann Intern Med 90: 317-323

Cavaliere R, Di Filippo F, Moricca G, Santori F, Varahese A, Pantano FP, Cassanelli A, Aloe L, Monticelli G (1982) Hyperthermic perfusion for treatment of tumors of the extremities. Chemotherapy 1: 278-287

Dewhirst MW, Sim DA, Wilson S, de Young D, Parsells JL (1983) Correlation between initial and long term responses of spontaneous pet animal tumors to heat and radiation or radiation alone. Cancer Res 43: 5735-5741

Elkon D, Dabio H, McGrath HE, Baker DG (1981) Temperature-dependent inhibition of murine granulocyte-monocyte precursors. Cancer Res 41: 1812-1816

Fauser AA, Messner HA (1978) Granuloerythropoietic colonies in human bone marrow, peripheral blood and cord blood. Blood 52: 1243-1248

Hahn GM (1983) Hyperthermia to enhance drug delivery. In: Chabner BA (ed) Rational basis for chemotherapy, UCLA symp on molecular and cellular biology-new series, vol. 4. UCLA symposium on the rational basis for chemotherapy, Keystone, CO 1982. Liss, New York, pp 427-436

Neumann HA, Fabricius HA, Engelhardt R (1982) Moderate whole-body hyperthermia in combination with chemotherapy in the treatment of small cell carcinoma of the lung: a pilot study. Natl Cancer Inst Monogr 61: 427-429

O'Donnel JF, McKoy WS, Makuch RW, Bull JM (1979) Increased in vitro toxicity to mouse bone marrow with 1,3-bis (2-chloroethyl) 1-nitrosourea and hyperthermia. Cancer Res 39: 1547-2549

Parks LC, Ninaberry D, Smith DP, Neely WA (1979) Treatment of far advanced bronchogenic carcinoma by extracorporally induced systemic hyperthermia. J Thorac Cardiovasc Surg 78: 883-892

Pettigrew RT, Galt JM, Ludgate CM, Smith AN (1974) Clinical effects of whole-body hyperthermia in advanced malignancy. Br Med J 21: 679-682

Till JE, McCulloch EA (1961) Direct measurement of the radiation sensitivity of normal mouse bone marrow cells. Radiat Res 14: 213-222

Combined Heat and X-Ray Toxicities in Intestine and Skin

S. P. Hume

MRC Cyclotron Unit, Hammersmith Hospital, Ducane Road,
London W12 OHS, Great Britain

Introduction

In combined heat and X-ray treatments, hyperthermia may have a direct, cytotoxic action or can act solely to enhance radiation damage. In vivo, the gross expression of thermal damage occurs much earlier than radiation damage so that the two modes of action can be studied separately and any interaction more clearly identified.

Direct Thermal Damage

The differences in the time courses for the expression of thermal and X-irradiation injuries are very clearly seen in skin. In mouse tail skin, for example, whereas the peak of the radiation reaction occurs approximately 20 days after irradiation, thermal damage (maximally expressed as moist desquamation accompanied by severe erythema and oedema) peaks 1–2 days after treatment (Hume and Myers 1984). It has been postulated that the threshold and size of peak of the radiation response are a function of the number of epithelial stem cells killed and that the lag period represents the transit time of the proliferating but non-clonogenic cells through the basal layer (Al-Barwari and Potten 1979). If this is the case, then the reasons for the differences in time course become very apparent when we use an experimental tissue with a high degree of spatial organisation, with distinct proliferative and non-proliferative but functional regions.

Such a tissue is small intestine. The two mucosal compartments, crypts and villi, are lined with epithelium but, whereas in crypts these cells have the ability to proliferate, in villi the epithelium is post-mitotic and functional. After irradiation, the reduction in size and number of villi is due to the lack of replacement of functional epithelial cells from the proliferative compartment in the crypts and takes several days to be maximally expressed (Quastler 1956). After hyperthermia, however, villus injury, resulting in a transient reduction in the absorptive surface, is maximally expressed only 4–6 h after treatment (Michalowski 1981). Damage to the villus compartment includes the production of conical and rudimentary villi and the

Recent Results in Cancer Research, Vol. 109

stacking of enterocytes, individual cells showing signs of abnormalities in their cell membranes, nuclei and cytoplasmic components (Carr et al. 1982).

Hyperthermia does have a cytotoxic effect on the clonogenic compartment of the mucosa but, again contrasting with radiation injury, the crypts are lost in an apparently "all-or-none" manner (Hume et al. 1979). The loss is very rapid, being complete by 6 h, and there is no recovery in crypt number for at least 3 weeks. The relative susceptibilities of crypt and villus epithelium have been assessed by labelling with tritiated thymidine and measuring the loss of label following hyperthermia given at times when either the label is still in the crypts or when the majority of the heavily labelled cells have moved to the villus tips (Hume et al. 1983). Both the labelling studies and histological examination indicate that the non-proliferative villus enterocytes are more susceptible to thermal injury than the crypt cells.

From intestine studies, we can suggest that thermal injury is manifest as a result of the death of post-mitotic functional cells, in addition to intermitotic death of proliferative cells. How much of this effect is due to a direct action on the epithelial cells remains unclear. There is some evidence to suggest a stromal involvement, in particular that microcirculatory disturbances contribute to the expression of thermal injury in vivo (recently reviewed by Reinhold and Endrich 1986). In small intestine, 2 h after hyperthermia, histological examination reveals not only stacked, rounded enterocytes but also collapse of the villus stroma, suggestive of a contribution of stromal-epithelial boundary disruption, possibly related to oedema (Kamel et al. 1985). At a more macroscopic level, using a benzidine stain for haemoglobin, Falk (1983) has quantitated the effect of heat on vasculature by measuring the total length of the visible venous tree and reports the disappearance of capillaries as the earliest sign of a vasculature disturbance, followed by loss of progressively larger vessels. Falk (1983) also reports a gradient of sensitivity from the inner layer of the jejunum to the outer. As illustrated in Fig. 1, the reduction in

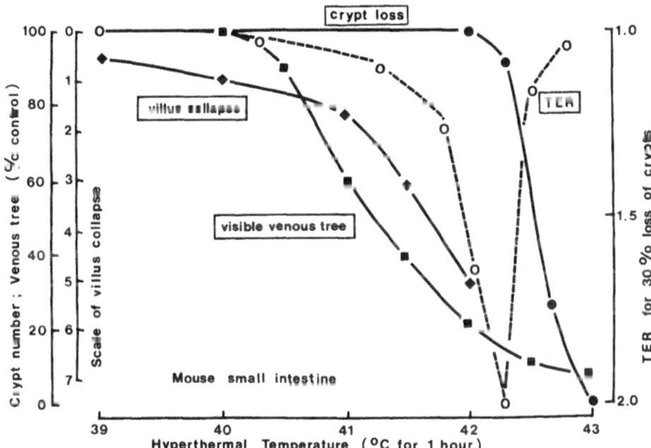

Fig. 1. Dose-response curves for crypt number (●) (from Hume and Marigold 1981), villus collapse (◆) (from Kamel et al. 1985) and visible venous tree (■) (from Falk 1983) measured in mouse small intestine following 1 h of heating. Crypt number was assessed at 1 day, villus collapse at 2 h and the venous tree immediately after treatment. Also shown are TER values (○), calculated for an iso-effect of 30% crypt loss taken from crypt survival curves obtained 4 days after graded doses of X-rays (from Hume and Marigold 1981)

visible venous tree correlates well with thermal damage to the villi, the more sensitive indicator of mucosal injury.

If the cytotoxic effect of hyperthermia in vivo is related to circulatory disturbances, one might expect to exacerbate thermal damage by vascular changes following other modalities, for example radiation, and this will be considered later.

Thermoradiosensitisation

As mentioned earlier, hyperthermia may be used to enhance the effects of ionising radiation. The degree of enhancement, quantified as the thermal enhancement ratio, or TER, is illustrated in Fig. 1 for the clonogenic crypt survival assay for radiation damage to small intestine. As can be seen, TER increases with treatment temperature up to a maximum value. In intestine, when thermal damage to the crypts is expressed directly, the ability of heat to enhance radiation damage is lost (Hume and Marigold 1981). The reason for this is not clear.

Many of the characteristics of thermoradiosensitisation are well defined but here are briefly described with respect to rodent skin and small intestine:

1. The time course of expression of radiation injury is not altered by combining the radiation with mild hyperthermia. The type of injury is qualitatively similar, heat apparently acting only to reduce the dose required for a given effect (e.g. Law et al. 1984).
2. In small intestine, the effect of heat is primarily on the shoulder of the radiation survival curve. When the combined treatment is given following a subthreshold primary heat treatment, the tissue develops thermotolerance to the combined modality treatment, resulting in a lower TER value. The X-ray sensitivity itself is not affected using intervals of up to 5 days between priming and test treatments (Marigold and Hume 1982).
3. Thermotolerance may also develop during chronic or prolonged hyperthermia, in intestine for example after approximately 1 h of heating at temperatures in the range 41.0°-42.3° C (Hume and Marigold 1985). Limiting the hyperthermal treatments to those subthreshold for gross injury, thermoradiosensitisation increases linearly with duration of hyperthermia for temperatures in the range 42.3°-44.0° C. As a result, if the whole of the temperature range is considered, i.e. 41.0°-44.0° C, then the thermoradiosensitisation iso-effect curve relating heating time to temperature is biphasic, with the transition occurring between 41.8° and 42.0° C. The time-temperature relationships for thermoradiosensitisation are similar to those for direct thermal injury and, at least in the higher temperature range, may allow the calculation of "biologically equivalent" heat treatments in a manner similar to that suggested for direct thermal injury.
4. In skin, heat given during or immediately before X-rays is more effective than when given immediately afterwards (e.g. Law et al. 1984). This is not true for all tissues, for example small intestine, where there is no effect of sequence (Hume and Marigold 1981). Where the effect does occur, there is probably a modifying influence of the first treatment on non-target surrounding tissues. For example, heat given prior to X-rays may cause an increase in blood flow at the time of irradiation, reducing the degree of radiobiological hypoxia. The hypothesis can

Table 1. Thermal enhancement of X-ray or "7.5 MeV" neutron damage in rodent normal tissue. (From Hume et al. 1982 and Law et al. 1984)

Tissue and end-point	Hyperthermal temperature for 1 h (° C)	Sequence	TER		RBE
			X-rays	Neutrons	
Ear skin	–	–	–	–	1.8
(mean of 3	43.0	R-H	1.8	1.5	1.5
iso-effects)	43.0	H-R	3.4	2.0	1.1
Foot skin	–	–	–	–	1.6
(average reaction days 8-46)	42.0	H-R	1.7	1.3	1.1
Baby rat cartilage	–	–	–	–	2.3
(30% stunting)	42.0	H-R	1.4	1.5	2.5
	43.0	H-R	1.7	1.7	2.3
Mouse jejunum	–	–	–	–	2.0
(30% crypt survival)	41.8	H-R	1.4	1.4	1.9

be tested by giving fast neutrons instead of X-rays since the protection by hypoxia is less for high LET (linear energy transfer) radiations. One might then expect the effect of sequence to be less for neutron irradiation and this is indeed what is found. In Table 1 for skin, we can see the marked effect of sequence using X-irradiation but a weaker effect using cyclotron-produced neutrons. When heat was given first, the TER for X-rays was higher than that for neutrons. There was no difference in neutron and X-ray TER values in intestine, a tissue unlikely to be hypoxic.

5. As the treatments are separated in time, the thermoradiosensitisation is eliminated, in intestine by 4 h for both sequences. For skin, there appears to be a longer lasting effect when heat is given before radiation but, again, this may have an indirect component (reviewed by Hume and Field 1978).

Combined Cytotoxicities

As the interval between irradiation and hyperthermia is further increased into days and weeks, additional interactions may occur. In mouse tail skin, for example, whereas 44.0° C for 30 min given 3 days after X-rays has no effect on the radiation response, the same treatment when given 6 or more days after X-rays results in a severe skin reaction, much greater than the individual responses following either treatment given separately (Hume and Myers 1984). Using an interval of 9 days, i.e. giving heat close to the time of expression of the gross radiation response, it could be seen that both the thermal and the radiation responses were increased, in a dose-dependent manner, although the times for peak reaction were not significantly altered by the additional treatment.

Although there was little evidence of thermal injury over the time of expression of the radiation injury, it was suggested that the increase in the radiation reaction was due to an increase in residual thermal injury at the time of expression of the gross radiation response. The increased thermal response was probably due to progressing radiation injury not yet manifest as overt damage. This is plausible if one takes into account the stromal component of thermal injury discussed earlier.

Effect of Residual Radiation Injury

When heat is given *after* the time of expression of the radiation reaction, the tissue may again show an increased thermal response. In skin, this enhancement of thermal sensitivity is very long-lasting but in intestine is a transient phenomenon (Hume and Marigold 1982). The difference in the tissue responses may be real or may simply be related to the different primary X-ray doses. In intestine, the enhancement of thermal damage is characterised by an increase in slope of the dose-response curve, as illustrated in Fig. 2, and, interestingly, is limited to temperatures of 43° C and below, that is, to temperatures below the transition in the Arrhenius curve. This is apparent from the lack of effect of prior radiation on the tissue response to 44° C illustrated in Fig. 2 but is shown more clearly in the Arrhenius plot of Fig. 3.

As mentioned earlier, the biphasic nature of the Arrhenius curve for heat inactivation in vitro is thought to result from the development of thermotolerance during prolonged hyperthermia. It is, therefore, plausible that the shift in the Arrhenius curve is due to a change in the kinetics of thermotolerance development in pre-irradiated tissue. However, as can be seen from Fig. 2, the development of thermotolerance, here indicated by the plateau in the dose-response curves for crypt loss, is not prevented by prior irradiation. This does not exclude the possibility that the rate of development of thermotolerance is changed and this is being investigated at present.

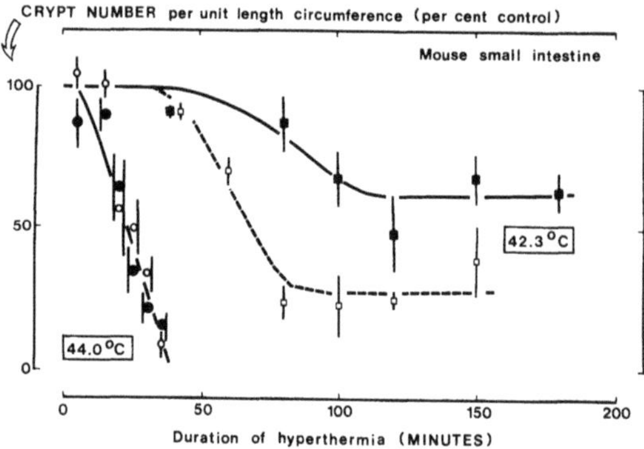

Fig. 2. Dose-response curves for crypt loss in mouse small intestine following hyperthermia at either 42.3° or 44.0° C for the times indicated. The *closed symbols* are for single heat treatment given locally to an exteriorised loop of jejunum (for the heating technique, see Hume et al. 1979). The *open symbols* are for heat given 10 days after 9 Gy of X-rays (240 kVp) given in situ to the abdomen. The data points are means with standard errors from at least six mice

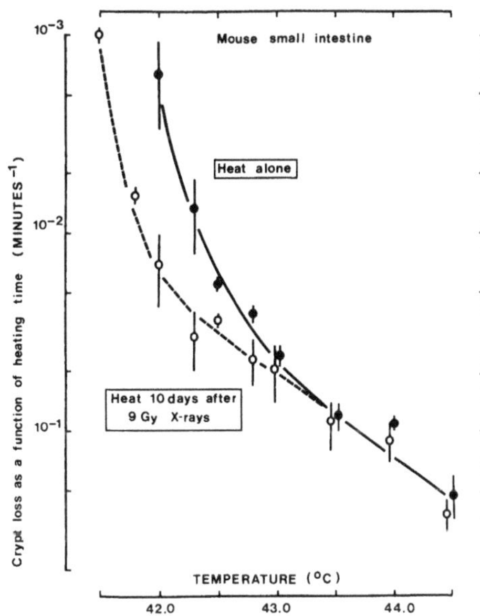

Fig. 3. "Arrhenius" plot for crypt loss in mouse small intestine. The "rate" values on the *ordinate axis* were calculated from log:linear regressions of dose-response curves for crypt survival assayed 1 day after hyperthermia. Examples of such curves are given in Fig. 2 and the *open* and *closed symbols* refer to the treatment described in the legend to Fig. 2. The *error bars* represent the standard error

Table 2. Thermal enhancement ratio[a] in mouse tail

Tissue response	Quantitation	TER_9 level of assessment	Hyperthermia (° C for 30 min)		
			43.0	44.0	44.5
Early reaction (up to 21 days)	Area of moist desquamation	50% per tail	1.00	1.10	1.16
Prolonged, chronic reaction (3 months)	Prolonged breakdown or necrosis	50% occurrence	1.00	1.10	1.17
Late reaction 6.5-11 months)	"Late" necrosis/ atrophy of distal tail	50% occurrence	1.00	1.08	1.17

[a] Hyperthermia was given 9 days after X-irradiation to the whole of the tail. Thermal enhancement ratios are therefore referred to as TER_9.

Late Responses

Results from both intestine and skin would suggest that "late" tissue responses following X-irradiation are not exacerbated by a progressing or latent heat reaction following an acute thermal exposure. As a consequence, TER values for "late" radiation reactions which may occur many months after the initial exposure can be predicted from the degree of enhancement of the acute radiation response (Hume and Myers 1985). This is illustrated in Table 2 for mouse tail skin, using a thermal enhancement value calculated from radiation dose-response curves obtained when heat was given just prior to the time of expression of injury, as discussed earlier. The same is, however, true for mouse ear skin when TER values are calculated from thermal enhancement of radiation response resulting from a combined treatment where heat is given immediately after X-irradiation (Law et al. 1985).

References

Al-Barwari E, Potten CS (1979) A kinetic model to explain the time of appearance of skin reaction after X-rays or ultraviolet light irradiation. Cell Tissue Kinet 12: 281-289

Carr KE, Hume SP, Marigold JCL, Michalowski A (1982) Scanning and transmission electron microscopy of the damage to small intestinal mucosa following X-irradiation or hyperthermia. Scan Electron Microsc I: 393-402

Falk P (1983) The effect of elevated temperature on the vasculature of mouse jejunum. Br J Radiol 56: 41-49

Hume SP, Field SB (1978) Hyperthermic sensitization of mouse intestine to damage by X-rays: the effect of sequence and temporal separation of the two treatments. Br J Radiol 51: 302-307

Hume SP, Marigold JCL (1981) The response of mouse intestine to combined hyperthermia and radiation: the contribution of direct thermal damage in assessment of the thermal enhancement ratio. Int J Radiat Biol 39: 347-356

Hume SP, Marigold JCL (1982) Increased hyperthermal response of previously irradiated mouse intestine. Br J Radiol 55: 438-443

Hume SP, Marigold JCL (1985) Time-temperature relationships for hyperthermal radiosensitisation in mouse intestine: influence of thermotolerance. Radiother Oncol 3: 165-171

Hume SP, Myers R (1984) An unexpected effect of hyperthermia on the expression of X-ray damage in mouse skin. Radiat Res 97: 186-199

Hume SP, Myers R (1985) Acute and late damage in mouse tail following hyperthermia and X-irradiation. Int J Hyperthermia 1: 349-357

Hume SP, Marigold JCL, Field SB (1979) The effect of local hyperthermia on the small intestine of mouse. Br Radiol 52: 657-662

Hume SP, Myers R, Field SB (1982) A comparison of thermal enhancement ratios for fast neutron and X-irradiation of two normal tissues in rodents. Br J Radiol 55: 151-155

Hume SP, Marigold JCL, Michalowski A (1983) The effect of local hyperthermia on non-proliferative, compared with proliferative, epithelial cells of the mouse small intestinal mucosa. Radiat Res 94: 252-262

Kamel HMH, Carr KE, Hume SP Marigold JCL (1985) Structural changes in mouse small intestinal villi following lower body hyperthermia. Scan Electron Microsc 2: 849-858

Law MP, Morris CC, Field SB (1984) The response of mouse skin to hyperthermia combined with fast neutrons or X-rays. Int J Radiat Biol 46: 17-24

Law MP, Ahier RG, Somaia S (1985) Thermal enhancement of radiation damage in previously irradiated skin. Br J Radiol 58: 161-167

Marigold JCL, Hume SP (1982) Effect of prior hyperthermia on subsequent thermal enhancement of radiation damage in mouse intestine. Int J Radiat Biol 42: 509-516

Michalowski A (1981) Effects of radiation on normal tissues: hypothetical mechanisms and limitations of in situ assays of clonogenicity. Radiat Environ Biophys 19: 157-172

Quastler H (1956) The nature of intestinal radiation death. Radiat Res 4: 303-320

Reinhold HS, Endrich B (1986) Tumour microcirculation as a target for hyperthermia. Int J Hyperthermia 2: 111-137

Toxic Effects of Irradiation or Doxorubicin in Combination with Moderate Whole-Body Hyperthermia on Bone Marrow in Rats

W. Hinkelbein, M. Birmelin, D. Menger, and R. Engelhardt

Abteilung Strahlentherapie, Radiologische Klinik, Albert-Ludwigs-Universität, Hugstetter Straße 55, 7800 Freiburg, FRG

Introduction

The therapeutic benefit that accrues from combining hyperthermia with other cancer treatment modalities implies enhancement of tumor control but not of normal tissue damage. In experimental tumor models the interactions between heat and cytostatic drugs (Bertino et al. 1984) or irradiation (Mooibroek et al. 1984; Dewhirst et al. 1985) are well known. However, only a few studies have been performed in normal tissues (Hume et al. 1983; Law et al. 1985), especially in critical organs for defined treatment regimes.

In our department moderate whole-body hyperthermia (WBH) is combined with chemotherapy or irradiation (Hinkelbein et al. 1981; Engelhardt et al. 1983) in clinical studies. For this reason we examined specific side-effects of doxorubicin and irradiation on bone marrow, which is a critical organ for both these treatments. We used a rat model to assess the histological alterations caused by heat, doxorubicin, irradiation, and the combined treatments.

Materials and Methods

Animals

Male Wistar rats aged 7-10 days (body weight 80 g) were used in all experiments. Each group of animals investigated consisted of at least ten rats.

Hyperthermia

Whole body hyperthermia at 41° C was induced by microwaves (Siretherm 609: 434 MHz, 200 W, Pyrodor applicator) on day 0. Five rats could be treated simultaneously; this required a distinct distribution of the animals and dummies ("dielectric rats") in the treatment cage in order to achieve a homogeneous linear temperature rise in all rats (Fig. 1). Power distribution ranged from 55.5 to 91.0 mW/cm^2

Recent Results in Cancer Research, Vol. 109

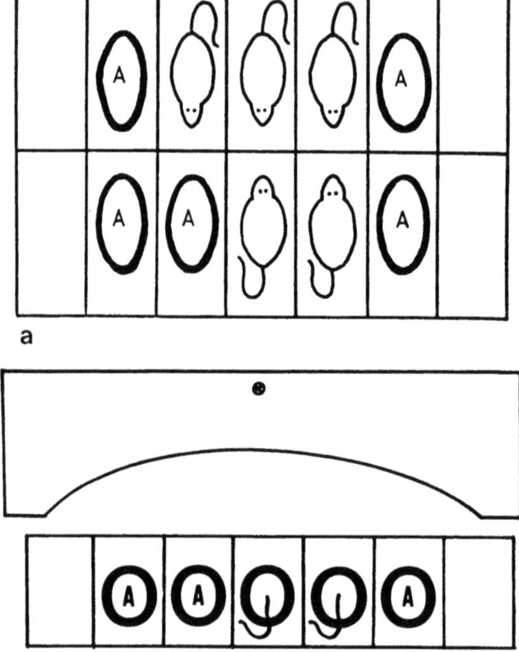

Fig. 1. **a** Arrangement of the rats and dielectric phantoms (*A*, saline-filled water bags) in the treatment cage to obtain a homogeneous electromagnetic field and temperature. **b** Design of the WBH treatment setup

depending on the body weight. Rectal temperature was measured with a thermistor. Within 20 min, the temperature rose from 37.1° ±0.3° C to 41.0° ±0.4° C. This treatment temperature was maintained for 10 (H1) or 20 min (H2).

Doxorubicin

Doxorubicin 6 mg/kg body weight dissolved in saline was injected into a tail vein on day 0. Another dose of 80 mg/kg was given on day 14 (Doroshow et al. 1979). All rats treated with the cytostatic drug alone (D) were killed by anoxia on day 21. The first injection of doxorubicin was followed within 30 min by WBH lasting 10 or 20 min after treatment. A temperature of 41° C was reached (DH1 and DH2 respectively) in all animals receiving thermochemotherapy. Control groups were treated with equal amounts of physiological saline (C).

Radiotherapy

Total body irradiation (TBI) with 3.5 Gy was applied only once, on day 0, using a telecobalt unit (RT) and the same treatment cage as was used for heat treatment. The animals receiving radiothermotherapy were irradiated immediately after hyperthermia (10 min hyperthermia: HRT1; 20 min hyperthermia: HRT2). All rats treated with TBI were killed on day 7 by nitrogen.

Histological Examinations

On days 21 (D, H1, H2, DH1, DH2) and 7 (RT, H1, H2, HRT1, HRT2) the animals were killed by N_2 anoxia. The right femur was removed and prepared according to Burkhardt (1966) and stained with Giemsa and Gomori.

Results

Figures 2a and b show the bone marrow of untreated rats (C) with normal cellularity and numerous megakaryocytes. WBH alone produced in both regimens (H1 and H2) identical nonspecific irritation expressed by an eosinophilic and macrophagic reaction and slight interstitial edema (Fig. 3a, b).

TBI alone (RT) led to an extensive loss of megakaryocytes, distinct interstitial edema, and a decrease in erythropoiesis (Fig. 4a, b). These radiation effects were intensified by 10 min prior hyperthermia (HRT1), with severe damage of bone marrow with vacuolation and interstitial bleeding (Fig. 5). The combination of TBI and 20 min prior WBH (HRT2) surprisingly seemed to "protect" the bone marrow against radiotoxic effects: all injuries were less pronounced than after after TBI alone (Fig. 6).

Doxorubicin alone (D) produced focal necroses with a minor eosinophilic and plasmocytic reaction and slight edema (Fig. 7a, b). When doxorubicin was combined with WBH, stronger cell loss was evident following 10 min heat exposure (DH1) than with doxorubicin alone (Fig. 8), while after 20 min heat exposure (DH2) there was very severe destruction with interstitial bleeding (Fig. 9). All morphological changes are summarized in Table 1.

Table 1. Synopsis of the bone marrow effects of all treatment regimens tested

Morphological effects	Treatment								
	C	H1	H2	RT	HRT1	HRT2	D	DH1	DH2
Interstitial edema	–	++	++	+++	++++	++	+	++	++
Eosinophilic reaction	–	+++	+++	+	+	+	+	+	+
Macrophagic reaction	–	+++	+++	–	–	–	+	–	–
Plasmocytic reaction	–	–	–	–	–	–	+++	+	+
Cellularity	+/–	+/–	+/–	––	–––	–	–	––	–––
Erythropoiesis	+/–	+/–	+/–	––	––	–	–	–	––
Granulopoiesis	+/–	+/–	+/–	+/–	–	+/–	–	–	––
Megakaryocytes	+/–	+/–	+/–	–––	–––	––	+/–	–	––
Vacuolation	–	–	–	+	++	+	+	++	+++
Interstitial bleedings	–	–	–	–	++	–	–	++	+++

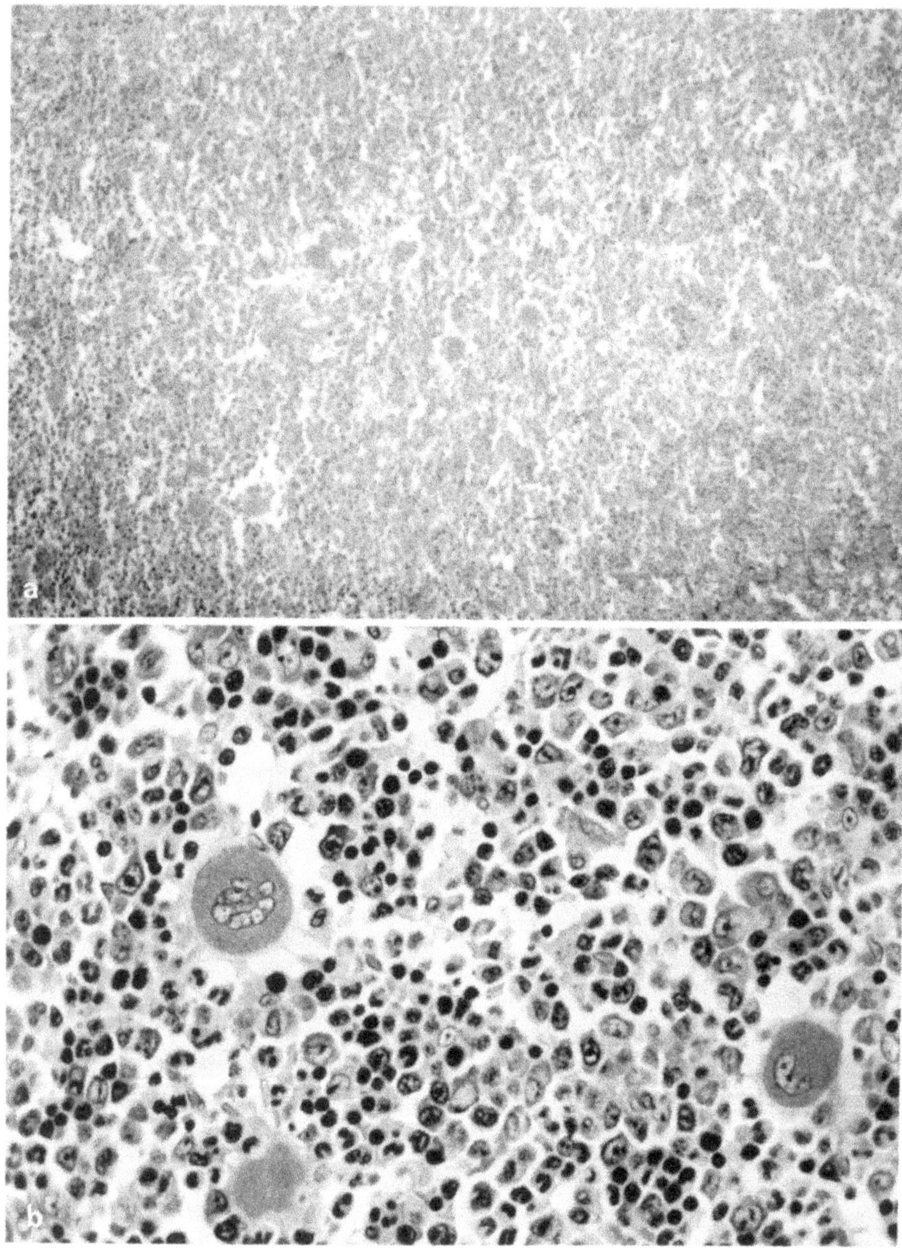

Fig. 2a, b. Bone marrow of untreated rats, with numerous megakaryocytes and normal cellularity. **a** Gomori argentation, × 40; **b** Giemsa, × 180

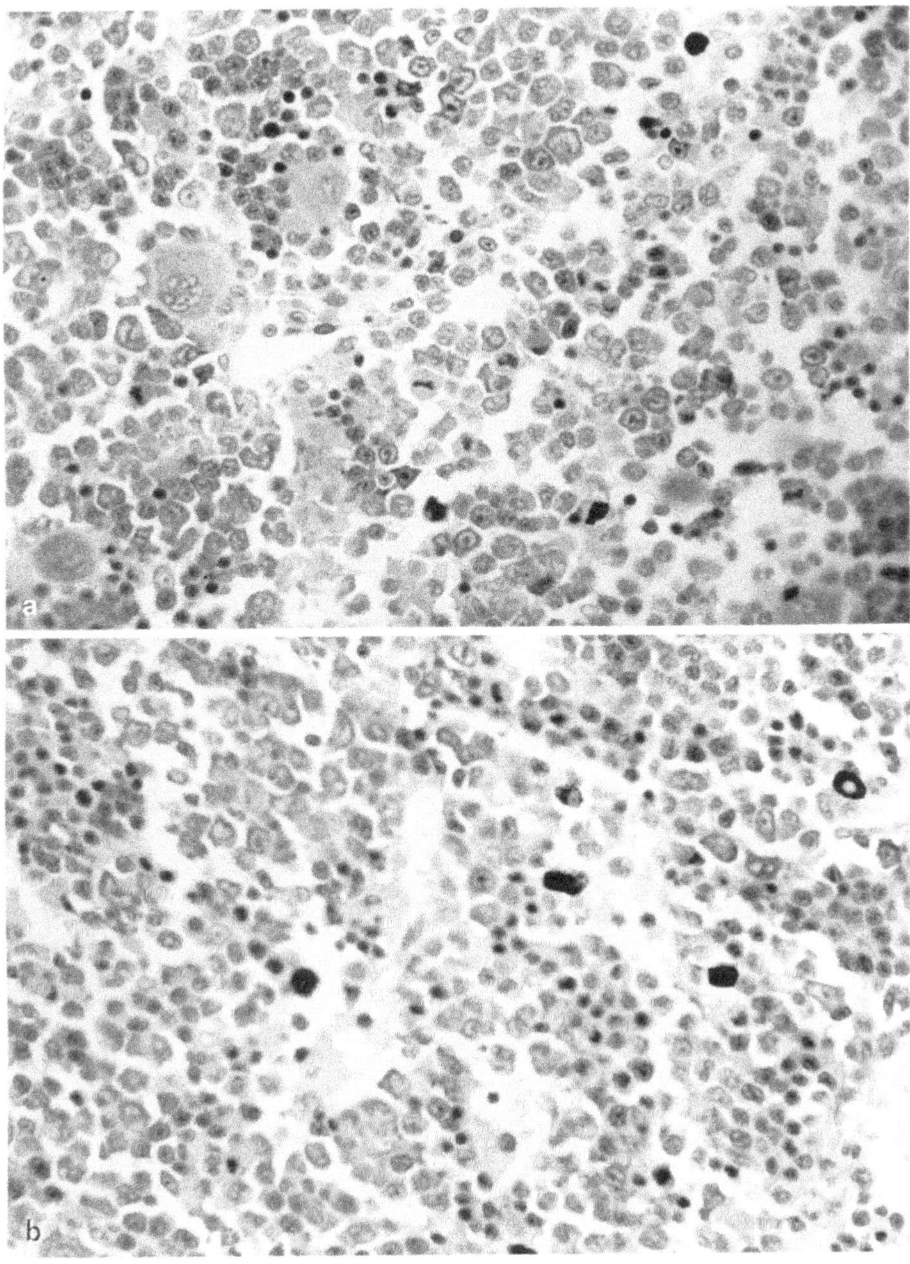

Fig. 3a, b. Bone marrow after WBH at 41° C alone. **a** Heat treatment for 10 min (H1). Immigration of eosinophilic leukocytes and pigment-loaded macrophages. The extracellular space is increased because of interstitial edema. Giemsa, × 180. **b** Heat treatment for 20 min (H2). Giemsa, × 180

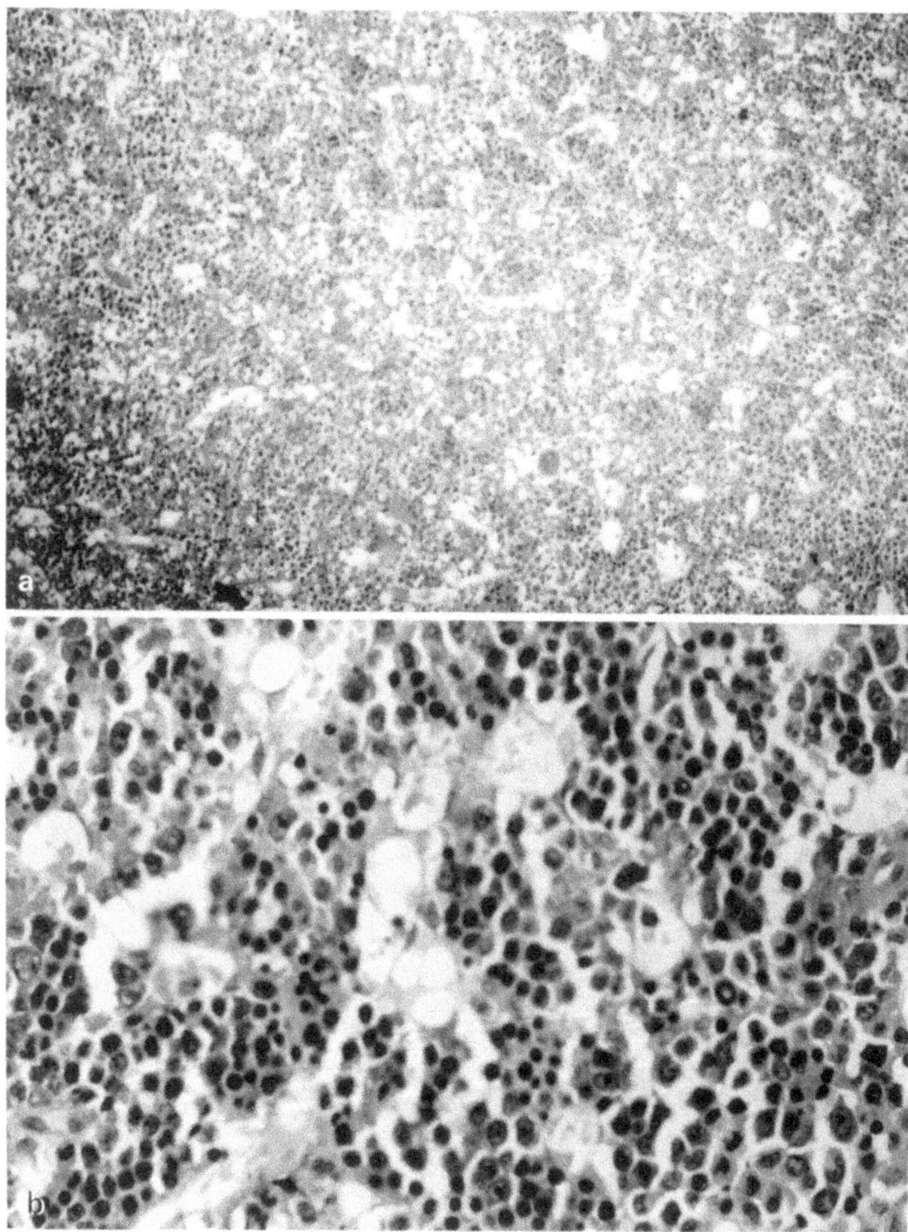

Fig. 4 a, b. Bone marrow damage after TBI alone with 3.5 Gy (RT). Extensive loss of megakaryocytes, interstitial edema, and a decrease in cellularity (mainly caused by a decrease in erythropoiesis). **a** Gomori argentation, × 40; **b** Giemsa, × 180

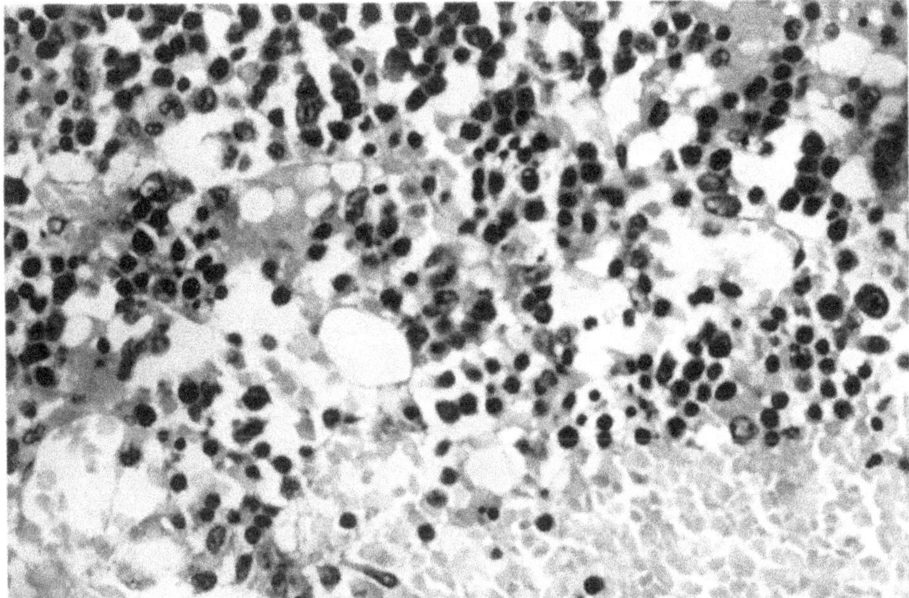

Fig. 5. TBI (3.5 Gy) after 10 min hyperthermia (HRT1). Severe bone marrow damage with vacuolation caused by necroses, interstitial edema, and interstitial bleeding. The ramaining cells appear with dark pyknotic nuclei. Giemsa, × 180

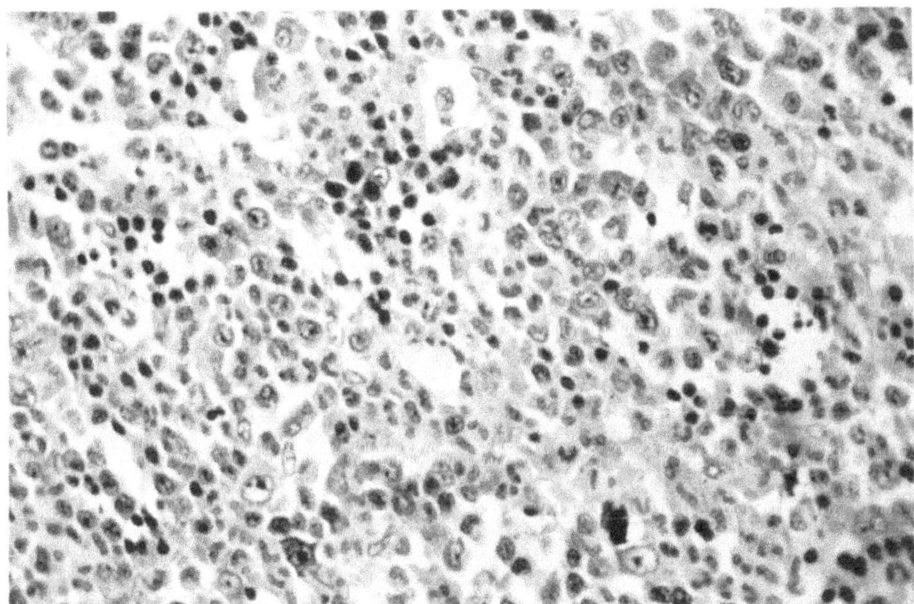

Fig. 6. Combination of TBI (3.5 Gy) and 20 min WBH at 41° C (HRT2). Only a few cells have pyknotic nuclei; there is slight interstitial edema, no bleeding, and no vacuolation. Giemsa, × 180

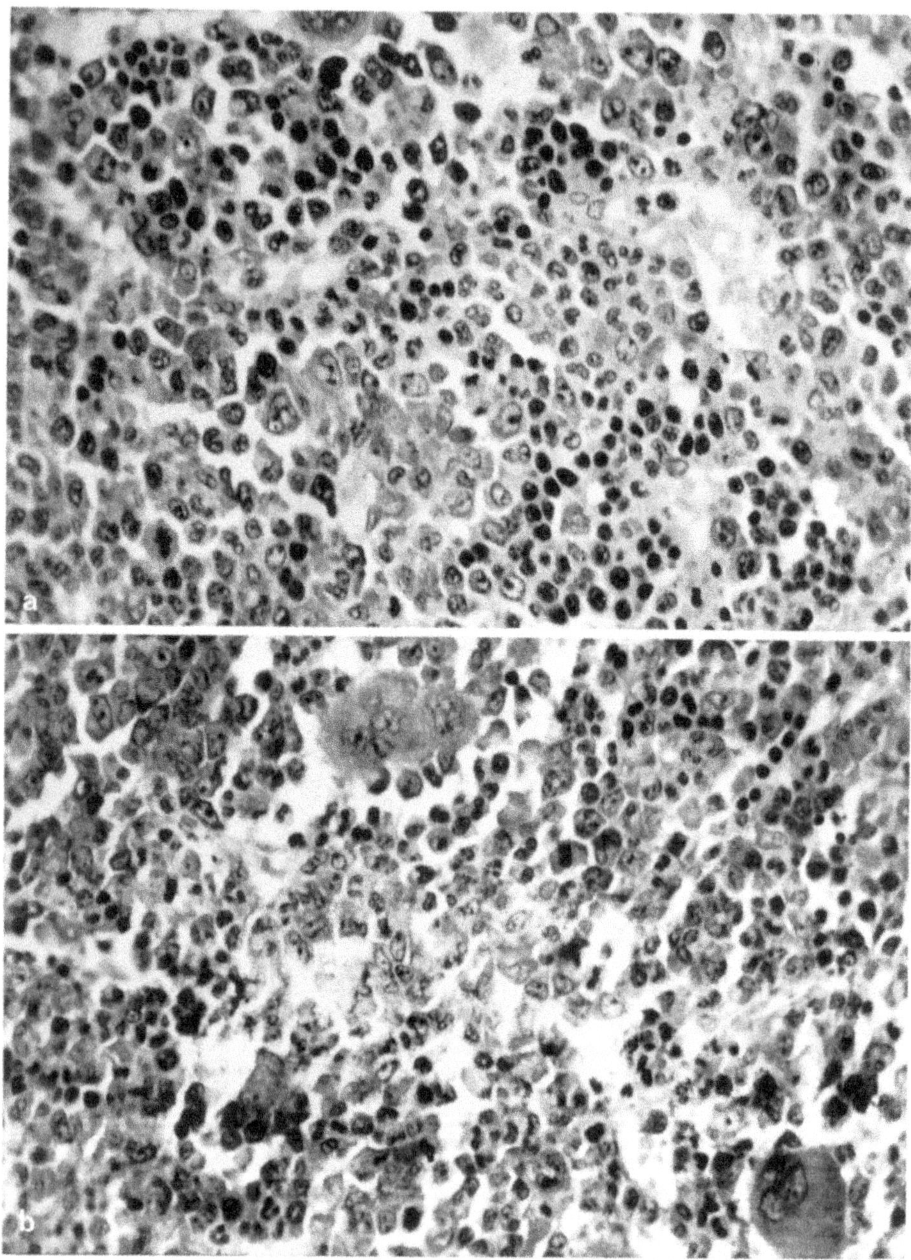

Fig. 7 a, b. Bone marrow after doxorubicin alone (D). Focal necroses with slight interstitial edema and some immigration of eosinophilic leukocytes and plasmocytes. **a, b** Giemsa, × 180

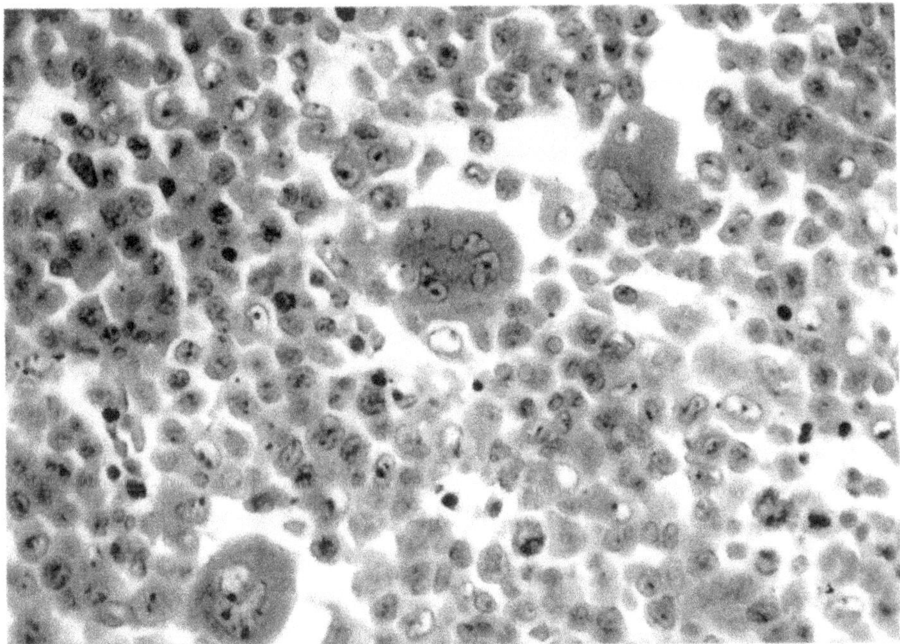

Fig. 8. Therapy with doxorubicin and 10 min WBH at 41° C (DH1). Marked cell loss with beginning vacuolation and interstitial edema. Gomori argentation, × 180

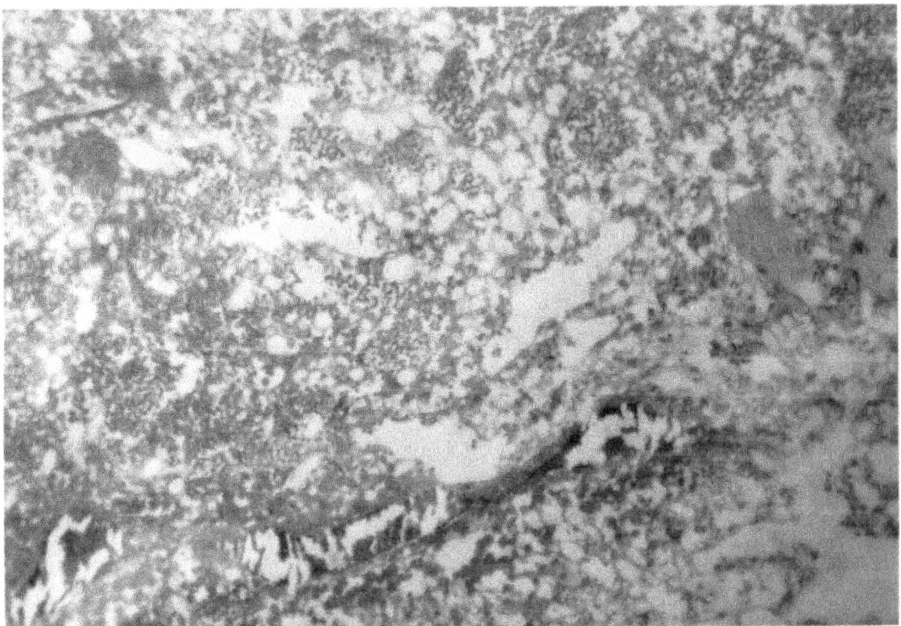

Fig. 9. Therapy with doxorubicin and 20 min WBH at 41° C (DH2). Severe destruction of bone marrow with marked vacuolation and bleeding. Gomori argentation, × 40

Discussion

We surprisingly found that even the low "thermal doses" used are able to produce nonspecific changes in the bone marrow. The early work on microwave effects on the hemopoietic system (Deichmann et al. 1964; Rotkovská and Vacek 1972) was unfortunately done without temperature measurement. Even 10-min exposure to only 41° C leads to strong enhancement of the bone marrow damage caused by TBI. This we regard as a radiosensitizing effect, for proliferation of cultured bone marrow stem cells is inhibited only at temperatures higher than 41.5° C (Tribukait 1978; Elkon et al. 1981, 1984; Sabio et al. 1981). Doubling the heat exposure time unexpectedly caused no enhancement of radiation damage; in fact the lesions were less marked. The reason might be a complex phenomenon of regulation in our whole-body system, but a real protective effect to the bone marrow cannot be excluded. Interestingly, after very similar microwave exposure Rotkovská et al. (1981) found radioprotection of the bone marrow, as shown by evaluation of the CFUs. However, it must in any case be pointed out that very small changes in the thermal dose can produce marked and unforeseeable effects when hyperthermia and radiotherapy are employed in conjunction.

When chemotherapy with doxorubicin was combined with WBH we found a dose-dependent enhancement of bone marrow toxicity; i.e., the longer the exposure time to WBH (at our small thermal doses), the greater the toxicity. There is a clear synergy between hyperthermia and doxorubicin in malignant cell lines (Dahl 1982; Roizin-Towle et al. 1982) at higher temperatures.

We know that other cytotoxic drugs also enhance the bone marrow injury caused by hyperthermia (Honess and Bleehan 1982). Docorubicin exerts its cytotoxicity by intercalating with DNA (Zunino et al. 1972) and a membrane mechanism (Tritton et al. 1978). The effectiveness of the drug is strongly influenced by its intracellular uptake and retention (Sirotnak et al. 1979). Hahn et al. (1975) reported that when doxorubicin chemotherapy was combined with hyperthermia there was synergistic cytotoxicity on mouse mammary carcinoma cells because much more of the drug was able to enter the cells at 43° C than at 37° C. However, cells became resistant to further killing by doxorubicin after heat exposure times of more than 30 min (Mizuno et al. 1980). The complexity and importance of temperature effects are indicated by Morgan and Bleehan's (1981) demonstration of heat-induced drug tolerance to doxorubicin after 1 h at 43° C but greatly enhanced cell killing after 6 h at 42° C.

Rose et al. (1979) could not detect enhancement of chemotherapeutic activity using single doses and short heat exposure in a panel of transplanted mouse tumors. In contrast to these findings, with our double-dose scheme we can show the amplification of bone marrow toxicity at low-temperature and short-exposure hyperthermia. We explain this by an increase in influx of the drug, for Nagaoka et al. (1986) have shown an increase in intracellular uptake even at 39° C. In their experiments with liver slices Dodion et al. (1986) did not see any effect of hyperthermia on the metabolism of doxorubicin.

In conclusion it must be stated that in clinical practice we should be cautious of combining systemic application of doxorubicin and heat because of possible severe side-effects.

References

Bertino JR, Kowal CD, Klein ME, Dombrowski J, Mini E (1984) The potential for chemotherapy and hyperthermia. In: Vaeth JM, Meyer J (eds) Hyperthermia and radiation therapy/chemotherapy in the treatment of cancer. Front Radiat Ther Oncol 18: 162–170

Burkhardt R (1966) Preconditions of histological preparation to the clinical histology of bone marrow and bone. II. A new method for the histological preparation of bone marrow and bone. Blut 14: 40–46

Dahl O (1982) Interaction of hyperthermia and doxorubicin on a malignant, neurogenic rat cell line (BT4 C) in culture. Nat Cancer Inst Monogr 61: 251–254

Deichmann WB, Miale J, Landeen K (1964) Effect of microwave radiation on the hemopoietic system of the rat. Toxicol Appl Pharmacol 6: 71–77

Dewhirst MW, Sim DA, Forsyth K, Grochowski KJ, Wilson S, Bicknell E (1985) Local control and distant metastases in primary canine malignant melanomas treated with hyperthermia and/or radiotherapy. Int J Hyperthermia 1: 219–234

Dodion P, Riggs CE, Akman SR, Bachur NR (1986) Effect of hyperthermia on the in vitro metabolism of doxorubicin. Cancer Treat Rep 70: 625–629

Doroshow JH, Locker GJ, Myers CE (1979) Experimental animal models of adriamycin cardiotoxicity. Cancer Treat Rep 63: 855–860

Engelhardt R, Neumann H, Hinkelbein W, Adam G, Weth R, Löhr GW (1983) Clinical studies in thermochemotherapy with whole-body hyperthermia. In: Spitzy KH, Karrer K (eds) Proceedings, 13th international congress of chemotherapy. Egermann, Vienna, TOM 18, pp 41–46

Elkon D, Sabio H, Mc Grath HG, Baker DG (1981) Temperature-dependent inhibition of murine granulocyte-monocyte precursors. Cancer Res 41: 1812–1815

Elkon D, Sabio H, Pinizzotto M, Sigrudsson M, Baker DG (1984) Effect of hyperthermia on murine myeloid precursors. Cancer 54: 1973–1976

Hahn GM, Braun J, Har-Kedar I (1975) Thermochemotherapy: synergism between hyperthermia (42–43° C) and adriamycin (or bleomycin) in mammalian cell inactivation. Proc Natl Acad Sci USA 72: 937–940

Hinkelbein W, Neumann H, Engelhardt R, Wannenmacher M (1981) Combined treatment of NSCLC with radiotherapy and moderate whole-body hyperthermia. Strahlentherapie 157: 301–304

Honess DJ, Bleehan NM (1982) Sensitivity of normal mouse marrow and RIF-1 tumor to hyperthermia combined with cyclophosphamide or BCNU: a lack of therapeutic gain. Br J Cancer 46: 236–248

Hume SP, Marigold JCL, Michalowski A (1983) The effect of local hyperthermia on non proliferative, compared with proliferative, epithelial cells of the mouse small intestinal muscosa. Radiat Res 94: 252–261

Law MP, Ahier RG, Somaia S (1985) Thermal enhancement of radiation damage in previously irradiated skin. Br J Radiol 58: 161–167

Mizuno S, Amagai M, Ishida A (1980) Synergistic cell killing by antitumor agents and hyperthermia in cultured cells. Gann 71: 471–478

Mooibroek J, Zywietz F, Dikomey E, Jung H (1984) Thermotolerance kinetics and growth pattern changes in an experimental rat tumor (R1 H) after hyperthermia. In: Overgaard J (ed) Hyperthermic oncology vol 1. Taylor and Francis, London, pp 215–218

Morgan JE, Bleehan NM (1981) Response of EMTG multicellular tumor spheroids to hyperthermia and cytotoxic drugs. Br J Cancer 43: 384–391

Nagaoka S, Kawasaki S, Sasaki K, Nakanishi T (1986) Intracellular uptake, retention and cytotoxic effect of adriamycin combined with hyperthermia in vitro. Gann 77: 205–211

Roizin-Towle L, Hall EJ, Capuanol L (1982) Interaction of hyperthermia and cytotoxic agents. Nat Cancer Inst Monogr 61: 149–152

Rose WC, Veras GH, Laster WR, Schabel FM (1979) Evaluation of whole-body hyperthermia as an adjunct to chemotherapy in murine tumors. Cancer Treat Rep 63: 1311-1325

Rotkovská D, Vacek A (1972) Effect of high frequency electromagnetic field upon haematopoetic stem cells in mice. Folia Biol (Praha) 18: 292-297

Rotkovská D, Vacek A, Bartonicková A (1981) Therapeutic effect of microwaves on radiation damage to haematopoiesis. Strahlentherapie 157: 677-681

Sabio H, Elkon D, Baker DG (1981) Effect of hyperthermia on murine myeloid proliferation. Proc Am Assoc Cancer Res 22: 238

Sirotnak FM, Chello PL, Brockman RW (1979) Potential for exploitation of transport system in anticancer drug design. Methods Cancer Res 16: 381-447

Tribukait B, Söderström S, Beran M (1978) Survival, repair and pH-dependence in hyperthermically treated murine and human bone marrow stem cells. In: Streffer C (ed) Hyperthermia and radiation. Urban and Schwarzenberg, Baltimore, pp 181-182

Tritton TR, Murphree SA, Sartorelli AC (1978) Adriamycin. A proposal on the specificity of drug action. Biochem Biophys Res Commun 84: 802-808

Zunino F, Gambetta R, Di Marco A, Zaccara A (1972) Interaction of daunomycin and its derivatives with DNA. Biochim Biophys Acta 277: 489-498

Cardiotoxicity of Moderate Whole-Body Hyperthermia, Doxorubicin, and Combined Treatment in Rats

M. Birmelin, W. Hinkelbein, W. Oehlert, and M. Wannenmacher

Abteilung für Innere Medizin IV, Dialysestation, Medizinische Universitätsklinik, Hugstetter Straße 55, 7800 Freiburg, FRG

Introduction

In clinical practice hyperthermia should enhance the cytotoxic effects of other cancer therapy modalities on tumors while not increasing side-effects on normal tissues. Interactions between hyperthermia and cytostatic drugs (Hahn 1982; Honess and Bleehen 1985; Neumann et al. 1985) on malignant cell lines or in experimental tumor models are well known, but only a few studies have been performed with defined treatment regimens in normal tissues (Overgaard and Suit 1979), especially in critical organs. In order to elucidate various toxic effects induced by combined therapy involving moderate whole-body hyperthermia (mWBH) and cytostatic drugs (thermochemotherapy, TCT) we examined specific side-effects of doxorubicin and/or mWBH.

One of the clinically most important side-effects of doxorubicin is cardiotoxicity (Bristow et al. 1981), which limits the application of the anthracycline derivate. Although TCT involving doxorubicin and moderate WBH has been used in clinical investigations (Engelhardt 1983), no experimental data are available on the cardiotoxic effects of this treatment. In this study concerning cardiotoxicity a rat model was used to evaluate the histological alterations caused by hyperthermia, doxorubicin, and combined treatment.

Material and Method

Male Wistar rats (80 g) were used in all experiments. WBH was induced by microwaves. Besides measurements of core temperature (colon), constant electromagnetic field was also checked by direct measurements. Within 20 min the temperature was raised from 37.1° ± 0.3° C to 41.0° ± 0.4° C. This treatment temperature was maintained for 10 (H_1) or 20 min (H_2). In all animals receiving doxorubicin (D) a dose of 6 mg/kg body weight was injected intravenously on day 0, and another dose of 8 mg/kg body weight on day 14. Rats were killed by anoxia on day 21. This regimen was used to reflect the so-called subacute cardiotoxicity (Doroshow et al. 1979) and thus to cast some light on the chronic cardiotoxicity of

Recent Results in Cancer Research, Vol. 109

this cytostatic antibiotic. In the modality, TCT doxorubicin administration was followed by WBH within 30 min, lasting for 10 (DH_1) or 20 min (DH_2). On day 21, the heart was removed and after embedding, HE, azan, and PAS staining was performed.

Results and Discussion

Hyperthermia with 10 Minutes' Exposure (H_1). Heat treatment at 41° C for 10 min showed no tissue damage to heart muscle except in one animal in which focal subepicardiac inflammation and vacuolation were caused by single cell death (Fig. 1).

Hyperthermia with 20 Minutes' Exposure (H_2). This treatment caused damage in all animals, with subepi- and subendocardiac single and grouped cell death. Inflammatory reactions, interstitial fibrosis, edema, vacuolation, and acute hyperemia causing vasodilatation were also seen after this therapy (Fig. 2).

Doxorubicin (D). This cytostatic drug mainly produced subendocardiac single cell death, sarcolysis, and focal inflammation; these side-effects occurred in more than 50% of the treated animals. Some hearts displayed massive ectatic vessels, bleedings, and intravascular thrombosis. In 30% perivascular edema and vacuolation, interstitial infiltrates, and mesenchymal activation expressed as increased mitosis were found. Azan staining demonstrated expanded scars which were more often in a subepicardiac than a subendocardiac location (Fig. 3).

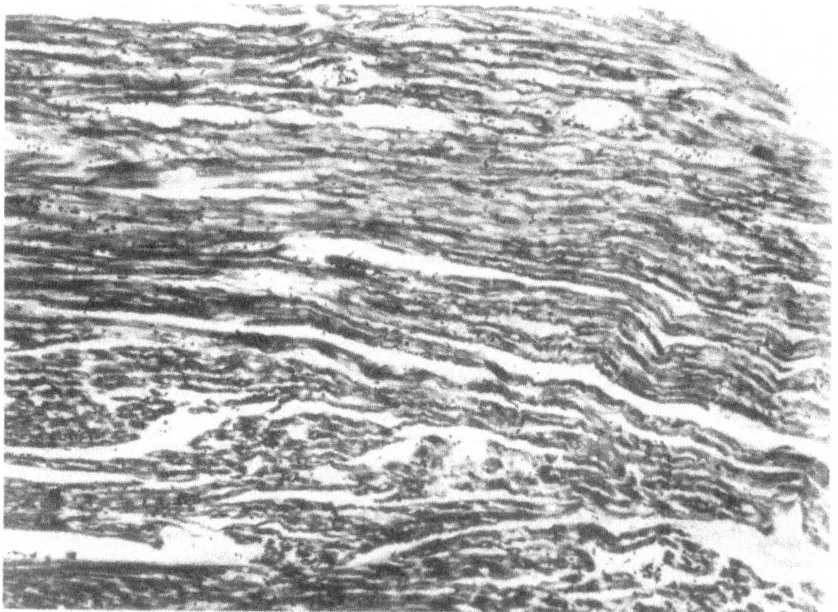

Fig. 1. Cardiac muscle after hyperthermia with 10 min exposure (H_1). HE, × 20

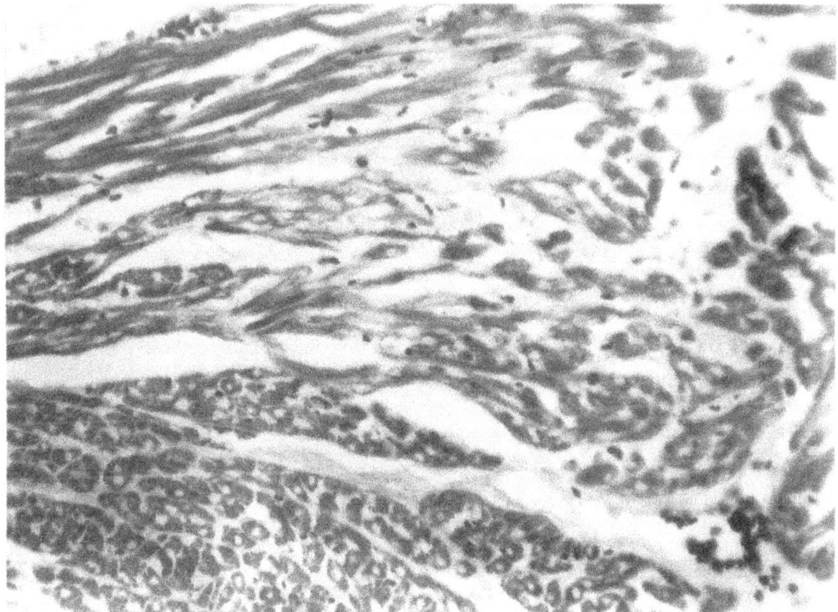

Fig. 2. Cardiac muscle after hyperthermia with 20 min exposure (H_2). Azan, × 100

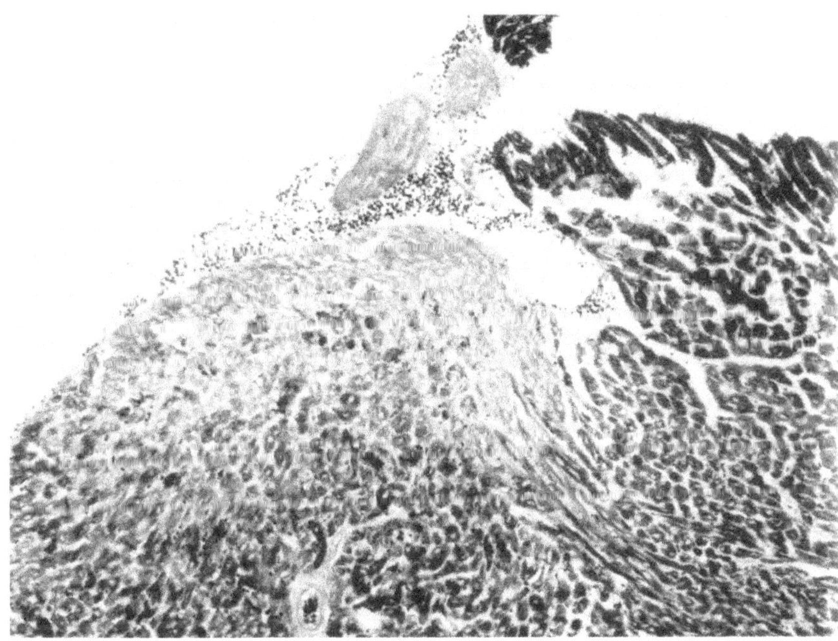

Fig. 3. Cardiac muscle after doxorubicin treatment (D). Azan, × 20

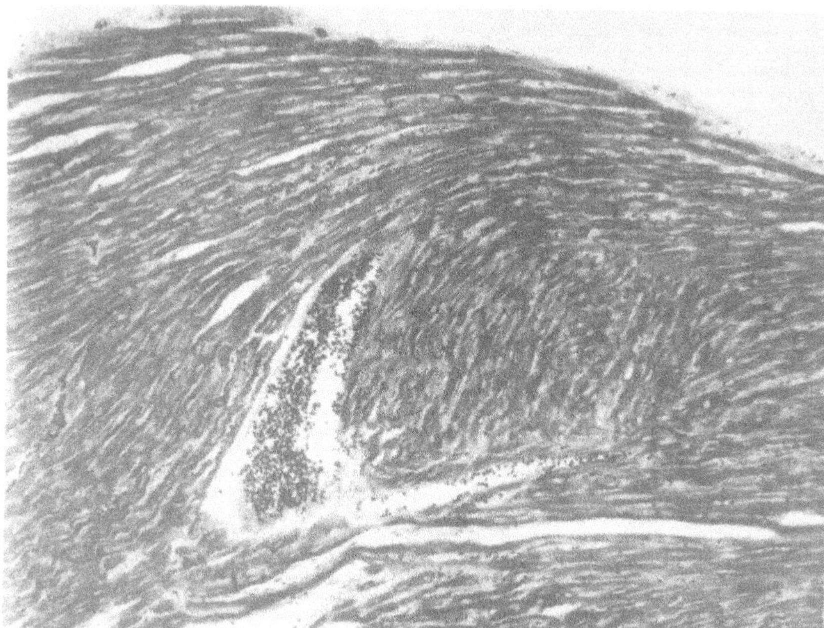

Fig. 4. Cardiac muscle after TCT with 10 min hyperthermia (DH_1). HE, × 20

TCT with 10 Minutes' Hyperthermia (DH_1). Which this regimen disseminated compact inflammatory paravascular infiltrates and gross interstitial edema were found in all animals, and in some hearts there was even interstitial bleeding. Necrotic muscle fibers were substituted by fibrotic network. The lesions were again more often subepi- than subendocardiac, but the scars were imposed as stripes. The striated structure of the heart muscle, however, was never destroyed (Fig. 4).

TCT with 20 Minutes' Hyperthermia (DH_2). All lesions described above were also found with this regimen, but they were much more serious (Fig. 5).

Nearly all results regarding heat injuries on normal tissues have been acquired at "high" temperatures (42.5° C and higher) (Overgaard 1983). The few investigations on the effects of lower temperature levels have involved experiments dealing with the toxicity of radarradiation, mostly without defined temperature monitoring. No experimental data are available on the heat damage to cardiac muscle; on the other hand, today potentially cardiotoxic drugs are used in combination with hyperthermia in clinical practice. All of the effects on cardiac muscle found in this study were induced by a very low "thermal dose." In conclusion all the results demonstrate that:

1. Surprisingly, at a temperature (mWBH) of "only" 41° C cardiac lesions dependent on exposure time were found which morphologically were similar to those found after administration of the cardiotoxic drug doxorubicin alone (D).
2. The combined treatment (TCT) was able to enhance the damage to the cardiac muscle by the increasing exposure time of mWBH. While the cardiotoxic side-

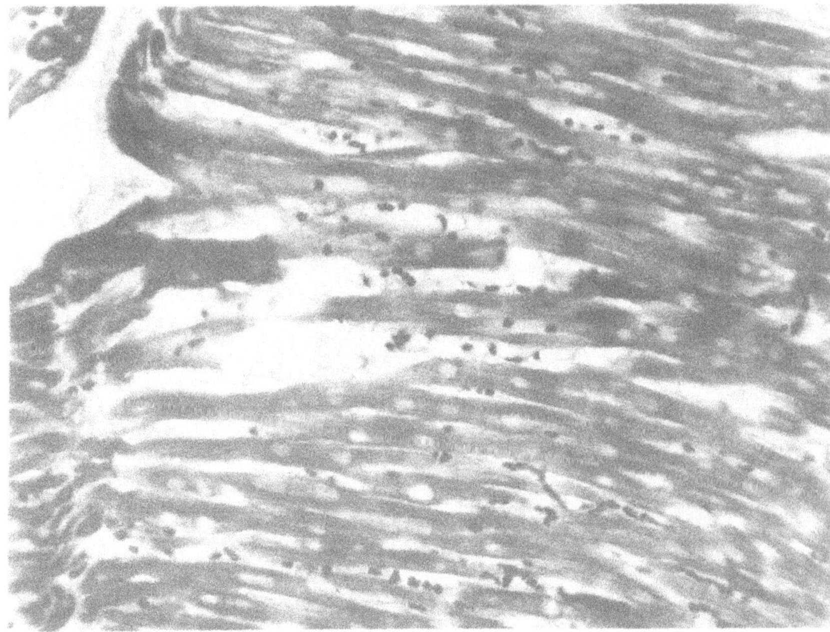

Fig. 5. Cardiac muscle after TCT with 20 min hyperthermia (DH_2). Azan, × 250

Table 1. Summary of the tissue alterations caused by the different therapy modalities

Histological findings	H_1	H_2	D	DH_1	DH_2
Single cell necrosis	(+)	+	+	+ +	+ + +
Focal necrosis	–	+	(+)	+ +	+ + +
Inflammatory reactions	–	+	+ +	+(+)	+ + +
Scars	–	+	·	+(+)	+ + +
Interstitial edema	–	(+)	+ +	+ +	+ + +
Ectatic vessels	–	+ +	(+)	+	+ +
Thrombus formation, intravascular	–	–	+	+	+
Interstitial bleeding	–	–	+ +	+	+ +
Distribution of the morphological changes	Focal	Focal	Focal	Disseminated	Disseminated

H_1, hyperthermia with 10 min exposure; *H_2*, hyperthermia with 20 min exposure; *D*, doxorubicin application only; *DH_1* and *DH_2*, the combinations of the afore mentioned regimens as TCT.

effects and the dependent morphological changes caused by doxorubicin are well known (Bristow et al. 1981), the reported histological changes after mWBH are assumed to be hypoxic lesions due to increased oxygen requirement although "thermal damage" to the cardiac muscle cannot definitely be ruled out.

By way of summary, the main types of tissue damage caused by the different modalities are shown in Table 1.

References

Bristow MR, Mason JW, Billingham ME, Daniels JR (1981) Dose effect and structure function relationships in doxorubicin cardiomyopathy. Am Heart J 102: 709-718

Doroshow JH, Locker GJ, Myers CE (1979) Experimental animal models of adriamycin cardiotoxicity. Cancer Treat Rep 63: 855-860

Engelhardt R (1983) Clinical trials on thermo-chemotherapy (TCT), TCT in small cell carcinoma of the lung. Strahlentherapie 159: 371-372

Hahn GM (1982) Thermal enhancement of the actions of anticancer agents. In: Hahn GM (ed) Hyperthermia and cancer. Plenum, New York, pp 55-86

Honess DJ, Bleehen NM (1985) Potentiation of mephalan by systemic hyperthermia in mice: therapeutic gain for mouse lung microtumours. Int J Hyperthermia 1: 57-68

Neumann HA, Fiebig HH, Löhr GW, Engelhardt R (1985) Effects of cytostatic drugs and 40.5° C hyperthermia on human clonogenic tumor cells. Eur J Cancer Clin Oncol 21: 515-523

Overgaard J (1983) Histopathologic effects of hyperthermia. In: Storm FK (ed) Hyperthermia in cancer therapy. Hall, Boston, pp 163-164

Overgaard J, Suit HD (1979) Time-temperature relationship in hyperthermic treatment of malignant and normal tissue in vivo. Cancer Res 39: 3248-3253

Preclinical Hpyerthermia in Animal Tumors and Malignant Cell Lines

*Effects of Hyperthermic Treatments on Malignant Cells and Animal Tumors: Introductory Remarks**

C. Streffer

Institut für Medizinische Strahlenbiologie, Universitätsklinikum Essen, Hufelandstraße 55, 4300 Essen, FRG

Introduction

The action of hyperthermia differs in many ways from the mechanism of other cytotoxic agents, like ionizing radiation or chemotherapeutic drugs. One of the most remarkable characteristics is the very fast expression of molecular and metabolic alterations during or after a heat treatment. While inhibition of DNA, RNA, and protein synthesis is observed only several hours or even days after X-irradiation (Streffer 1969), such effects already occur during heating of cells at 42° -43° C (Hahn 1982; Streffer 1982). Protein synthesis appears to be even more thermosensitive than DNA synthesis, while the opposite is true for the response to ionizing radiation. Hpyerthermia apparently induces conformational changes in complex macromolecular structures like multienzyme complexes which lead to the inactivation of the biological function. Conformational changes of proteins seem to be highly significant in this connection (Streffer 1985). Lepock and his associates (1982, 1983) have shown that such changes are important for the hyperthermic damage to membranes, although the cooperativity between proteins and lipids with changes in fluidity should not be neglected (Yatvin et al. 1982).

Conformational changes of proteins could also explain the damage to cytoskeletal structures and to the mitotic spindle fibers with the high thermosensitivity of cells in mitosis (Coss et al. 1982). An interesting proposal has been made by Burdon (1985), namely that shock proteins may stabilize cytoskeletal structures and in this way contribute to the development of thermotolerance. The thermosensitivity of protein conformation would also explain the pH dependence of the hyperthermic effect on cell killing. With the lowering of the pH, the protonation of ionic groups in proteins changes and as a consequence further conformational alterations are introduced or facilitated.

The microenvironment and the pH of cells in tissues and tumors are largely determined by metabolic and physiological factors. It has been shown that cells in culture become more thermosensitive when the pH decreases (Gerweck and Ri-

* These investigations have been supported by the Bundesminister für Forschung und Technologie, Bonn.

Recent Results in Cancer Research, Vol. 109

chards 1981). As a decreased pH has been observed in many experimental tumors, it has been suggested that tumors are more thermosensitive than normal tissues. Further, it has been assumed that hyperthermia decreases the pH to even lower values by metabolic processes, especially by the production of lactate (von Ardenne 1980). However, comparatively few experimental studies of this kind have been performed and the data do not show an increase of lactate in all cases. Especially when the lactate level is already high in the untreated tumor, no further increase is observed (Table 1) (Hengstebeck 1983). The metabolic investigations with adenocarcinoma show that the metabolic sources of energy (glucose and lipids) decrease and the lactate level is also slightly decreased, but that a remarkable increase in the lactate/pyruvate ratio occurs which indicates induction of hypoxia within the tumor (Table 1) (Hengstebeck 1983; Tamulevicius et al. 1984).

Similar findings have been observed by us in xenografts of human melanomas on nude mice (Mirtsch and Streffer unpublished data). After local hyperthermia at 43° C for 30 min, only a slight increase in lactate occurred in one of the xenografts (MeWo), while in the second (MHB) the lactate level was doubled (Fig. 1). In both tumors the lactate/pyruvate ratio increased appreciably. It is of special interest to

Table 1. Metabolites in a transplanted adenocarcinoma (μmol/g tissue) in a C57 BL mouse immediately after local hyperthermia (43° C, 60 min). (Hengstebeck 1983)

Metabolite	Control	Hyperthermia
Glucose	3.2	1.0
Glucose-6-phosphate	1.1	0.6
Glycerol-3-phosphate	0.39	0.52
Lactate	14.6	12.9
Lactate/pyruvate	39	66
β-Hydroxybutyrate	0.09	0.25

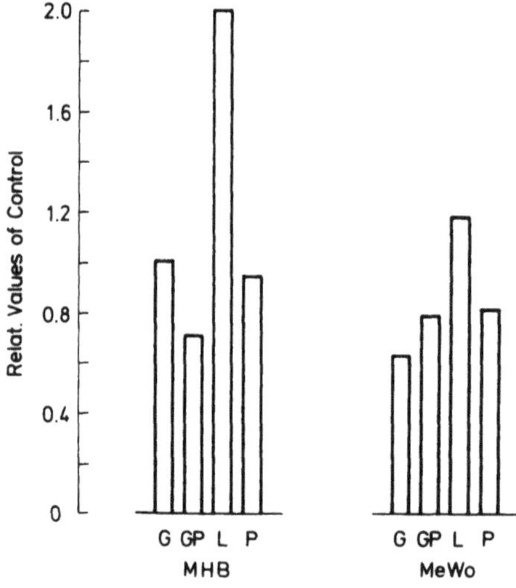

Fig. 1. Glycolytic metabolites in xenografts of two human melanomas (*MHB* and *MeWo*) on athymic nude mice after local hyperthermia at 43° C for 30 min. The data are presented as relative values of the controls. *G*, glucose; *GP*, glucose-6-phosphate; *L*, lactate; *P*, pyruvate

compare such effects after treatment of cells in vitro and of tumors in situ. Therefore the same human melanoma cells were grown in vitro or as a xenograft on nude mice and treated with hyperthermia. In the cells in vitro lactate and also the lactate/pyruvate ratio decreased. However, in the xenograft a slight increase in lactate and especially in the lactate/pyruvate ratio occurred (Table 2). The metabolites were determined by enzymatic techniques coupled to NAD^+ or NADH (Hengstebeck 1983). These data showed that hyperthermia per se does not induce an accumulation of lactate within the melanoma cells. However, from the tumor the produced lactate must be transported to the liver through the blood (Fig. 2). If the blood flow is reduced, an increase in lactate will occur in the tumor. The enhancement of lactate decreases the pH and as a consequence the blood flow will be reduced further (Vaupel et al. 1983). Through these processes an "autocatalytic" mechanism leads to an enhanced reaction. However, the reduced blood flow also reduces the glucose supply from the liver to the tumors (Fig. 2). Thus an interesting interplay occurs between these factors which will modify the thermosensitivity of the cells.

Von Ardenne (1980) proposed giving a glucose load in combination with hyperthermia in order to accelerate these biochemical changes and to increase the thermosensitivity of the tumor by decreasing the pH. Dickson and Calderwood (1979) observed an increase in lactate after large glucose injections in a rat tumor. The same phenomenon was found by Hengstebeck (1983) in a mouse tumor. In these studies it was especially remarkable that the lactate/pyruvate ratio was increased for a long period (Fig. 3). This effect is an indication that long-lasting hypoxia is induced by hyperthermia in the tumor, especially when employed in combination

Table 2. Metabolites in human melanoma cells (in vitro) and in xenografts from the same cells on nude mice after hyperthermia (HT) (43° C; 60 min). (Mirtsch and Streffer, unpublished results)

Metabolite	Cells in vitro		Xenografts	
	Co	HT	Co	HT
	(fmoles/cell)		(µmol/g tissue)	
Lactate	16.4	11.2	6.6	7.8
Pyruvate	1.44	2.16	0.25	0.20
Lactate/pyruvate	11.4	5.2	26.4	39.0

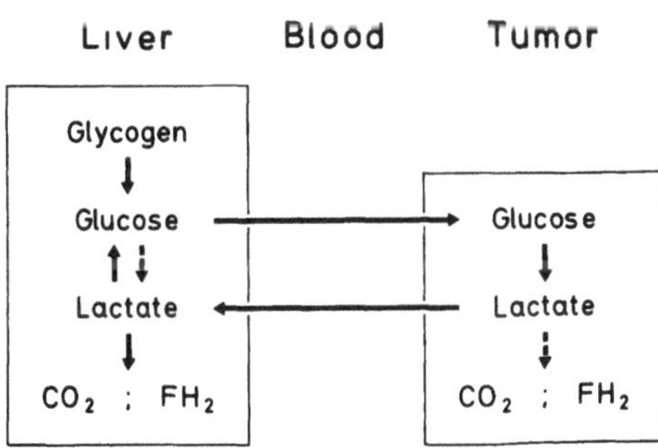

Fig. 2. Flow diagram for transport of metabolites between liver and tumor

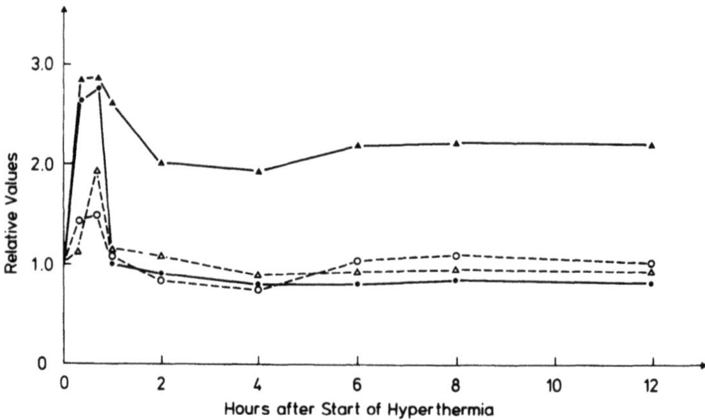

Fig. 3. Lactate/Pyruvate ratio in mouse liver and adenocarcinoma after local heating for 60 min at 43° C or after injection of 6 mg/g body wt. glucose plus heating. △, liver heating alone; ○, tumor heating alone; ●, liver heating plus glucose; ▲, tumor heating plus glucose

with glucose. From these data it can be concluded that for a combined therapeutic modality of ionizing radiation plus hyperthermia, heating should always follow the radiation in order to avoid irradiation of the tumor during a period of heat-induced hypoxia, although such generalizations have to be made with some caution.

In general it looks as if these metabolic alterations can modify the microenvironment in tumors and through this mechanism alter the cellular response after a hyperthermic treatment. However, more data are needed in order to correlate the metabolic changes with the cell-killing effect of hyperthermia and to elucidate the underlying mechanisms.

In clinical studies local hyperthermia is most frequently used in combination with ionizing radiation. It has been demonstrated that the mechanism of hyperthermia as a radiosensitizing agent differs clearly from that of a cytotoxic agent (Hahn 1982; Dewey 1984; Leeper 1985). While hyperthermia alone does not induce chromosomal aberrations in resting cells or in G_1-phase cells, it enhances the number of chromosomal aberrations remarkably when it is used in close connection with irradiation (Hahn 1982). Further, it has been demonstrated that the recovery from sublethal radiation damage and the repair of radiation-induced DNA single strand breaks are considerably reduced by hyperthermia (Ben Hur et al. 1974; Dikomey 1982). Therefore it has been proposed and also demonstrated that the radiosensitization by heat is very effective in cells with a broad shoulder in the dose effect curve (Fig. 4). The degree of radiosensitization is apparently dependent on the D_q-value of the dose effect curve (Streffer et al. 1984). Under these conditions it would be very useful to develop methods for a rapid test in order to select tumors with cell lines which have a high capacity for recovery. Such tumors are usually relatively radioresistant and might be good candidates for combined treatment. When the same total radiation doses are compared, the survival of cells is higher after fractionated X-irradiation than after single X-irradiation owing to intracellular recovery. This fractionation effect is completely suppressed when each dose is followed by hyperthermic treatment (Fig. 5).

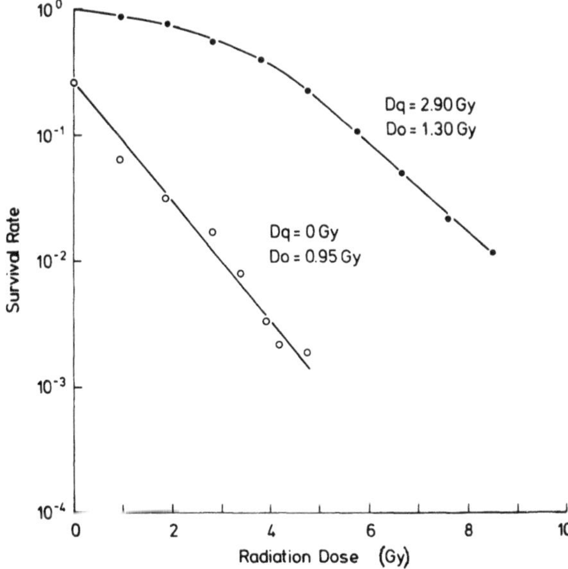

Fig. 4. Survival (CFU) of human melanoma cells (Be 11) after X-irradiation alone (●) and after X-irradiation plus heating for 3 h at 42° C (○). The cells were treated 24 h after the start of the culture and plated directly after treatment

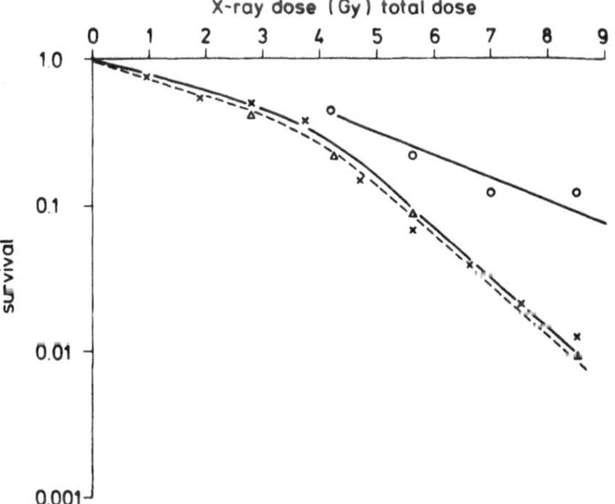

Fig. 5. Survival (CFU) of human melanoma cells (Be 11) after X-irradiation and X-irradiation plus heat. x, single doses of X-irradiation; ○, three equal doses of X-rays; △ three doses of X-rays, each followed by 1 h heating at 42° C (the latter data are corrected for three times heating for 1 h at 42° C alone). The interval between the treatments was 24 h

After irradiation a block of cells in the G_2-phase is usually observed (Alper 1979). This G_2-block can be prolonged or shifted to later periods by the additional hyperthermic treatment. As the extent of cell killing is dependent on the cell cycle phase after irradiation as well as after hyperthermia, knowledge of these effects is important and more data are needed under these conditions. Comparatively few studies have been performed with fractionated treatment which have considered effects on the cell cycle.

Prolonged or fractionated heat treatments can induce thermotolerance (Hahn 1982). This phenomenon is usually studied after heat treatment alone. If thermotolerance were also to develop for the radiosensitizing effect, it would disturb the therapeutic efficiency of a fractionated combined treatment. Some investigations have shown that the development of thermotolerance is less when hyperthermia is used as a radiosensitizing agent (Streffer et al. 1984). However, it has also been observed that thermotolerance occurs with combined treatments (Nielsen 1984). It has been proposed that radiosensitization is reduced by thermotolerance in the low radiation dose range but it is not altered by thermotolerance in the high dose range (Dewey 1984). This question is essential for the clinical use of hyperthermia in combination with ionizing radiation, as clinical treatments are performed using fractionated schedules. More data are needed in order to solve this important question for the optimal treatment schedule.

References

Alper T (1979) Cellular radiobiology. Cambridge University Press, Cambridge

Ben-Hur E, Elkind MM, Bronk BV (1974) Thermally enhanced radioresponse of cultured Chinese hamster cells. Nature 238: 209-211

Burdon RH (1985) Heat shock proteins. In: Overgaard J (ed) Hyperthermic oncology, vol II. Taylor and Francis, London, pp 223-230

Coss RA, Dewey WC, Bamburg JR (1982) Effects of hyperthermia on dividing Chinese hamster ovary cells and on microtubules in vitro. Cancer Res 42: 1059-1071

Dewey WC (1984) Interaction of heat with radiation and chemotherapy. Cancer Res (Suppl) 44: 4714s-4720s

Dickson J, Calderwood SK (1979) Effect of hyperglycemia and hyperthermia on the pH, glycolysis and respiration of the Yoshida sarcoma in vivo. JNCI 63: 1371-1381

Dikomey E (1982) Effect of hyperthermia at 42° C and 45° C on repair of radiation-induced DNA strand breaks in CHO cells. Int J Radiat Biol 41: 603-614

Gerweck LE, Richards B (1981) Influence of pH on the thermal sensitivity of cultured human glioblastoma cells. Cancer Res 41: 845-849

Hahn GM (1982) Hyperthermia and cancer. Plenum, New York

Hengstebeck S (1983) Untersuchungen zum Intermediärstoffwechsel in der Leber und in einem Adenocarcinom der Maus nach Hyperthermie. Dissertation, Universitäts-Gesamthochschule, Essen

Leeper DB (1985) Molecular and cellular mechanisms of hyperthermia alone or combined with other modalities. In: Overgaard J (ed) Hyperthermic oncology 1984. Vol. 2. Taylor and Francis, London, pp 9-40

Lepock JR (1982) Involvement of membranes in cellular responses to hyperthermia. Radiat Res 92: 433-438

Lepock JR, Cheng KH, Al-Qysi H, Kruuv J (1983) Thermotropic lipid and protein transitions in Chinese hamster lung cell membranes: relationship to hyperthermic cell killing. Can J Biochem Cell Biol 61: 421-427

Nielsen OS (1984) Fractionated hyperthermia and thermotolerance. Dan Med Bull 31
Streffer C (1969) Strahlen-Biochemie. Springer, Berlin Heidelberg New York
Streffer C (1982) Aspects of biochemical effects by hyperthermia. Natl Cancer Inst Monogr 61: 11-16
Streffer C (1985) Metabolic changes during and after hyperthermia. Int J Hyperthermia 1: 305-319
Streffer C, van Beuningen D, Uma Devi P (1984) Radiosensitization by hyperthermia in human melanoma cells: single and fractionated treatments. Cancer Treat Rev 11: 179-185
Tamulevicius P, Würzinger U, Luscher G, Streffer C (1984) Lipid metabolism in mouse liver and adenocarcinoma following hyperthermia. In: Overgaard J (ed) Hyperthermic oncology 1984. Vol. 1. Taylor and Francis, London, pp 23-26
Vaupel P, Müller-Klieser W, Otte J, Manz R, Kallinowski F (1983) Durchblutung, Sauerstoffversorgung des Gewebes und pH-Verteilung in malignen Tumoren nach Hyperthermia. Pathophysiologische Grundlagen und Einfluß verschiedener Hyperthermiedosen. Strahlentherapie 159: 73-81
von Ardenne M (1980) Hyperthermia and cancer therapy. Adv Pharmacol Chemother 10: 137-138
Yatvin MB, Cree TC, Elson CE, Gipp JJ, Tegmo I-M, Vorpahl JW (1982) Probing the relationship of membrane "fluidity" to heat killing of cells. Radiat Res 89: 644-646

Hyperthermia and Microcirculatory Effects of Heat in Animal Tumors

B. Endrich

Allgemeinchirurgische Abteilung, Kreiskrankenhaus Sinsheim,
Akademisches Lehrkrankenhaus der Universität Heidelberg, Alte Waibstadter Straße 2,
6920 Sinsheim, FRG

Introduction

Up to the present, much attention in cancer research has been focussed on biological changes of malignant cells in vitro when they are treated with hyperthermia. Very little is known how and to what extent the in vivo environment in which these cells are lodged will affect the therapeutic outcome. As a consequence of functional as well as morphological differences of microvascular beds in neoplastic tissue, attempts were made recently to exploit the possibility of enhancing the efficacy of tumor therapy by affecting the microcirculation. Some encouraging results were obtained, and the combination of hyperthermia and conventional tumor treatment began to attract an increasing number of investigators because nutritionally deprived and hypoxic tumor cells appeared to be particularly sensitive to heat (Overgaard and Bichel 1977; Overgaard and Nielsen 1980; Overgaard 1981; Rhee 1984; for a review see Streffer 1985; Vaupel et al. 1983). The extent and etiology of vascular damage in tumors and the possible clinical impact are still subjects of controversy. It is the aim of this paper to:

1. Describe the typical features of a tumor microcirculation as reported in the literature
2. Summarize the changes occurring in the tumor microcirculation as a result of hyperthermia
3. Discuss the mechanism(s) involved in vascular damage

Features of the Tumor Microcirculation

The characteristics of a tumor microcirculation have been summarized by several authors and are listed in Table 1. According to Vaupel et al. (1980) and Vaupel (1982), the nutritional deficiency in tumors is a consequence of the low and inhomogeneous blood flow. This factor, brought about by the growth of tissue, tends to cause progressive underperfusion which is counteracted only to some extent by the process of neovascularization (Endrich et al. 1979a, 1982a; Oda et al. 1984; Simpson and Fraser 1983; Warren 1979). On the other hand, the tumor capillaries

Recent Results in Cancer Research, Vol. 109

Table 1. Characteristics of the tumor microcirculation. (According to Warren 1979; Vaupel et al. 1983; Hammersen et al. 1983, 1985; Reinhold and Endrich 1986)

Nutritional deficiency
Areas with hypoxia/anoxia
Areas with low pH
Necrotic regions
Heterogeneous microarchitecture
Chaotic vascular alignment
Elongated or compressed capillaries
Microaneurysms
Intravascular thrombi formation
Inhomogeneous flow and tissue perfusion
Areas with high perfusion
Areas with low flow state
Arteriovenous shunting
Alterations within the vessel wall
Endothelial edema
Lack of endothelial lining
Partial lack of a basement membrane
Blood cell penetration/extravasation

are highly permeable because along these vascular channels the endothelium is discontinuous, the basal lamina is not present, and plasma and possibly cellular elements pass directly into the tissue (Hammersen et al. 1983, 1985). A consequence of this pathological alteration is the transmission of the capillary hydraulic pressure in toto to the tissue fluid (Oda et al. 1984) without any hindrance from oncotic effects which are present in the normal microcirculation. The direct hydraulic connection between the capillary system and the interstitium causes the tissue pressure to be high and very likely to be identical to the mean capillary hydrostatic pressure (Oda et al. 1984). The presence of abnormal rheological conditions coupled with the possibility of very high rates of fluid exchange makes the tumor microcirculation a system which cannot be analyzed in terms of transport properties conventional for normal tissues. Moreover, the fact that blood flow varies greatly from region to region reflects the necessity to analyze the terminal vascular bed of experimental tumors at the level of single capillaries. Today, this can be accomplished utilizing intravital microscopy and quantitative television techniques (Intaglietta et al. 1975).

In conjunction with transparent skin fold chambers (for a review see Endrich et al. 1980), a chaotic microarchitecture could be visualized even in very small tumors (Fig. 1); these in vivo studies revealed that any rhythmic contraction of arterioles feeding a tumor (spontaneous arteriolar vasomotion) disappears during earliest tumor growth, suggesting that this microvascular bed is exhausting its full dilatory reserve from the very beginning (Endrich et al. 1979a, b, 1982a, b). Consequently, *the viscosity of blood becomes a limiting factor of tissue perfusion*. In malignant tumors, prestasis, stasis, rouleaux formation of erythrocytes, and blood cell aggregation were frequently described, indicating a "degradation" of blood to a reticulated suspension with extremely low fluidity that can be fully abolished whenever rouleaux structures straddle bifurcations within the tumor microvascula-

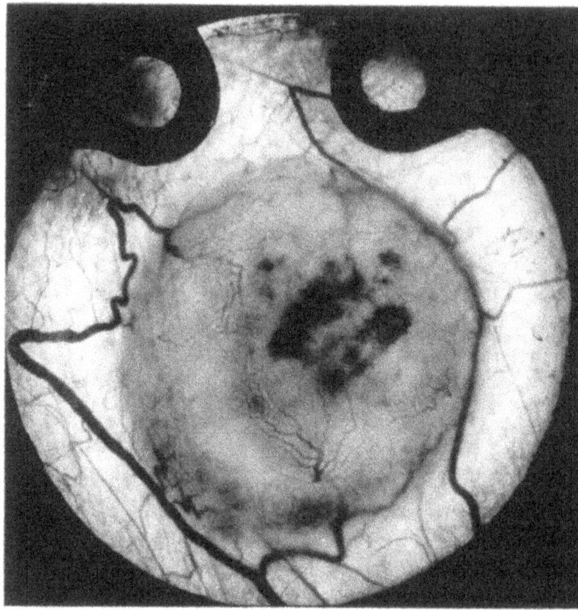

Fig. 1. The amelanotic melanoma A-Mel-3 seven days after tumor implantation. Note the chaotic microarchitecture at the edge of the tumor which grew in a transparent skin fold chamber. ca. × 8

ture or completely obstruct the lumen of a tapering vessel of smaller diameter (Gullino et al. 1982; Müller-Klieser and Vaupel 1984; Vaupel 1982). Moreover, a recent, systematic analysis of the vascular ultrastructure in malignant tumors revealed abnormalities of both new and preexisting vessels (for a review see Hammersen et al. 1983, 1985).

One consistent finding, derived from human and experimental tumors, has been the greatly reduced rate of nutritive tissue perfusion, and as a consequence of the persisting low flow state, tissue hypoxia. This indicates that an apparently redundant terminal vascular bed is functionally inefficient, probably because of its elevated intravascular resistance (Endrich et al. 1982a, 1986) which in turn does not permit a sufficient perfusion of nutritional tumor capillaries.

Changes in the Tumor Microcirculation upon Hyperthermia

While applying hyperthermia in malignant tumors, a circulatory system is to be treated in which the intravascular resistance is abnormally high. This specific feature might explain other pathological changes that are observed in malignant tumors such as a reduced capillary blood flow and tissue hypoxia. Furthermore, if the temperature is gradually increased, it has been a consistent finding that the microcirculatory function is changed from a slightly enhanced tumor blood flow during moderate hyperthermia into a state of total circulatory dysfunction as soon as a critical temperature is exceeded (Berg-Blok and Reinhold 1984; Dewhirst et al. 1984; Dickson and Calderwood 1980; Song et al. 1980a, b). This critical temperature is likely to be different for different tumors. In general, however, the micro-

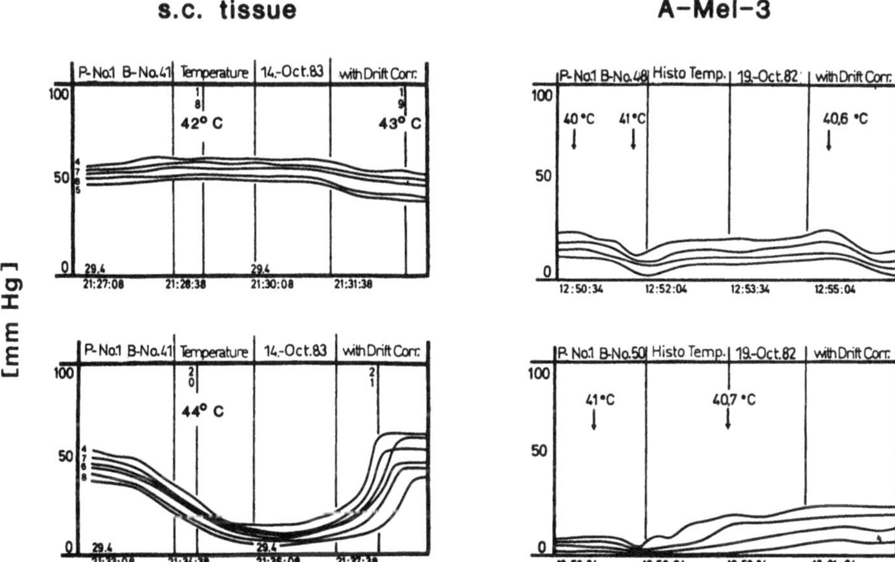

Fig. 2. Original registration of local PO_2 (platinum multiwire electrode). A decrease was noted in the normal microcirculation (s.c. tissue and skeletal musculature) at a temperature of 44° C while in the tumor (amelanotic melanoma A-Mel-3 of the hamster) the local PO_2 already decreased at a temperature above 40° C

circulation of experimental tumors cannot tolerate elevated temperatures as well as the normal microcirculation (Dudar and Jain 1984; Endrich and Hammersen 1986; Scheid 1961). In Fig. 2, an original registration of local PO_2, a difference of approximately 3° C is demonstrated in temperature at which PO_2 decreases in the normal and in the tumor microcirculation. Such a difference has been observed by several investigators (Berg-Blok and Reinhold 1984; Dickson and Calderwood 1980; Dudar and Jain 1984; Pence and Song 1986; Reinhold et al. 1978) since Scheid first noticed in 1961 that the tumor microvasculature was more sensitive to the effects of heat. Hyperthermia itself not only causes alterations in the growth rate of the malignant tissue portion but also affects the microarchitecture and microangiodynamic parameters, which in turn will lead to a further increase in capillary flow resistance. This effect constitutes a limiting factor which modulates tumor growth and impairs the action of those curative and palliative procedures that depend upon the blood supply for their effectiveness, such as radiation, chemotherapy, and hyperthermia.

Evidence is also found in the literature that vascular collapse may take place during hyperthermia in human tumors as well. Storm et al. (1979) treated intraabdominal sarcomas with a 13.56-MHz electromagnetic system at a temperature of ca. 50° C for 15-30 min. After five treatment regimens, there seemed to be pronounced intravascular congestion as suggested from histological sections. Recently, Reinhold and Endrich (1986) reported similar observations during whole body hyperthermia when they added local hyperthermia. During the first days after the treatment of a recurrent, large mammary carcinoma, extensive necrosis and microvascular damage were seen in the tumor as well as in the overlying skin. Similar conclusions could be derived from the reports by Karino et al. (1984) and others (for a review see Reinhold and Endrich 1986). However, there appeared to be large and significant variations in the temperature needed to induce microvascular thrombosis and tissue necrosis. Therefore, it seems necessary to carry out a systematic determination of the heat dose (dependent on time and temperature) which is required:

1. To achieve microvascular dysfunction in various tumors
2. To establish the usefulness of this effect.

Moreover, precise knowledge of the mechanism(s) underlying a heat-induced microvascular breakdown is of utmost importance.

Mechanisms of Heat-Induced Microvascular Dysfunction in Malignant Tumors

Possible mechanisms of heat-induced microvascular dysfunction which could finally result in complete occlusion of tumor capillaries throughout the tumor are listed in Table 2 for experimental tumors.

Recent experimental data (Endrich and Hammersen 1986) obtained with stepwise temperature increments suggest that a temperature as low as 42.5° C could induce stasis in tumor capillaries within only 15-30 min. It is likely not only that the heating method itself has a significant impact on tumor destruction, but also that the tumor type, the rate of heating, and the "assay method" used to determine the flow decrease will greatly affect the data obtained (Reinhold and Endrich 1986). With regard to the latter, it should be noted that electronic flow measurements at the level of a single capillary, in which the perfusion rate is observed to decrease, are the most sensitive method for evaluating a cessation of flow in experimental

Table 2. Mechanisms of hyperthermia-induced microvascular stasis in tumors. (From Badylak et al. 1985; Dewhirst et al. 1984; Eddy 1980; Endrich 1979b; Endrich and Hammersen 1986; Lee et al. 1985; Pence and Song 1986; Reinhold et al. 1978; Reinhold and Endrich 1986; Vaupel et al. 1980, 1983; von Ardenne 1981)

I. Changes at the vessel wall
Destruction of endothelial cells
Leukocyte and platelet sticking
II. Changes in blood rheology
Decrease in erythrocyte flexibility
Aggregation of erythrocytes
Thrombosis in capillaries
Fibrin formation
III. Changes in microhemodynamics
Further increase in microvascular resistance
Decrease in the arteriovenous pressure gradient
Arteriolar constriction
Edema formation
Arteriovenous shunting

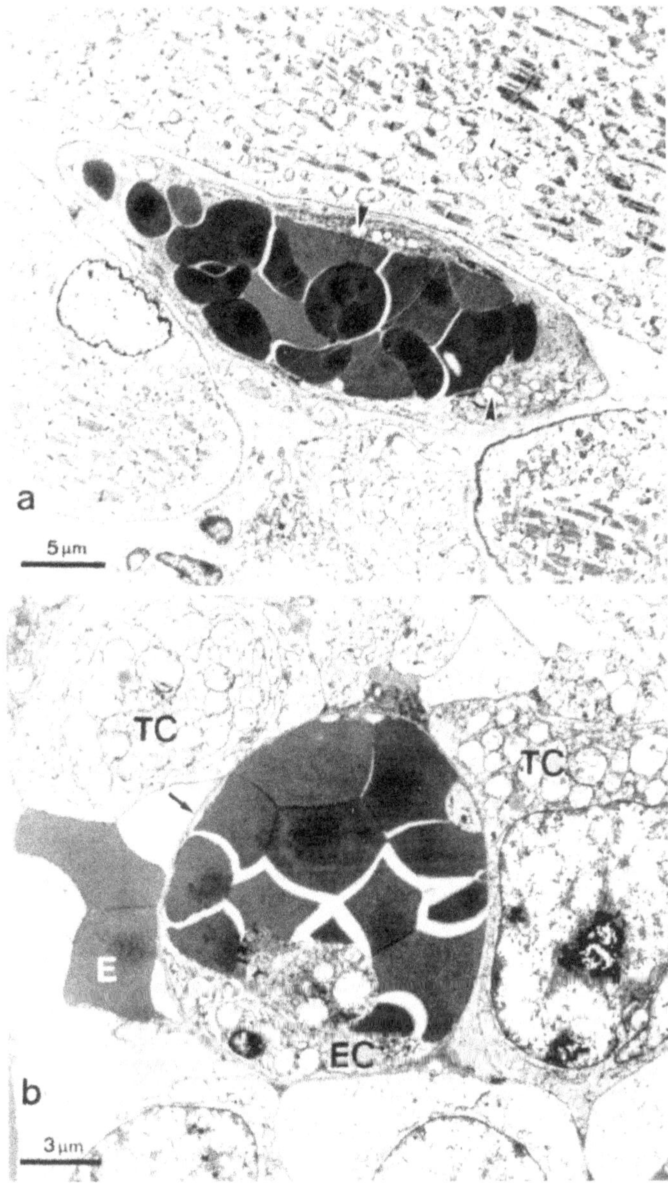

Fig. 3a, b. Electron micrographs of the microcirculation in a dorsal skin fold chamber of the hamster. **a** s.c. tissue; **b** amelanotic melanoma A-Mel-3; hyperthermia of 42.5° C was employed for 40 min. In **a**, skeletal muscle fibers are almost completely destroyed. The capillary located in the *center* of the picture is packed with erythrocytes while the endothelium is still intact. However, it reveals quite a few destroyed mitochondria (—▬). By contrast, the capillary in **b** is found between strongly damaged tumor cells *(TC)*; it retains only fragments of the endothelium and basal lamina (←—). Some erythrocytes *(E)* are found outside the capillary wall texture between tumor cells. *EC*, possibly part of an endothelial cell

animals. Even the use of such techniques is justified because Dewhirst et al. (1984) indicated that the "vascular stasis temperature" will depend not only on the rate of heating but also on the type of the vessel and the microvascular segment under observation.

Figure 3 demonstrates some of the ultrastructural changes that occur after 40 min at a temperature of 42.5° C in the amelanotic melanoma A-Mel-3 of the hamster. Erythrocyte aggregation in tumor vessels was observed as soon as 10 min after reaching a temperature of 42.5° C. This was accompanied by severe tissue hypoxia and swelling of mitochondria in tumor cells but very little degenerative change at the capillary endothelium. Sticking of leukocytes to the vessel wall has also been reported (Endrich 1979b). It should be noted that, upon hyperthermia, specific morphological changes, particularly at the vessel wall, will be observed much later than intravascular capillary stasis, which appears rather quickly (Emami et al. 1980, 1981; Emami and Song 1984). Moreover, arteriolar constriction in experimental tumors has been observed *after stasis in the microcirculation* became evident. This will result in a further reduction of nutritive capillary flow.

Therefore, it is likely that changes in blood flow and rheology initiate the response of the microvascular bed to a heat stimulus. Based on earlier in vitro data

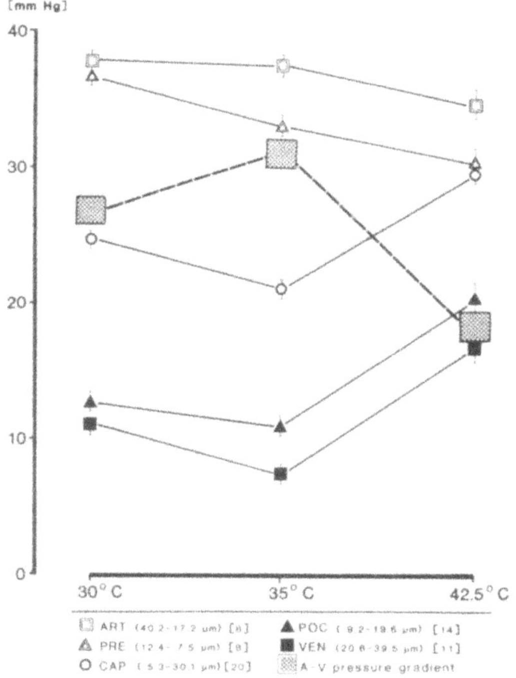

Fig. 4. Intravascular pressures for different segments of the microcirculation of the amelanotic melanoma A-Mel-3. The vessels were categorized according to Zweifach (1974) in arterioles *(ART)*, precapillaries *(PRE)*, capillaries *(CAP)*, postcapillaries *(POC)*, and venules *(VEN)*. In *brackets* are the number of single determinations for each microvascular segment; the pressure measurements were carried out using the servo-nulling technique as described by Wiederhelm et al. (1964)

reported by Schmid-Schönbein et al. (1975), von Ardenne (1981, 1986) has proposed the concept that at a low pH, erythrocytes will lose their flexibility and subsequently occlude the capillary bed in tumors. This hypothesis has been criticized recently for the following reasons:

1. Using intravital microscopy, stiffened erythrocytes have never been seen in a tumor microcirculation.
2. According to in vitro data reported by Crandall et al. (1978) and Vaupel et al. (1980), the time interval at which a red cell will become rigid is of the order of 20 min at a pH of 6.5. In vivo, however, only a few minutes are available for red cells to pass the capillaries in a tumor.
3. Recent work by Schmid-Schönbein et al. (1984) suggests that only subpopulations of erythrocytes, ca. 10%, may be stiffened at a very low pH, and this number seems too small to explain complete capillary occlusion as observed by intravital microscopy.

Vascular stasis, however, is prominent in conditions of low perfusion pressure (Schmid-Schönbein et al. 1984), suggesting that intravascular, hemodynamic changes initiate the microvascular dysfunction and congestion during hyperthermia. In fact, our own recent data indicate that the factors governing hyperthermia-induced vascular stasis are a combination of rheological, intravascular, and endothelial alterations that are preceded by local changes of the microvascular pressure gradient (Endrich and Hammersen 1986; Reinhold and Endrich 1986).

Figure 4 strongly supports this view because the arteriolar-venular pressure gradient was found to be much lower during hyperthermia of 42.5° C. From the data

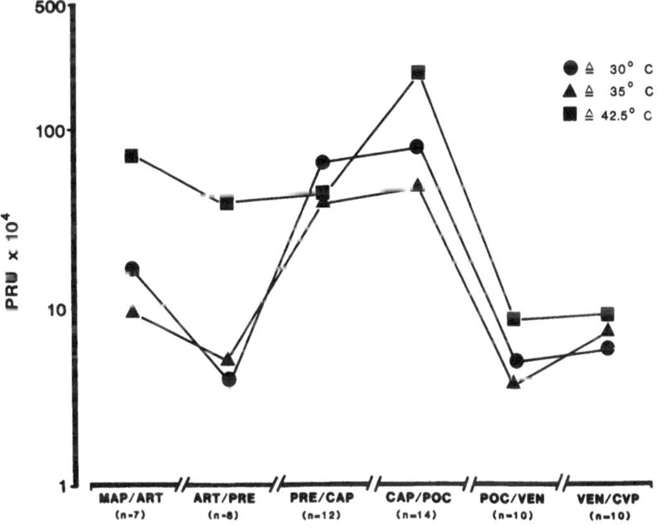

Fig. 5. Segmental resistance in the terminal vascular bed of the amelanotic melanoma A-Mel-3 of the hamster. This parameter was calculated from the systemic pressure as well as the local microvascular pressure and flow according to Ohm's relationship. Note that the change in resistance is most pronounced in arterioles/precapillaries and postcapillaries. For further explanation see Fig. 4

regarding systemic pressures, local microvascular pressure, and flow, the segmental microvascular resistance can be calculated. Figure 5 demonstrates that a disproportionate increase in precapillary and venular resistance was found upon local hyperthermia in the amelanotic melanoma A-Mel-3 of the hamster. This elevation is a result of both the significant increase in venular pressure and the severe reduction in flow throughout the microcirculation. We propose that this change in local microvascular resistance will subsequently initiate the arteriolar constriction in tumor vessels because vascular smooth muscle can be stimulated to contract after the intravascular pressure/resistance is enhanced. This occurs in much the same manner that stretching of other smooth muscle cells leads to their contraction (Johnson 1980). Any elevation of venous pressure causes a sustained increase in precapillary resistance. Consequently, the precapillary wall tension is higher, resulting in vasoconstriction (Fig. 6). By contrast, the reduction in flow occurring at the same time should lead to a metabolite accumulation which is a stimulus to vasodilation. Apparently, the stimuli provided by the low PO_2, the low pH, and the flow reduction are not strong enough to overcome the vasoconstriction seen. Therefore, a myogenic mechanism seems a very likely explanation for the phenomenon observed in Fig. 6.

It should further be noted that vascular smooth muscle cells are "tension receptors" rather than „length receptors." This finding (Johnson 1980) is of particular importance in considering vascular smooth muscle response since the circumferential wall tension of vessels varies with the intravascular pressure as well as with the vessel radius according to the La Place relationship $(T = P \times r)$. Any increase in microvascular pressure would lead to an elevation of wall tension which in turn would elicit a myogenic contraction. As the contraction and the reduction in the vessel radius become evident, wall tension will decrease.

The mechanism proposed here incorporates a negative feedback system that limits the magnitude of contraction elicited by pressure elevation. Since a fair number of preexisting arterioles feed the tumor, one can assume that this control system is still operating in many regions of the tumor; it is geared to maintain a rather constant wall tension with the vessel radius decreasing in proportion to the pressure increase.

Summary and Clinical Relevance of the Data

A great number of studies have shown that tumor blood flow can be reduced by hyperthermia to a larger extent than blood flow in normal tissue. While the great majority of data on experimental tumors show a decrease and even a total lapse in blood flow within the microcirculation, the results are far less conclusive for human tumors during or after hyperthermia (Wike-Hooley et al. 1984). From our own recent study, however, it can be concluded that by reducing venous outflow and capillary circulation, the heating of a tumor could be facilitated. To achieve a greater benefit for tumor destruction, the control of local tumor temperature is of utmost importance (Table 3) because at a temperature of app. 41° C a difference in tumor temperature of ± 1° C will generate a totally different reaction in the tumor microcirculation. Moreover, no significant changes in microvascular flow are seen

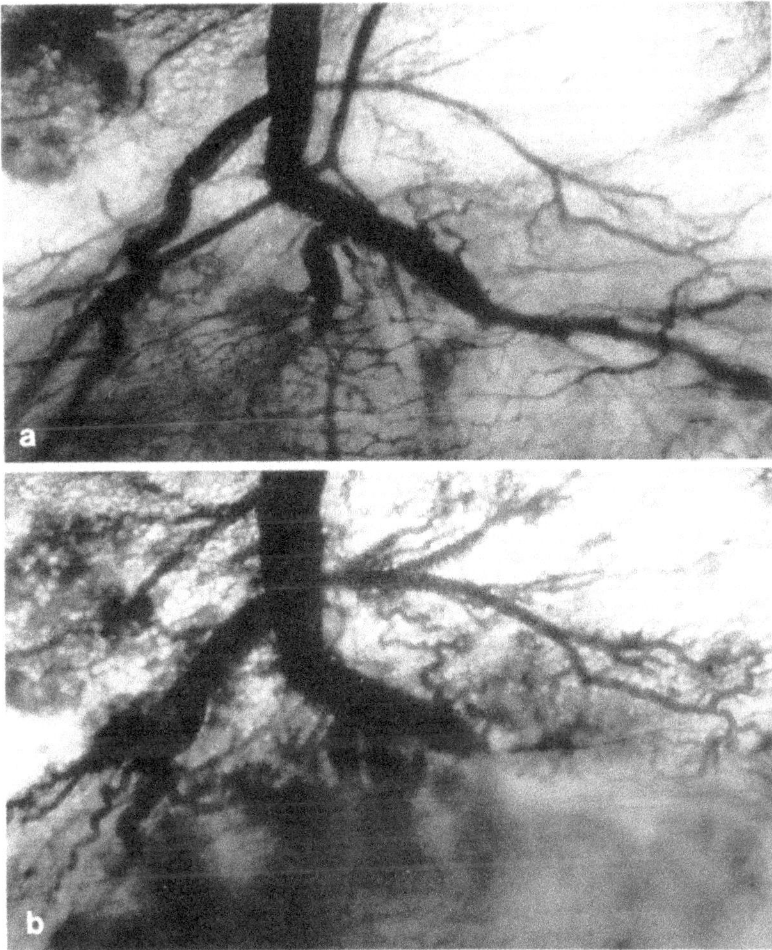

Fig. 6a, b. Effect of local hyperthermia on the microcirculation of the amelanotic melanoma A-Mel-3 in a dorsal skin fold chamber. Even 72 h after hyperthermia, the arteriolar constriction which occurred after ca. 30 min at a tumor temperature of 42.5° C still persisted, leading to necrosis in the center of the tumor (**b**). The accompaniing vein, which is draining the tumor, is still dilated, showing only sluggish blood flow. × 50

Table 3. Treatment of tumors by hyperthermia: conclusions derived from experimental data

1. The measurement of *tumor temperature* seems of critical importance.
2. Mild hyperthermia (< 40° C) should be applied as an adjuvant measure (perfusion) only.
3. Arteriolar constriction and capillary stasis temporarily exclude experimental tumors from the systemic circulation.
4. Quick and pronounced microvascular dysfunction at temperatures above 42° C might suggest the use of hyperthermia after radiation therapy.

at a temperature range between 35° and 40° C (Endrich and Hammersen 1986); thus, when using moderate hyperthermia in conjunction with chemotherapy one should aim not to exceed a tumor temperature of 40° C.

Finally, if hyperthermia is used as a "cytotoxic measure" with the temperature increased to more than 41.5° C, a sudden collapse of the tumor microcirculation is likely to occur. Due to specific morphological features of this microvessel network, it seems possible that such a circulatory breakdown can selectively be stimulated and utilized to intensify the local hyperthermic treatment.

References

Badylak SF, Babbs CF, Skojac TM, Voorhees WD, Richardson RC (1985) Hyperthermia-induced vascular injury in normal and neoplastic tissue. Cancer 56: 991-1000

Berg-Blok AE, Reinhold HS (1984) Time-temperature relationship for hyperthermia induced stoppage of the microcirculation in tumors. Int J Radiat Oncol Biol Phys 10: 737-740

Crandall ED, Critz AM, Osher AS, Keljo DJ, Forster RE (1978) Influence of pH on elastic deformability of the human erythrocyte membrane. Am J Physiol 235: 269-278

Dewhirst M, Gross JF, Sim D, Arnold P, Boyer D (1984) The effect of rate of heating or cooling prior to heating on tumor and normal tissue microcirculatory flow. Biorheology 21: 539-558

Dickson JA, Calderwood SK (1980) Temperature range and selective sensitivity of tumors to hyperthermia: a critical review. Ann NY Acad Sci 335: 180-205

Dudar TE, Jain RK (1984) Differential response of normal and tumor microcirculation to hyperthermia. Cancer Res 44: 605-612

Eddy HA (1980) Alterations in tumor microvasculature during hyperthermia. Radiology 137: 515-521

Emami B, Song CW (1984) Physiological mechanisms in hyperthermia: a review. Int J Radiat Oncol Biol Phys 10: 289-295

Emami B, Nussbaum GH, TenHaken RK, Hughes WL (1980) Physiological effects of hyperthermia: response of capillary blood flow and structure to local tumor heating. Radiology 137: 805-809

Emami B, Nussbaum GH, Hahn N, Piro AJ, Dritschilo A, Quimby F (1981) Histopathological study on the effects of hyperthermia on microvasculature. Int J Radiat Oncol Biol Phys 7: 401-405

Endrich B, Hammersen F (1986) Morphologic and hemodynamic alterations in capillaries during hyperthermia. In: Anghileri LJ, Robert J (eds) Hyperthermia in cancer treatment, vol II. CRC, Boca Raton, Florida, pp 17-47

Endrich B, Reinhold HS, Gross JF, Intaglietta M (1979a) Tissue perfusion inhomogeneity during early tumor growth in rats. JNCI 62: 387-395

Endrich B, Zweifach BW, Reinhold HS, Intaglietta M (1979b) Quantitative studies of microcirculatory function in malignant tissue: influence of temperature on microvascular hemodynamics during the early growth of the BA 1112 rat sarcoma. Int J Radiat Oncol Biol Phys 5: 2021-2030

Endrich B, Asaishi K, Götz A, Meßmer K (1980) Technical report. A new chamber technique for microvascular studies in unanesthetized hamsters. Res Exp Med (Berl) 177: 125-134

Endrich B, Götz A, Meßmer K (1982a) Distribution of microflow and oxygen tension in hamster melanoma. Int J Microcirc Clin Exp 1: 81-99

Endrich B, Hammersen F, Götz A, Meßmer K (1982b) Microcirculatory blood flow, capillary morphology and local oxygen pressure of the hamster amelanotic melanoma A-Mel-3. JNCI 68: 475-485

Gullino PM, Jain RK, Grantham FH (1982) Relationship between temperature and blood supply or consumption of oxygen and glucose by rat mammary carcinomas. JNCI 60: 519-533

Hammersen F, Osterkamp-Baust U, Endrich B (1983) Ein Beitrag zum Feinbau terminaler Strombahnen und ihrer Entstehung in bösartigen Tumoren. Prog Appl Microcirc 2: 15-51

Hammersen F, Endrich B, Meßmer K (1985) The fine structure of tumor blood vessels. I. Participation of non-endothelial cells in tumor angiogenesis. Int J Microcirc Clin Exp 4: 31-43

Intaglietta M, Silverman NR, Tompkins WR (1975) Capillary flow velocity measurements in vivo and in situ by television method. Microvasc Res 10: 165-179

Johnson P (1980) The myogenic response. In: Bohr DF, Somlyo AP, Sparks HV (eds) Handbook of physiology, vol II/2. American Physiological Society, Bethesda, Maryland, pp 409-442

Karino M, Koga S, Maeta M, Hamazoe R, Kumane T, Oda M (1984) Experimental and clinical studies on effect of hyperthermia on tumor blood flow. In: Overgaard J (ed) Hyperthermic oncology, vol I. Taylor and Francis, London, pp 173-176

Lee SY, Song CW, Levitt SH (1985) Change in fibrinogen uptake in tumors by hyperthermia. Eur J Cancer Clin Oncol 21: 1507-1513

Müller-Klieser W, Vaupel P (1984) Effect of hyperthermia on tumor blood flow. Biorheology 21: 529-538

Oda T, Lehmann A, Endrich B (1984) Capillary blood flow in the amelanotic melanoma of the hamster after isovolemic hemodilution. Biorheology 21: 509-520

Overgaard J (1981) Effect of hyperthermia on the hypoxic fraction in an experimental mammary carcinoma in vivo. Br J Radiol 54: 245-249

Overgaard J, Bichel P (1977) The influence of hypoxia and acidity on the hyperthermic response of malignant cells in vitro. Radiology 123: 511-514

Overgaard J, Nielsen OS (1980) The role of tissue environmental factors on the kinetics and morphology of tumor cells exposed to hyperthermia. Ann NY Acad Sci 335: 254-278

Pence DW, Song CW (1986) Effects of heat on blood flow. In: Anghileri LJ, Robert J (eds) Hyperthermia in cancer treatment, vol II. CRC, Boca Raton, Florida, pp 1-16

Reinhold HS, Endrich B (1986) Tumor microcirculation as a target for hyperthermia. Int J Hyperthermia 2: 111-137

Reinhold HS, Blachiewicz B, Berg-Blok A (1978) Decrease in tumor microcirculation during hyperthermia. In: Streffer C (ed) Cancer therapy by hyperthermia and radiation. Urban and Schwarzenberg, Baltimore, pp 231-232

Rhee JG, Kim TH, Levitt SH, Song CW (1984) Changes in acidity of mouse tumor by hyperthermia. Int J Radiat Oncol Biol Phys 10: 393-399

Scheid P (1961) Funktionelle Besonderheiten der Mikrozirkulation im Karzinom. Bibl Anat 1: 327-335

Schmid-Schönbein H, Volger E, Weiss J, Brandhuber M (1975) Effect of O-β-(hydroxyethyl)-rutosides on the microrheology of human blood under defined flow conditions. Vasa 4: 263-270

Schmid-Schönbein H, Singh M, Malotta H, Leschke D, Teitel P, Driessen G, Scheidt-Bleichert H (1984) Subpopulations of rigid red cells in hyperthermia and acidosis: effect on filtrability in vitro and on nutritive capillary perfusion in the mesenteric microcirculation. Int J Microcirc Clin Exp 3: 497

Simpson JG, Fraser RA (1983) Angiogenese in malignen Tumoren. Prog Appl Microcirc 2: 1-14

Song CW, Kang MS, Rhee JG, Levitt SH (1980a) Effect of hyperthermia on vascular function in normal and neoplastic tissues. Ann NY Acad Sci 335: 35-47

Song CW, Kang MS, Rhee JG, Levitt SH (1980b) The effect of hyperthermia on vascular function, pH and cell survival. Radiology 137: 795-803

Storm FK, Harrison WH, Elliott RS, Morton RL (1979) Normal tissue and solid tumor effects of hyperthermia in animal models and clinical trials. Cancer Res 39: 2245-2251

Streffer C (1985) Metabolic changes during and after hyperthermia. Int J Hyperthermia 1: 305-319

Vaupel P (1982) Einfluß einer lokalisierten Mikrowellenhyperthermie auf die pH-Verteilung in bösartigen Tumoren. Strahlentherapie 158: 168-173

Vaupel P, Ostheimer K, Müller-Klieser W (1980) Circulatory and metabolic responses of malignant tumors during normothermia and hyperthermia. J Cancer Res Clin Oncol 98: 15-29

Vaupel P, Müller-Klieser W, Otte J, Manz R, Kallinowski F (1983) Blood flow, tissue oxygenation, and pH distribution in malignant tumors upon localized hyperthermia. Basic pathophysiological aspects and the role of various thermal doses. Strahlentherapie 159: 73-81

von Ardenne M (1981) Krebs-Mehrschritt-Therapie - Stand der Forschung. Deutsches Ärzteblatt 33: 1560-1568

von Ardenne M (1986) The present developmental state of cancer multistep therapy (CMT): selective occlusion of cancer tissue capillaries by combining hyperglycemia with two stage regional or local hyperthermia using the CMT Selectotherm technique. In: Anghileri LJ, Robert J (eds) Hyperthermia in cancer treatment, vol III. CRC, Boca Raton, Florida, pp 1-24

Warren BA (1979) Tumor angiogenesis. In: Petersen HI (ed) Tumor blood circulation. CRC, Boca Raton, Florida, pp 49-75

Wiederhelm CA, Woodbury JW, Kirk ES, Rushmer RF (1964) Pulsatile pressure in the microcirculation of the frog's mesentery. Am J Physiol 207: 173-176

Wike-Hooley JL, Zee J, Rhoon GC, Berg AP, Reinhold HS (1984) Human tumor pH changes following hyperthermia and radiation therapy. Eur J Cancer Clin Oncol 20: 619-623

Zweifach BW (1974) Quantitative analysis of microcirculatory structure and function. I. Analysis of pressure distribution in the terminal vascular bed in cat mesentery. Circ Res 34: 843-857

Importance of the Glutathione Level and the Activity of the Pentose Phosphate Pathway in Cellular Heat Sensitivity

A. W. T. Konings

Department of Radiopathology, State University of Groningen, Bloemsingel 1, 9713 BZ Groningen, The Netherlands

Introduction

Since the initial observations by Mitchell et al. (1983) and Konings and Penninga (1983), several publications have tried to link the level of cellular reduced glutathione (GSH) to heat sensitivity and to the capacity of the cell to develop thermotolerance. The current article critically reviews the reports on this topic, in order to reach a conclusion with respect to the general importance of GSH. Furthermore, the possible role of the pentose phosphate pathway (PPP) will be discussed. Before individual publications on hyperthermia are analyzed, some general information is given on established relations of GSH and PPP with the metabolic state of the cell in normal situations and under conditions of oxidative stress.

As discussed in the chapter on "Membranes as Targets for Hyperthermic Cell Killing", at the moment the most probable primary molecular targets seem to be the proteins in the plasma membrane of the cell. Because of damage to these molecules, intermediary metabolism can be affected such that cells will die as a result of alterations in critical structures or metabolic activities distinct from the plasma membrane, e.g., on the level of chromatin.

A three-stage sequence of events may be formulated as follows: primary damage →intermediary metabolism →critical structures; for example: plasma membrane, Ca^{2+} homeostasis, chromatin. Modulation of heat sensitivity (e.g., by endogenous glutathione) may take place at all three stages.

The application of heat may possibly be considered as one of the many ways known to impose oxidative stress on cells and tissues, such as processes associated with inflammatory responses, ischemia, and injuries resulting from intracellular metabolism of chemicals and drugs. Oxidative stress may be denoted as a disturbance in the pro-oxidant/antioxidant systems in favor of the former. Elevation of temperature increases many metabolic reactions, including those connected with the formation of active species of oxygen, essential for oxygen-dependent organisms to survive at physiological temperatures. Because of this rise in temperature cellular defense mechanisms may become overwhelmed and redox systems are shifted to the more oxidized state. If this happens during and after hyperthermia, sensitization for heat damage may be expected by compounds that either produce

Recent Results in Cancer Research, Vol. 109

toxic oxygen-related species or (partially) eliminate the defense system. There are several indications in the literature that damage by reactive oxygen species (O_2^-, $HO\cdot_2$,H_2O_2, $HO\cdot$, $RO\cdot$, $ROO\cdot$) resembles and potentiates heat damage.

Kapp and Hahn (1979) observed thermosensitization by the sulfhydryl compounds 2-aminoethylisothioureum (AET) and β-mercaptoethylamine (cysteamine), agents able to generate free radicals leading to reactive oxygen species under aerobic conditions. Issels et al. (1984) showed that the described heat sensitization could be prevented by the addition of catalase, suggesting the involvement of hydrogen peroxide. The latter compound sensitizes cells for hyperthermia (Freeman et al. 1985b) and induces heat resistance in bacteria (Morgan et al. 1986). One of the enzymes participating in the defense system, superoxide dismutase (SOD), has been found to be increased after a hyperthermic treatment (Loven et al. 1985).

Relation of Oxidative Stress to Cellular GSH Content and PPP Activity

The counteraction of hazardous reactions initiated by reactive oxygen species may take place at the level of prevention, interception, or repair. It comprises nonenzymatic scavengers and quenchers denoted by the term antioxidants, as well as enzymatic systems. Vitamin E (α-tocopherol), vitamin C (ascorbate), and GSH are well known naturally occurring antioxidants. SOD, GSH peroxidases, and catalase are important enzymes active in the cell against free radical damage. A number of additional, or ancillary systems are also very important, especially the regeneration of GSH as catalyzed by GSSG (glutathione disulfide) reductase and the system to provide the reducing equivalents in the form of NADPH to this system. The PPP has an active role in supplying NADPH. This coenzyme is also necessary to form endogenous polyols from aldo-sugars. According to a publication by Henle et al. (1982) these polyols might be crucial in heat sensitivity and thermotolerance. So, as indicated in Fig. 1, the PPP plays a central role in the regeneration of GSH from GSSG as well as by the formation of polyols. Glucose (an aldo-sugar) may be converted into fructose (a keto-sugar) by aldose reductase and sorbitol dehydrogenase. This is a pathway that bypasses the control points of hexokinase and phos-

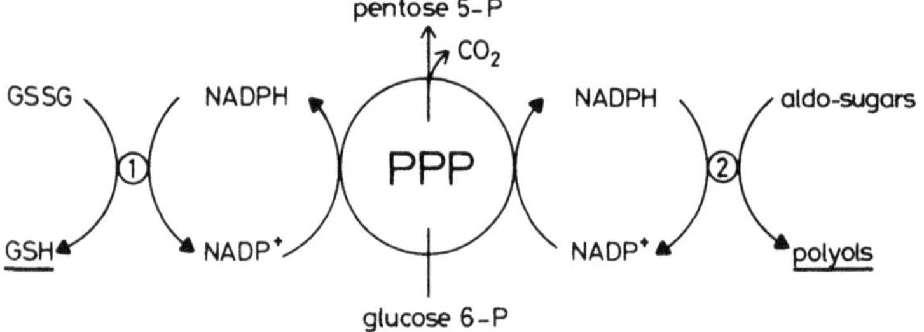

Fig. 1. Schematic presentation of the central role of pentose phosphate pathway *(PPP)* and NADAPH in the generation of reduced glutathione *(GSH)* from oxidized glutathione *(GSSG)* and of polyols from aldo-sugars. Reaction *(1)* is catalyzed by glutathione reductase, reaction *(2)* by aldose reductase. (Konings and Penninga 1985)

phofructokinase in glucose metabolism and involves oxidation of NADPH for the generation of polyols from aldo-sugars by aldose reductase [reaction (2) in Fig. 1]. Regeneration of reduced glutathione from oxidized glutathione is catalyzed by glutathione reductase [reaction (1) in Fig. 1] and is also dependent on the supply of NADPH. This cofactor is primarily produced by the PPP wherein glucose-6-phosphate is metabolized to pentose 5-phosphate and CO_2 by glucose-6-phosphate dehydrogenase and 6-phosphogluconate dehydrogenase concomitant with the production of the two molecules of NADPH. The glucose-fructose bypass is also called the sorbitol pathway or the polyol pathway and because of the usage and production of NADPH, this pathway and the PPP are mutually facilitative.

Hyperthermia may change the conformation of membrane-bound proteins and as such disturb membrane-related functions in the cell. Many enzymes (e.g., plasma membrane bound Ca^{2+} ATPase) contain sulfhydryl groups. A number of these enzymes are known to be modified with respect to their activity, by the formation of mixed disulfides with glutathione (N. Kosower and E. Kosower 1978):

$$\mathrm{GSH} + \mathrm{R}\begin{array}{l}\diagup \mathrm{S} \\ | \\ \diagdown \mathrm{S}\end{array} \rightleftharpoons \mathrm{R}\begin{array}{l}\diagup \mathrm{SSG} \\ \\ \diagdown \mathrm{SH}\end{array}$$

$$\mathrm{GSH} + \mathrm{R}\begin{array}{l}\diagup \mathrm{SSG} \\ \\ \diagdown \mathrm{S}\end{array} \rightleftharpoons \mathrm{GSSG} + \mathrm{R}\begin{array}{l}\diagup \mathrm{SH} \\ \\ \diagdown \mathrm{SH}\end{array}$$

The formation of mixed disulfides between glutathione and protein sulfhydryl groups might protect these groups from irreversible oxidation. In thise sense glutathione belongs to the group of preventive antioxidants. The cytoplasmic GSH content of various organs and tissues represents at least 80% of total nonprotein low-molecular-weight thiols present. Thiol-disulfide exchange is involved in the process of protein folding and as such in enzymatic regulation. Under conditions of oxidative stress, where the oxidized forms of thiols are increased with a concomitant decrease in the reduced forms, the mixed disulfide content should increase. Disulfide reduction or thiol oxidation may be one of the first steps in protein degradation. In this way GSH seems to function as a link between reduced and oxidized forms of protein thiols. Before a protein disulfide bond is closed or split, one of the corresponding SH groups is masked by mixed disulfide formation with glutathione.

As yet, no reports are known in the available literature concerning cellular content of mixed disulfides after a hyperthermic treatment. The assay of mixed disulfides is, however, not easy and moreover these compounds undergo fluctuations, especially with the nutritional status and other growth conditions of the cells. What has been measured by several groups of investigators is the level of GSH during and after hyperthermia.

Cellular GSH Level and Heat Sensitivity

Intrinsic Heat Sensitivity and Constitutive Levels of GSH

Depending on the cell type, the intracellular concentration of glutathione is maintained in the range of 0.5–10 mM (N. Kosower and E. Kosower 1978). Human fibroblasts contain 3–4 mM GSH; this is 30–40 nmol GSH per milligram cell protein. The turnover of this GSH is rapid, with a half-life of 1–1.5 h (Bannai 1983). Nearly all the glutathione is present in the reduced form (GSH) with less than 5% as GSSG. This ratio of reduced and oxidized glutathione is due to the thiol redox status maintained by intracellular glutathione reductase and NADPH. Continual endogenous production of reduced oxygen species, including hydrogen peroxides and lipid peroxides, creates a constant production of GSSG by the glutathione redox cycle. Intrinsic heat sensitivities of different cell lines appear not to correlate with constitutive levels of GSH. In this respect it has been shown that, for example, the surviving fraction for mouse fibroblasts after 40 min at 44° C was 0.090 and for Ehrlich ascites tumor (EAT) cells 0.003 (Konings and Ruifrok 1985), while the GSH concentrations in both cell lines were about the same (28 nmol/mg protein). Lilly et al. (1986) showed that a glutathione synthetase-deficient [GSH(−)] human fibroblast line containing only about 6% of the GSH content found in normal human fibroblasts was as heat sensitive as its normal counterpart. Shrieve et al. (1986) determined the GSH content of HA-1 Chinese hamster fibroblasts and of two heat-resistant mutants. It turned out that the cell line with the highest level of GSH was the most heat sensitive.

Cellular Level of GSH During and After Hyperthermia

The first reports concerning GSH concentration in cells during and after hyperthermia pointed to elevated levels (Mitchell et al. 1983; Konings and Penninga 1983). Although the increase in GSH in the experiments of Mitchell et al. (1983) using V79 cells was quite extensive (40%–80%), Konings and Penninga (1985) reported a smaller increase (0%–50%) in EAT cells and mouse fibroblasts. An example of heat-induced increase of GSH content is depicted in Fig. 2. After heating human fibroblasts, Lilly et al. (1986) found an increase in the GSH level from about 2.5 μg to about 7.5 μg/mg cellular protein. No increase in GSH was observed by Freeman et al. (1985 a) after heating CHO cells at 42° C. Shrieve et al. (1986) even reported a decrease in the GSH level after heating HA-1 cells at 43.5° C or at 45° C. This is illustrated in Fig. 3. Shrieve et al. (1986) are not the only ones to have observed a decrease in GSH after hyperthermia. Anderstam and Harms-Ringdahl (1986) used an in vivo system of mice bearing a mammary carcinoma. The GSH level (in the tumor cells) fell to about 30% of control levels when a subtoxic hyperthermia dose of 40 min at 43° C was applied. So, no consistent picture arises with respect to the effect of hyperthermia on cellular GSH content. The same conclusion may be drawn concerning the GSH level of thermotolerant cells. While Mitchell et al. (1983) reported an elevated level of GSH in thermotolerant cells, the work of Konings and Penninga (1984, 1985) showed that ther-

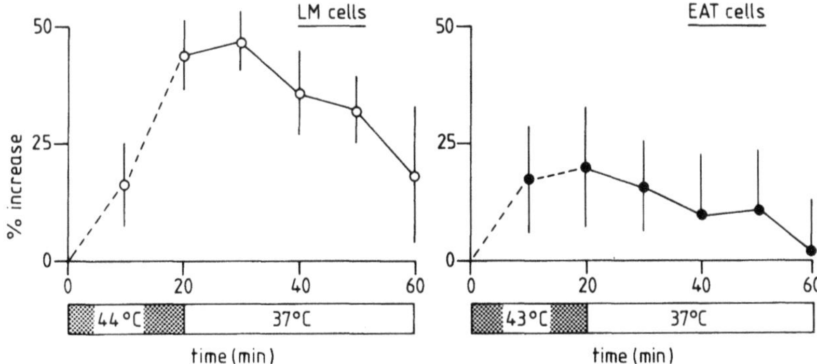

Fig. 2. Effect of hyperthermia of mouse fibroblast LM cells and EAT cells on the level of reduced glutathione (GSH). The cells were heated for 20 min at 44° or 43° C and incubated at 37° C for up to 60 min. Data are given as percentage above control value (GSH level of nonheated cells). Control concentrations were 29 ± 3 nmol/mg protein and 27 ± 3 nmol/mg protein for LM cells and EAT cells respectively. Mean ± standard deviation of three independent experiments. (Konings and Penninga 1985)

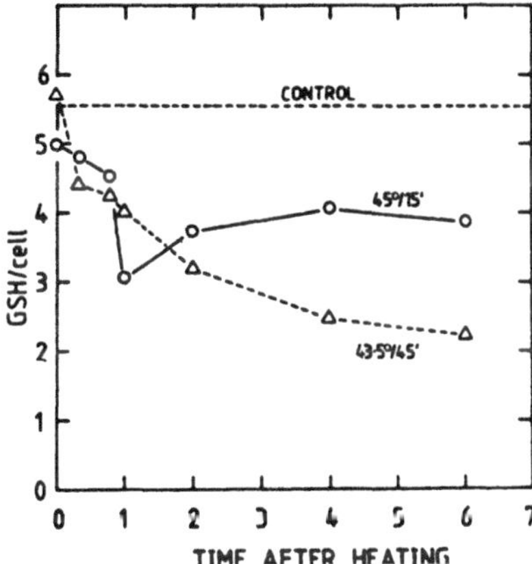

Fig. 3. GSH levels for HA-1 cells following heating. ○, 45° C/15 min.; △, 43.5° C/45 min. Results are from a single experiment. (Shrieve et al. 1986)

motolerant mouse fibroblasts and EAT cells contained less GSH. An observation similar to the last one was also reported by Shrieve et al. (1986) with HA-1 cells.

Effect of GSH Depletion on Thermosensitivity and Thermotolerance

The level of GSH in the cells may be lowered by different means. The two most popular ways to deplete GSH are treatment with diethylmaleate (DEM) and with DL-buthionine-*S*, *R*-sulfoximine (BSO). DEM is an agent that conjugates the thiol group of GSH by the action of glutathione transferase (Boyland and Chasseaud 1970). BSO is an inhibitor of γ-glutamylcysteine synthetase (Griffith and Meister 1979), an enzyme essential for the biosynthesis of glutathione. Depletion of GSH by DEM is rather rapid (<1 h), while it takes 6-10 h before low levels of GSH are reached when BSO is used. Although BSO is the preferred compound to use because of its higher specificity, not all cell lines may sufficiently be depleted by nontoxic doses of this inhibitor. The latter is the case for mouse fibroblast LM cells as reported by Konings and Penninga (1983, 1984, 1985). As shown in one of their papers (Konings and Penninga 1985), the highest nontoxic dose of DEM for mouse fibroblasts was 250 μM while GSH depletion (>95%) was already complete at 75 μM. When BSO was used the highest nontoxic dose was as low as 5 μM while at least 100 μM BSO was necessary for GSH depletion. The opposite situation was found for EAT cells; no nontoxic doses of DEM could be found for full (>95%) depletion of GSH. In the reported experiments DEM treatments were for 6 h and BSO treatments for 29 h.

Mitchell and Russo (1983) and Mitchell et al. (1983) as well as Konings and Penninga (1983, 1984, 1985) used DEM and BSO for GSH depletion. With both agents Mitchell and co-workers observed thermosensitization. Examples of the BSO treatments mentioned are given in Fig. 4. Note that survival after a hyperthermic treatment at 45.5° C (Fig. 4b) is only minimally influenced by BSO. At 42.5° C (Fig. 4a) BSO clearly sensitizes the cells for heat killing. After 6 h exposure of the

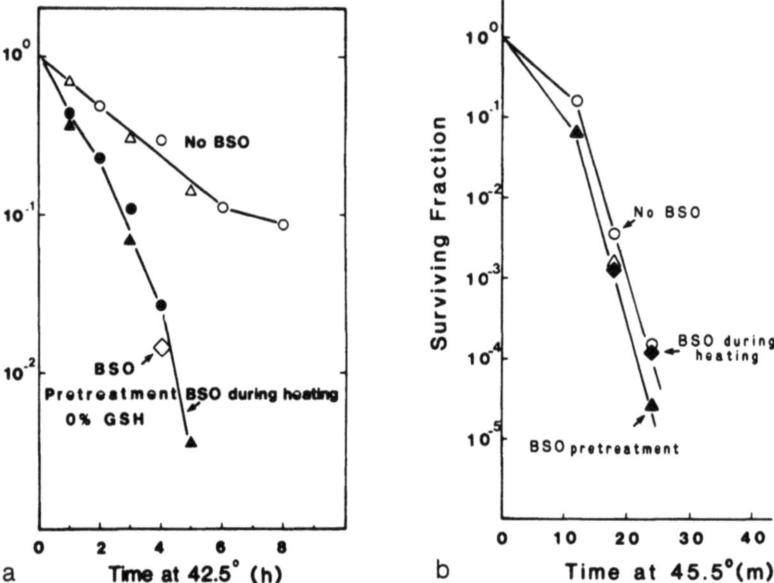

Fig. 4a, b. Survival of BSO-treated V79 cells as a function of time at **a** 42.5° C and **b** 45.5° C. Figure 4a represents an experiment where cells were exposured to 10 mM BSO only during heating periods, then washed free of drug and assayed for survival (●, ▲). Cells were pretreated for 4 h with 10 mM BSO, rinsed, and then heated (◇); GSH concentration following the pretreatment was <5%. Control non-drug-treated heat response (○, △). Figure 4b represents an experiment in which the cells were treated without drug (o), 10 mM BSO present during the heating periods (◆), or pretreated with 10 mM BSO for 4 h (GSH= <5% of controls), rinsed, and then heated at 45.5° C (▲). (Mitchell and Russo 1983)

control cells thermotolerance seems to have developed. No sign of thermotolerance is observed in the curve representing the combined treatment of BSO and hyperthermia, although no data after the 5-h point are supplied. When Russo et al. (1984) induced thermotolerance by a 12-min exposure at 45.5° C followed by a 10-h incubation at 37° C, less surviving cells were found in the thermotolerant BSO pretreated cells as compared to the normal thermotolerant cells. The same was found when a 43° C pretreatment was given. Complete inhibition was, however, never reported. There may be a problem with the interpretation of these data. Connected with the data discussed, no information is given on the direct effect of BSO on thermosensitivity. The BSO thermotolerance data are compared with the non-BSO control data! So it is possible that even more thermotolerance has been developed in the BSO treated cells if correction for direct BSO effects is included. It is not clear from the experiments of Mitchell and co-workers how the GSH level was influenced before and during the heat treatments and whether non-GSH thiols (especially protein-SH) were affected by the drug treatments.

This kind of data has been provided by Konings and Penninga (1985) and is shown in Table 1. In this table the effect of three different concentrations of DEM and BSO on the level of GSH and the non-GSH thiols is presented. The latter group is to be considered as protein thiols. When 50 μM DEM is used for 1 h, GSH depletion is complete (column a) and non-GSH thiols are hardly affected. After 6 h the GSH content of the cells starts to recover. This is not the case for 100 and 200 μM DEM. After 6 h the GSH content is still low and the level of non-GSH thiols has further decreased. For the BSO treatment the situation is equivalent for all three treatments. A tendency to a lower level of non-GSH thiols might be present. Figure 5 shows a time-course study of the treatment with 50 and 100 μM DEM. The treatment with 50 μM DEM is insufficient to keep a low GSH level for 6 h or more. After heating, the recovery of GSH in control cells was faster than the recovery in thermotolerant cells. Heating of the GSH-depleted cells at 44° C for different periods of time revealed that no enhanced thermosensitivity was observed with 50 and 100 μM DEM (Fig. 6a). When the cells received a heat

Table 1. Cellular levels of glutathione *(GSH)* and non-GSH thiols after treatment with different concentrations of DEM or BSO. (Konings and Penninga 1985)

Cell line	Depleting agent	GSH		Non-GSH thiols	
		a	b	a	b
LM cells	DEM 50μm	6±4	21+6	89± 9	98± 9
	DEM 100 μm	5±4	4±5	84± 6	75± 7
	DEM 200 μm	4±3	4±5	76+ 8	70± 8
EAT cells	BSO 0-5 mM	6±3	5±3	89±18	84±15
	BSO 1-0 mM	5±4	6±4	78±18	81±16
	BSO 10-0 mM	5±6	6±7	84±17	82±15

Data are given as percentage of the concentration of GSH and non-GSH thiols of untreated cells. Mean ± standard deviation of at least four independent experiments. *a*, 1 h after DEM treatment or 24 h after BSO treatment; *b*, 6 h after DEM treatment or 29 h after BSO treatment.

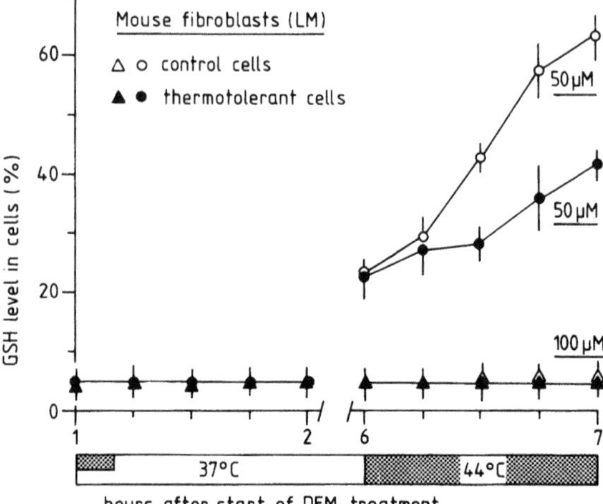

Fig. 5. The effect of a treatment with diethylmaleate *(DEM)* on the level of GSH in mouse fibroblasts at different times after the start of the treatment. The triggering of thermotolerant development was at 1 h after the start of the DEM treatment. At this time point GSH depletion was maximal for both doses of DEM. The plating efficiency (measure of toxicity) was not influenced by these treatments. This is a typical experiment. All *data points* are in triplicate and represent the mean ± SD. (Konings and Penninga 1985)

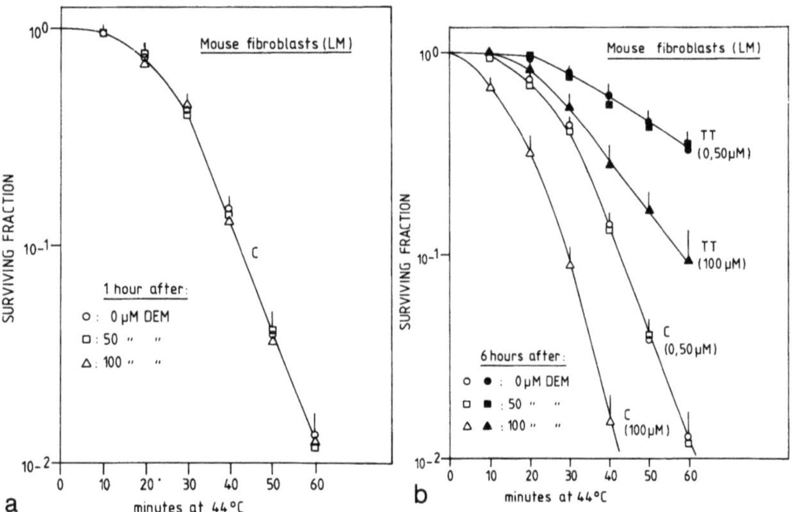

Fig. 6 a, b. The effect of GSH depletion by DEM on survival of mouse fibroblasts at different times after the start of the treatment. In **a**, survival after hyperthermia is indicated 1 h after the start of DEM treatment. In **b**, survival of control *(C)* and thermotolerant *(TT)* cells is given 6 h after the start of the DEM treatment. The level of GSH at these time points is indicated in Table 1 and Fig. 5. Data are given as the mean ± SD of at least five independent experiments. (Konings and Penninga 1985)

dose of 10 min at 44° C to trigger thermotolerance, 1 h after the start of the 50 μM DEM treatment (GSH < 5%), thermotolerance was developed in the normal way (Fig. 6b). For 100 μM DEM the situation was somewhat different. At 6 h after the start of the DEM treatment thermosensitivity was enhanced. Thermotolerance was expressed normally. The thermoresistance acquired for the control and 50 μM DEM-treated cells is comparable to the acquired resistance of the 100 μM DEM-treated cells. The higher thermosensitivity for both the normal and the thermotolerant 100 μM DEM-treated cells corresponds with the lower level of non-GSH thiols, probably being protein-SH (Table 1). It is concluded that the increased cellular sensitivity to heat after 6 h of 100 μM DEM is not related to the level of GSH and has probably to be explained as a secondary effect of the DEM treatment. So here we see that DEM can sensitize the cells for a heat treatment, just as observed by Mitchell and Russo (1983), but that this is not related to the GSH level, which was already maximally decreased. Again, as can be seen in Table 1, the DEM treatment has seriously affected the non-GSH thiols (75% of control), which probably is protein-SH. If the DEM-treated thermotolerant cells were compared with the untreated control cells, as was done by Russo et al. (1984), it looks as if thermotolerance is inhibited. However, such an evaluation is not fair, because then the toxic effect of DEM is only accounted for in the thermotolerant cells. Maximal GSH depletion with BSO in EAT cells requires an incubation time of 8–12 h with a dose of 0.5 mM. When reached, the low concentration of GSH is maintained for at least 30 h. As a routine a 24 h depletion time was allowed in these experiments before heating was started. As indicated in Table 1, 24 and 29 h after the start of the BSO treatment the levels of GSH were still below detection (< 5%). In Fig. 7 it can be seen that GSH depletion did not significantly affect thermosensitivity of the EAT cells. The BSO treatments used were all nontoxic for the cells. Thermotolerance development of BSO-treated cells was equal to the development in nontreated cells. At the higher doses of BSO there is a tendency to increased thermosensitivity at the highest heat dose (60 min at 43° C). In accordance with the

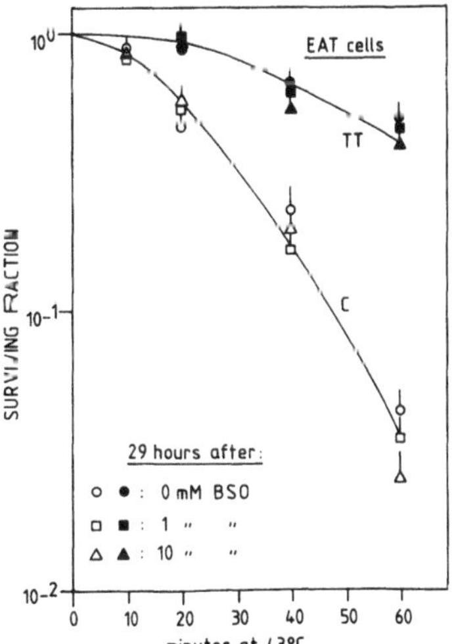

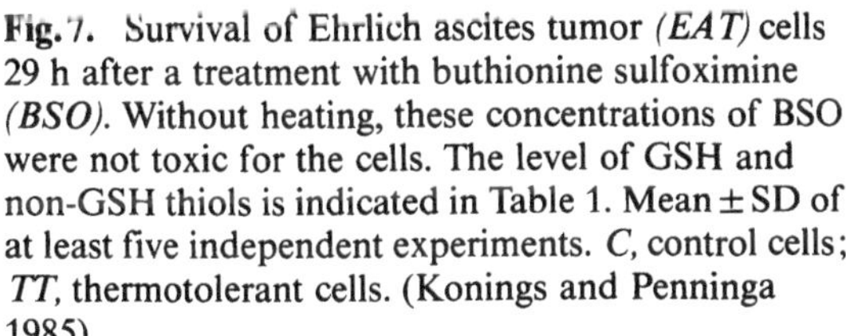

Fig. 7. Survival of Ehrlich ascites tumor *(EAT)* cells 29 h after a treatment with buthionine sulfoximine *(BSO)*. Without heating, these concentrations of BSO were not toxic for the cells. The level of GSH and non-GSH thiols is indicated in Table 1. Mean ± SD of at least five independent experiments. *C*, control cells; *TT*, thermotolerant cells. (Konings and Penninga 1985)

results of the experiments with the mouse fibroblasts, it is concluded that also for EAT cells, GSH depletion per se has no influence on thermosensitivity and on the capacity to develop thermotolerance.

Also in *E. coli* K1060 cells it was found (Konings et al. 1984) that a DEM treatment of cells could only sensitize for hyperthermia when toxic doses (20 mM) of DEM were used. Plating efficiency dropped from 80% to 20% and protein-SH was seriously affected (55% left) in these cases. Nontoxic doses of DEM could even protect the cells against heat damage. This is illustrated in Fig. 8. Oleic acid (18:1) substituted cells are less heat sensitive than linolenic acid (18:3) substituted cells, probably because of the higher membrane fluidity, as discussed earlier (Konings et al. 1984, Konings 1985, Konings and Ruifrok 1985). Treatment of the bacteria with 10 mM DEM lowered the GSH level to about 25% of control. One would expect that if oxidative stress is a major factor in heat killing of the bacteria that DEM treatment would especially sensitize the 18:3 substituted cells because these phospholipids are more vulnerable to lipid peroxidation (Konings et al. 1979).

DEM has also been used by Freeman et al. (1985b). In these experiments thermosensitization was observed after heating at 43° C but not at 45° C. BSO pretreated cells were found to be sensitized at 42° C. Freeman et al. (1985b) also reported that thermotolerance acquisition was reduced by DEM when the triggering dose was at 45° C but not at 43° C.

When HA-1 Chinese hamster fibroblasts and two heat-resistant mutants were pretreated with BSO (Shrieve et al. 1986), resulting in less than 10% GSH in the

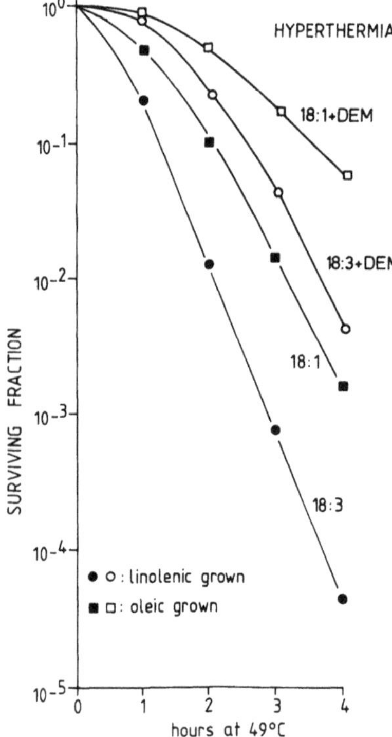

Fig. 8. Thermosensitivity of oleic acid (18:1) and linolenic acid (18:3) grown *E. coli* K1060 cells. Effect of a pretreatment with 10 mM diethylmaleate *(DEM)*. This is a nontoxic dose eliminating about 75% of nonprotein SH (GSH). (Konings et al. 1984)

control cells, and heated at 43.5° C, all three cell lines were sensitized to hyperthermic killing. This can be seen in Fig. 9a. It is interesting to note that especially the surplus resistance in the mutants is eliminated and almost none of the heat resistance in the parent line. As was mentioned earlier in this chapter, the intrinsic heat sensitivities did not correlate with constitutive GSH levels in these cells. So it must seriously be questioned whether the loss of the extra resistance in the mutants has anything to do with the GSH level. Figure 9b demonstrates that a mutant with a very low GSH content (about 6% of normal) has the same heat sensitivity as the parent line. Shrieve et al. (1986) could still observe full thermotolerance development after inhibition of GSH synthesis. When GSH levels were maintained at extremely low levels, however, the development of thermotolerance seemed partially inhibited. The latter effect, again, may possibly be accounted for by secondary effects of the BSO treatment. Figure 10 illustrates these experiments where the BSO effect on thermotolerance development was investigated. As can be seen in Fig. 10a, normal thermotolerance development covers about 3 logs (from 10^{-4} to 10^{-1}) and the BSO pretreated cells cover only about 2 logs during thermotolerance development.

Anderstam and Harms-Ringdahl (1986) concluded from their in vivo experiments that thermotolerance induction does not depend on, or cause, changes in intracellular GSH levels.

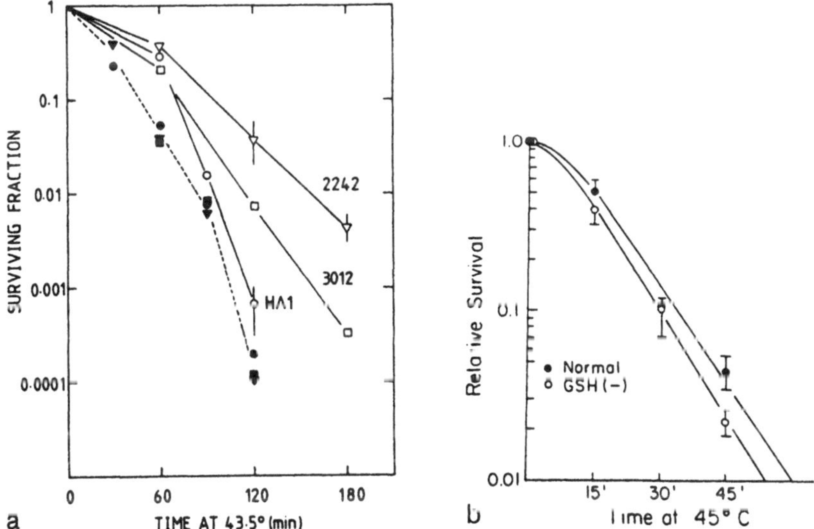

Fig. 9a, b. Heat sensitivity of HA-1 cells and two heat-resistant mutants (**a**) and of normal and GSH-deficient human fibroblasts (**b**). **a** Survival curves for HA-1 (○), 3012 (□), and 2242 (▽) following heating at 43.5° C. Survival curves for HA-1 (●), 3012 (■), and 2242 (▼) cells following exposure to 50 μM BSO for 12-14 h prior to heating at 43.5° C. *Points,* mean of two separate experiments for 2224 and HA-1 cells and the results of a single experiment for 3012 cells; *bars,* SD. Error bars omitted for BSO-treated points (Shrieve et al. 1986). **b** Heat sensitivity of normal and GSH(-) human fibroblasts. Each *point* is the mean ± SE of triplicate experiments. There is no significant difference in survival between GSH(-) and normal fibroblasts. (Lilly et al. 1986)

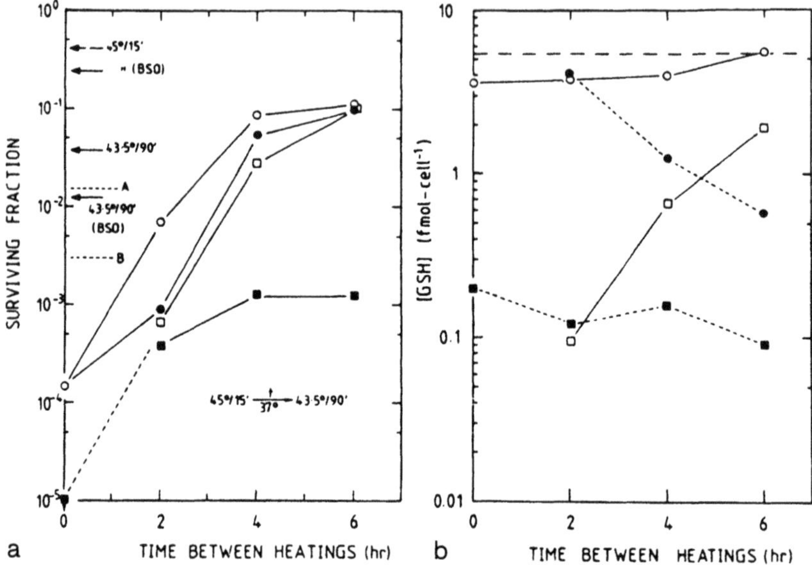

Fig. 10. **a** Survival of HA-1 cells following split-dose heating. A first dose of 45° C/15 min was followed by an interval (0–6 h) at 37° C and a second heating at 43.5° C/90 min. *Symbols:* ○, no BSO treatment; ●, 50 μM BSO present only during interval between heatings; □, 50 μM BSO present only for 12 h before first heating; ■, 50 μM BSO present for 12 h before first heating and during interval between heatings. *Arrows* indicate surviving fractions following single heat treatments. *A*, surviving fraction expected by multiplying that found following 45° C/15 min by that following 43.5° C/90 min.; *B*, same as *A* for BSO-pretreated cells. **b** Glutathione levels for cells treated as in **a**. GSH was measured before the second heating (i.e., all cells were heated at 45° C/15 min) at time 0. *Symbols:* same as in **a**. *Dashed line*, control level of GSH for HA-1 cells. The paired results from one of two replicate experiments are shown. (Shrieve et al. 1986)

The results of experiments with mammalian cells, as discussed in this section, are summarized in Table 2.

It must be concluded that the GSH level in eukaryotic cells may not be taken as a general determinant of heat sensitivity and the acquisition of thermotolerance.

Pentose Phosphate Pathway and Heat Sensitivity

No data are as yet available in the literature relating pentose phosphate pathway (PPP) activity with heat sensitivity and development of thermotolerance, except those of Konings and Penninga (1985). These will be discussed in this section. In order to measure the importance of PPP as compared with the citric acid cycle, the production of $^{14}CO_2$ from [1-^{14}C]glucose and [6-^{14}C]glucose was assayed. For both cell lines used (mouse fibroblasts and EAT cells) the yield of $^{14}CO_2$ from C6-labeled glucose was rather low in comparison with $^{14}CO_2$ from C1-labeled glucose, indicating a relative active PPP. Heating of mouse fibroblasts and EAT cells resulted in an increase of $^{14}CO_2$ production during the initial period of heating, fol-

Table 2. Relation of GSH levels with heat sentitivity and the development of thermotolerance

Authors	Cell lines	HT: °C	GSH level	GSH depletion			
				Agent	% GSH left	Heat sens.	TT dev.
Mitchell	V79	42.5	↑↑↑	DEM	< 5	+++	–
(1983-1985)	V79	42.5	↑↑↑	BSO	< 5	+++	–
	V79	45.5	↑↑↑↑	BSO	< 5	+	–
Konings	EAT	43.0	↑	BSO	< 5	0	0
(1983-1985)	Fibrobl.	44.0	↑↑	DEM	< 5	0	0
Freeman	CHO	42.0	0	BSO	33	++	ND
(1985)	CHO	43.0	↑	DEM	< 5	++	0
	CHO	45.0	*ND*	DEM	< 5	0	–
Shrieve	HA-1	43.5	↓	BSO	< 10	(0,++)	(0,–)
(1986)	Mutants						
Lilly	Fibrobl.-N	45.0	↑↑↑↑↑	*ND*	*ND*	*ND*	*ND*
(1986)	Fibrobl-GSH(–)	45.0	0	(Mutant)	6	0	0
Anderstam	Mamm. Ca.	43.0	↓↓	BSO	14	(0,+)	0(–)
(1986)	in vivo						

0, no effect; +, heat sensitization; –, inhibition of thermotolerance *(TT)* development; ↑, increased GSH level; ↓, decreased GSH level; *ND*, not determined

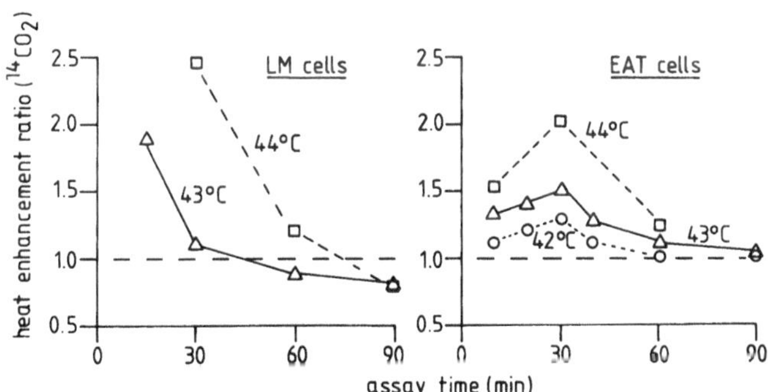

Fig. 11. Effect of hyperthermia on the production of $^{14}CO_2$ from [1-^{14}C]glucose in mouse fibroblast *(LM)* cells and in Ehrlich ascites tumor *(EAT)* cells. Data are expressed as the ratio between $^{14}CO_2$ evolving from heat treated and non-heat-treated cells. *Data points* are means of triplicate determinations of a typical experiment. The SD for each point was less than 20%. (Konings and Penninga 1985)

lowed by a decrease (Fig. 11). Hyperthermia for 30 min at 44° C caused an activation of glucose oxidation by a factor of 2.

When the $^{14}CO_2$ production was followed during the 37° C induction period of thermotolerance, an enhanced glucose oxidation was observed up to about 3-4 h after a triggering heat dose of 10 min at 44° C. A diminished PPP activity was present at later periods, starting about 4-5 h after the heat dose. In order to verify further the decrease in PPP activity of thermotolerant cells, $^{14}CO_2$ production was measured in control and thermotolerant cells 2 h after the addition of radioactive glucose and 7 h after the triggering heat dose applied to achieve the state of thermotolerance. The measurements were conducted over a period of 1 h every 20 min. Here also, thermotolerant fibroblasts had a lower PPP activity. Although the same tendency was observed for EAT cells the effect was much smaller. For both cell lines it must be concluded that the initially observed increase in $^{14}CO_2$ production is converted to a decrease when measured 7 h after the heat treatment. When thermotolerant mouse fibroblasts were heated for 30 min at 44° C, PPP activity increased again but the $^{14}CO_2$ production remained lower compared to heated control cells.

PPP activity of GSH-depleted cells was also examined. The development of thermotolerance was not inhibited under these circumstances, as was shown in Fig. 6 and 7, and therefore the study of the importance of an active PPP was of considerable interest. The DEM treatment of LM cells resulted in a severely decreased PPP activity while BSO treatment of EAT cells caused a slight increase (Fig. 12). Because both GSH-depleting actions did not disturb thermotolerance development, it must be concluded that an active PPP is not required for thermotolerance induction. When the GSH-depleted cells (DEM or BSO) were heated for 30 min at 44° C, PPP activity could still be activated. The extent of the increased $^{14}CO_2$ production was comparable to that observed for control cells, again indicating that the extent of glucose oxidation (PPP activity) is not dependent on the level of GSH.

As discussed earlier, it was also because of the interesting hypothesis of Henle et al. (1982), an active polyol pathway being necessary for the development of thermotolerance, that the PPP activity under conditions of GSH depletion was investigated. As postulated by Henle et al. (1982) an inhibition in metabolic flux through the PPP was expected to prevent or inhibit thermotolerance development

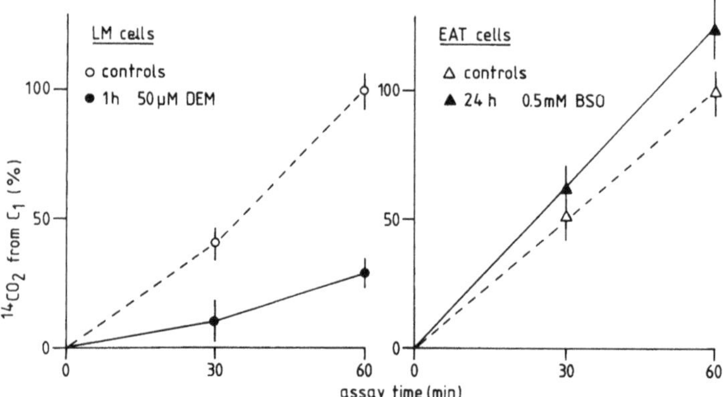

Fig. 12. Pentose phosphate pathway (PPP) activity in GSH-depleted cells. Depletion of mouse fibroblast *(LM)* cells was accomplished by a DEM pretreatment (50 μM) and of Ehrlich ascites tumor *(EAT)* cells by a pretreatment with BSO. DEM and BSO were also present during the PPP assay. GSH level was < 5%. $^{14}CO_2$ production from [1-^{14}C]glucose in the control cells after 1 h of incubation is taken as 100%. Data are given as the mean of three independent experiments. The *error bars* represent the standard deviation of the mean. (Konings and Penninga 1985)

because of a lack of NADPH necessary for polyol synthesis. However, the experiments reported in the current study clearly show that the magnitude of the glucose flux through the PPP is completely independent of the capacity to acquire thermoresistance. It is also shown that the PPP activity in thermotolerant cells is certainly not enhanced, which might be expected when the synthesis of endogenous polyols is important during the state of thermotolerance. Heating of thermotolerant cells does not give an extra burst of $^{14}CO_2$ development as compared with heating of control cells.

The initial burst in PPP activity might mean that the cellular redox potential is increased during the early moments of heat stress. This does not seem to be important for the triggering of thermotolerance, however, because DEM-treated cells have a low PPP activity and are equally able to become thermotolerant. In summary, the results of the investigations presented strongly indicate that neither a high level of GSH per se nor an active polyol pathway is a general prerequisite for the development of thermotolerance.

Oxidative Stress and Hyperthermia; Concluding Remarks

As mentioned earlier, GSH is involved in many metabolic activities of the cell, mostly concerned with redox reactions. The ratio of GSH/GSSG is coupled to the ratio of NADPH/NADP+ and just like the lactate/pyruvate and NADH/NAD+ ratios, they could be suitable indicators for oxygenation states in the cell (Streffer 1985). It must, however, be concluded from the discussions above, that either GSH is not a good monitor in these cases of oxidative stress or the latter phenomenon does not play a substantial role in heat killing.

The reported effects of hyperthermia on the level of cellular GSH are very diverse. This may have different causes. Cellular GSH content of cultured cells depends very much on the feeding conditions and the time elapsed since subculturing with fresh medium. The extracellular milieu may influence GSH synthesis and transport. Suspension cells may react differently to attached cells. Metabolic regulations involving GSH may be different in different cell lines. Furthermore, the severity of the heat treatment and the temperatures used seem to be important and different for different cell lines. An illustration of the latter remark is the following. For V79 cells it is found that the higher the temperature applied, the more did GSH accumulate in the cells (Mitchell and Russo 1983), while for EAT cells increasing temperatures did not result in a rise in GSH content (Konings and Penninga 1985). So cells that have lost their reproductive capacity do not always have higher levels of GSH. Whatever the reasons for the observed differences, it is obvious that the level of GSH is not a usable parameter to predict a hyperthermic response or to monitor the extent of heat damage to cells or tissues after the treatment.

The reported different effects of GSH-depleting agents on thermosensitivity and the development of thermotolerance are also very remarkable. From the discussion of the experiments analyzed in this article, it must be concluded that there is not a generally established relation between the level of GSH, heat sensitivity, and the capacity to develop thermotolerance. The actions of DEM and BSO as described in most of the work cited, have to be attributed to side-effects of the compounds used or to secondary effects of GSH depletion, e.g., redox reactions of other cellular compounds. On top of this, the reactions involved may depend on cell line, feeding conditions, and severity of the heat treatment. In this context Freeman et al. (1985b) reported that DEM treatments could only affect the development of thermotolerance in CHO cells when a relative high priming heat dose was given to the cells leading to about 50% dead cells!

The possible importance of the cellular GSH content in hyperthermia apparently fascinates many groups of investigators and this might be the reason why it is generally found difficult simply to conclude that there are no correlations, instead of using formulations like "cells severely depleted of GSH for a prolonged period are compromised in their ability to develop thermotolerance" (Shrieve et al. 1986) or only comment on those experiments where the compounds used have the desired effect (Freeman et al. 1985b).

Whether heat causes substantial oxidative stress in surviving cells is still an open question, which will probably be answered in the years to come. If so, it is not likely that GSH will be the candidate of choice to monitor these processes.

References

Anderstam B, Harms-Ringdahl M (1986) Relationship between cellular glutathione and hyperthermic toxicity in mammary carcinoma in mice. Int J Radiat Biol 50: 231-240

Bannai S (1983) Turnover of glutathione in human fibroblasts in culture. In: Sakamoto Y, Higashi T, Tateishi N (eds) Glutathione: storage, transport and turnover in mammals. Japan Sci Soc Press, Tokyo, VNO, Utrecht, pp 41-51

Boyland E, Chasseaud LF (1970) The effect of some carbonyl compounds on rat liver glutathione levels. Biochem Pharmacol 19: 1526-1528

Freeman ML, Malcolm AW, Meredith MJ (1985a) Decreased intracellular glutathione concentration and increased hyperthermic cytotoxicity in an acid environment. Cancer Res 45: 504-508

Freeman ML, Malcolm AW, Meredith MJ (1985b) Role of glutathione in cell survival after hyperthermic treatment of Chinese hamster ovary cells. Cancer Res 45: 6308-6313

Griffith OW, Meister A (1979) Potent and specific inhibition of glutathione synthesis by buthionine sulfoximine (*S-n*-butyl homocysteine sulfoximine). J Biol Chem 254: 7558-7560

Henle KJ, Nagle WA, Moss AJ, Herman TS (1982) Polyhydroxy compounds and thermotolerance: a proposed concatenation. Radiat Res 92: 445-451

Issels RD, Biaglow JE, Epstein L, Gerweck LE (1984) Enhancement of cysteamine cytotoxicity by hyperthermia and its modification by catalase and superoxide dismutase in Chinese hamster ovary cells. Cancer Res 44: 3911-3915

Kapp DS, Hahn GM (1979) Thermosensitization by sulfhydryl compounds of exponentially growing Chinese hamster cells. Cancer Res 39: 4630-4635

Konings AWT (1985) Development of thermotolerance in mouse fibroblast LM cells with modified membranes and after procaine treatment. Cancer Res 45: 2016-2019

Konings AWT, Penninga P (1983) Role of reduced glutathione in cellular heat sensitivity and thermotolerance. Strahlentherapie 159: 377-378

Konings AWT, Penninga P (1984) Role of reduced glutathione protein thiols and pentose phosphate pathway in heat sensitivity and thermotolerance. In: Overgaard J (ed) Hyperthermic oncology, vol 1. Taylor and Francis, London, pp 115-118

Konings AWT, Penninga P (1985) On the importance of the level of glutathione and the activity of the pentose phosphate pathway in heat sensitivity and thermotolerance. Int J Radiat Biol 48: 409-422

Konings AWT, Ruifrok ACC (1985) Role of membrane lipids and membrane fluidity in thermosensitivity and thermotolerance of mammalian cells. Radiat Res 102: 86-98

Konings AWT, Damen J, Trieling WB (1979) Protection of liposomal lipids against radiation induced oxidative damage. Int J Radiat Biol 35: 343-350

Konings AWT, Gipp JJ, Yatvin MB (1984) Radio- and thermosensitivity of *E. coli* K1060 after thiol depletion by diethylmaleate. Radiat Environ Biophys 23: 245-253

Kosower NS, Kosower EM (1983) Glutathione and cell membrane thiol status. In: Larson A et al. (eds) Functions of glutathione: biochemical, biophysical, toxicological, and clinical aspects. Raven, New York, pp 307-315

Lilly MB, Carroll AJ, Prchal J (1986) Lack of association between glutathione content and development of thermal tolerance in human fibroblasts. Radiat Res 106: 41-46

Loven DP, Leeper DB, Oberley LW (1985) Superoxide dismutase levels in Chinese hamster ovary cells and ovarian carcinoma cells after hyperthermia or exposure to cyclohexamide. Cancer Res 45: 3029-3033

Mitchell JB, Russo A (1983) Thiols, thiol depletion, and thermosensitivity. Radiat Res 95: 471-485

Mitchell JB, Russo A, Kinsella TJ, Glatstein E (1983) Glutathione elevation during thermotolerance induction and thermosensitization by glutathione depletion. Cancer Res 43: 987-991

Morgan RW, Christman MF, Jacobson FS, Storz G, Amer BN (1986) Hydrogen peroxide-inducible proteins in *Salmonella typhimurium* overlap with heat shock and other stress proteins. Proc Natl Acad Sci USA 83: 8059-8063

Russo A, Mitchell JB, McPherson S (1984) The effect of glutathione depletion on thermotolerance and heat stress protein synthesis. Br J Cancer 49: 753-758

Shrieve DC, Li GC, Astromoff A, Harris JW (1986) Cellular glutathione, thermal sensitivity, and thermotolerance in Chinese hamster fibroblasts and their heat-resistant variants. Cancer Res 46: 1684-1687

Streffer C (1985) Metabolic changes during and after hyperthermia. Int J Hyperthermia 1: 305-319

Potentiation of Hyperthermia by Lanthanum

L. Anghileri

Biophysics Laboratory, University of Nancy, 18 rue Lionnois, 54000 Nancy, France

Introduction

Lanthanum is a member of the series of rare earth metals that constitute a group of 15 transition elements (Group 3b) starting with lanthanum (atomic number 57) and ending with lutetium (atomic number 75). The ions of the lanthanide group have a high affinity for calcium-binding sites (Evans 1983). Some lanthanides' ions can replace calcium in a functional sense in biological systems. In interpreting the biological behavior of these cations, the concept of ionic exchange or replacement based on the ionic model of chemical bonding is of fundamental importance (Pauling 1960). According to this model, in an exchange reaction leading to a complex formation there are stability sequences that depend on the nature of the ligand as well as on the free energy order related to the radius ratio effect operating in that system. As a consequence, cations with similar atomic or ionic radii would be expected to bind to the same sites, but the binding would be expected to be stronger when the ion possesses a higher charge of valence. A typical example of this ionic exchange is the replacement of calcium by the lanthanides. In isomorphous replacement in minerals the radius is more important than the charge, but in biological systems a higher valence can play a more determinant role in this reaction in spite of the fact that the radius is an important factor. This seems to be the reason why lanthanides, having a radius size close to that of calcium but a higher valence, show excellent characteristics as competitors (probes) for calcium-binding sites (Lehninger 1970; Phillips and Williams 1966). On the other hand, in biological systems there is the possibility of steric fitting that can overcome differences in radius size (Fig. 1).

Biological Effects of Lanthanum

Effects at the Cellular Level

Lanthanum and other lanthanides at concentrations of 0.1-0.2 M inhibit active transport of calcium ion, mediated by respiratory linked substrates as well as by ATP hydrolysis, without affecting respiration and membrane-bound ATPase activ-

Recent Results in Cancer Research, Vol. 109

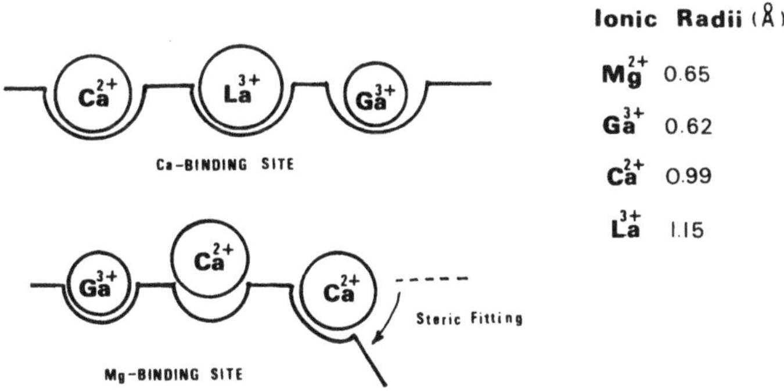

Fig. 1. Cation-binding site interactions

ity in bacteria (Agarwal and Kalra 1983). In tumor cells, lanthanum ion induces dramatic changes in cellular electrolyte content, and these changes are associated with a concomitant increase in membrane potential. The experimental evidence indicates that these effects of lanthanum ion may be the result of an interaction of lanthanum with the plasma membrane (Levinson et al. 1972).

Electron microscope studies on several tissues have demonstrated that lanthanum ion is bound to the external surface of cell membranes (Fahimi and Cotran 1971). Since these deposits appear restricted to the basement of the coat layer (Hoffstein et al. 1975), it seems likely that the lanthanum interaction region extends across the basement coat into the plasmalemma (Martinez-Palomo et al. 1973), where it interacts with the acidic groups of phospholipids (von Breeman and McNaughton 1970). However, the plasmalemma is enzymatically active (Nayler 1976) and among the enzymes present in the plasmalemma, sodium- and potassium-activated, magnesium-dependent ATPase is sensitive to various cations (Skou 1965), including calcium ion (Glick 1972). Lanthanum ion has shown a dose-dependent, competitive inhibitory effect on this enzyme, 100 times greater than that of an equimolar concentration of calcium ion (Nayler and Harris 1976). This phenomenon suggests that lanthanum ion acts in a different way to a calcium antagonist (Kass and Tsien 1975). A recent report (Luterbacher and Schatzmann 1983) has shown that lanthanum ion inhibits the calcium-ATPase pump of the red cell by arresting the protein in a phosphorylated form and thus blocking the transition from the first form of the protein to the second form, which performs ATP hydrolysis.

Systemic Effects

The pharmacological effects of lanthanum ion are determined by the route of administration, but in any case it acts as a direct calcifier (Calcergen) that does not precipitate calcium itself but provokes a calcification through the increase in calcium concentration at the site of injection when administered subcutaneously (Padmanabhan et al. 1963) or in a distant organ when administered systemically (parenterally). As a calcergen lanthanum ion draws calcium from the blood into the tissue. Parenterally administered lanthanum ion localizes mainly in liver (Durbin et al. 1956); consequently its effects on target tissue can be expected to differ according to whether it (a) is injected intraperitoneally, reaching the target tissue only after passing through the liver detoxication mechanisms, or (b) is in close contact with the target tissue (e.g., intratumoral application) before reaching the blood circulation. In order to minimize the calcergenic effects on other tissues, the organism provokes its chemical transformation in a chelated or insoluble form. In this way, as a natural defense mechanism reaction it reduces the effect of lanthanum ions on remote target areas. This type of effect is very important in determining the efficiency of lanthanum ion in in vivo hyperthermic killing of tumor cells.

Lanthanum and Hyperthermia

Lanthanum ion has shown weak in vivo tumor growth inhibition (Anghileri 1979), and the very interesting temperature-dependent cytotoxicity of lanthanum ions has been used to enhance hyperthermic killing of tumor cells (Anghileri et al. 1982, 1985a). At 4° C the tumor cells treated with lanthanum ion do not take up trypan blue, and the rate of dye inclusion increases with temperature (Fig. 2). This behavior seems to indicate that the physicochemical state of the plasma membrane, mainly controlled by the fluidity of the lipid bilayer, determines the interaction between lanthanum ion and the cell membrane. These experimental results also suggest that the target of its action must be in the area of the cell membrane poorly accessible and/or highly sensitive to changes in fluidity. This cytotoxic effect has been studied in vitro and in vivo. As evidence of tumor cells' loss of viability we have used the trypan blue inclusion test (this is not a true test of viability but an index of plasma membrane modifications), investigated the inhibition of cloning of cells, and studied in vivo tumor growth inhibition (Anghileri et al. 1983a). A direct relationship appears to exist between trypan blue inclusion and (a) lanthanum concentration and (b) temperature (Fig. 2). The cloning of HeLa S_3

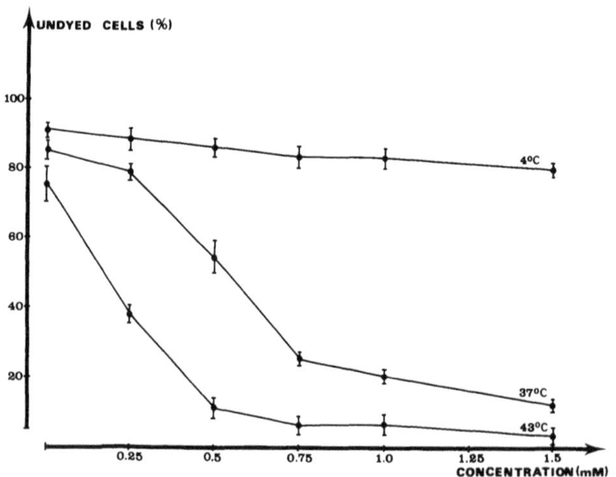

Fig. 2. Effects of temperature and lanthanum ion concentration on trypan blue inclusion by DS sarcoma cells

cells treated with hyperthermia was investigated in the presence or absence of lanthanum ions, and lanthanum was shown to enhance tumor cell lethality significantly (Figs. 3-5). When the effects of lanthanum on in vivo viability of tumor cells submitted to hyperthermia were studied, significant inhibition of tumor growth was observed (Fig. 6). To study the possible modifications of cell permeability provoked by lanthanum ion we used radioactive tracer methods. Lanthanum was shown to cause an important increase in ^{86}Rb release from cells preloaded with ^{86}RbCl, and the effect was slightly modified by temperature (Fig. 7) (Anghileri et al. 1985 a). There was also an important outflux of ^{32}P-labeled molecules present in tumor cells after 48 h in vivo tagging with ^{32}P-orthophosphate (Figs. 8, 9). Another technique used to determine permeability modifications of the cell plasma membrane was the uptake of carrier-free ^{67}Ga-citrate and of ^{59}Fe-citrate. DS sarcoma cells submitted to pretreatment with lanthanum ions took up considerably more radioactivity than control cells (Fig. 10).

Postirradiation treatment of tumor cells with 1 mM procaine plus hyperthermia has been reported to increase radiation lethality (Djordjevic and Szechter 1981). The effects of procaine seem to be achieved via an augmentation of cell membrane fluidity due to calcium ion replacement (Seeman 1972) and its interaction with the inner half of the bilayer containing the acidic phospholipids (Gordon et al. 1980). Lanthanum also displaces calcium ion (Williams 1971) and blocks in-

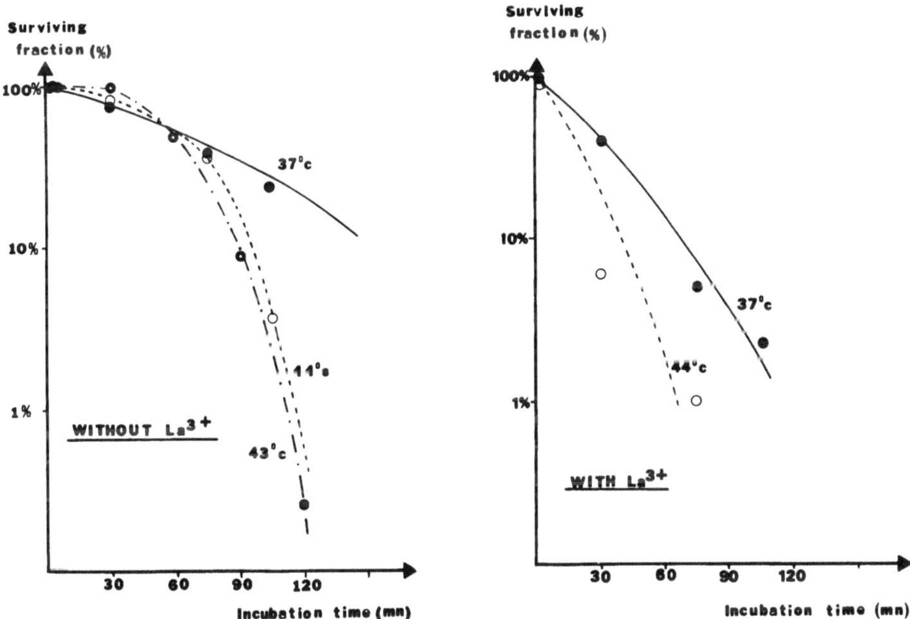

Fig. 3 *(left)*. Effects of incubation time on the surviving fraction of HeLa S_3 cells assayed by the cloning technique in the absence of lanthanum ion

Fig. 4 *(right)*. Effects of incubation time on the surviving fraction of HeLa S_3 cells assayed by the cloning technique in the presence of 1 mM lanthanum ion

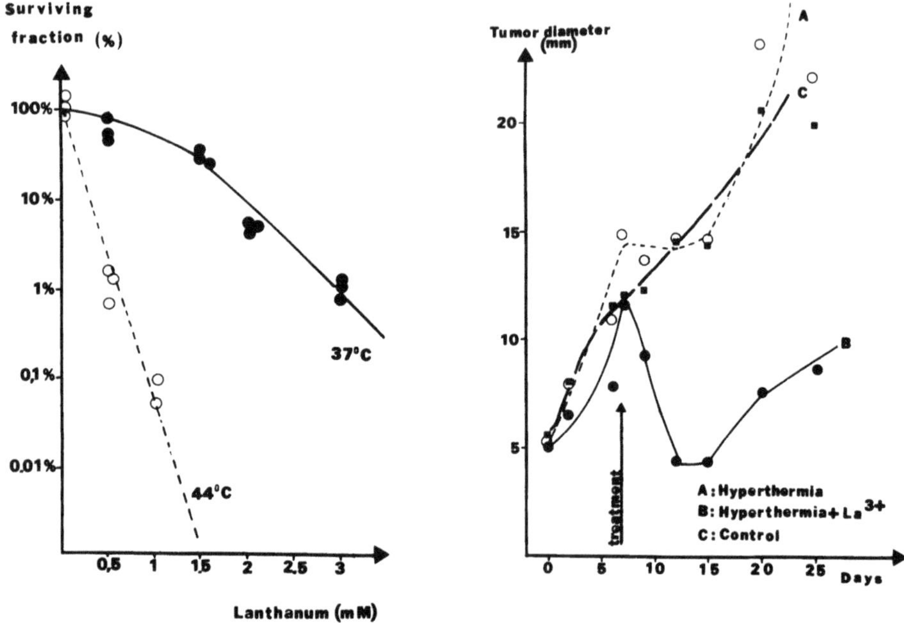

Fig. 5 *(left).* Effects of lanthanum ion concentration on the surviving fraction of HeLa S_3 assayed by the cloning technique after 1 h incubation at 37° C and 44° C

Fig. 6 *(right).* Tumor diameter evolution of rhabdomyosarcoma in C_3H bearing mice treated with hyperthermia and lanthanum (15 min 44° C, intratumoral injection of $LaCl_3$ to give 1 mM followed by 15 more minutes' hyperthermia) (mean value from eight to ten animal groups)

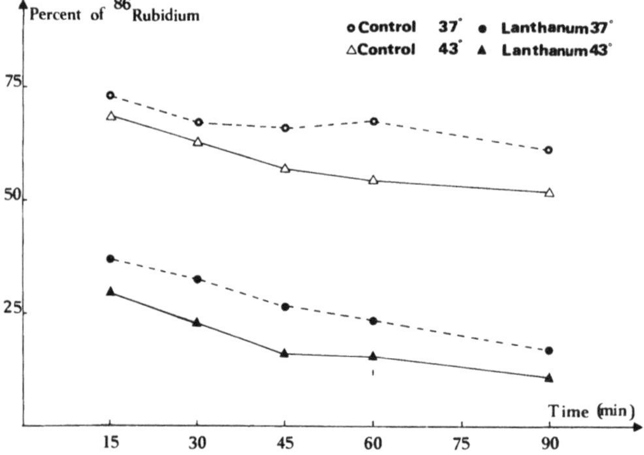

Fig. 7. Effects of hyperthermia and lanthanum on ^{86}Rb release from DS sarcoma cells previously loaded with ^{86}RbCl

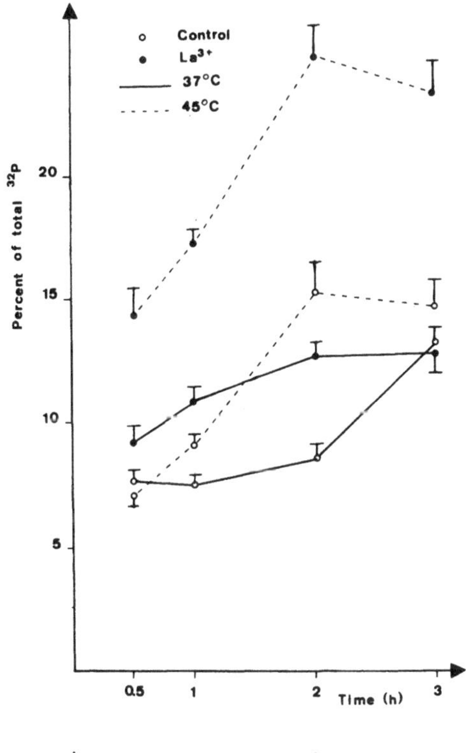

Fig. 8. ^{32}P-labeled molecules released from Ehrlich ascites tumor cells and present in the supernatant as trichloracetic acid soluble molecules after hyperthermia and hyperthermia plus 1 mM lanthanum (mean value ± SD of three incubations)

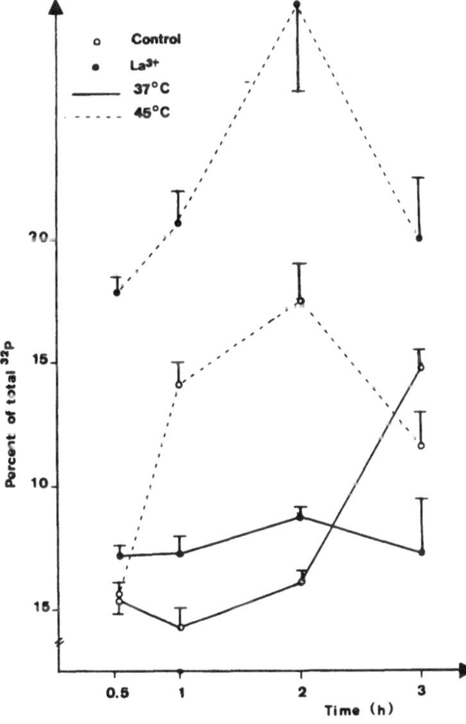

Fig. 9. ^{32}P-labeled molecules released from Ehrlich ascites tumor cells and present in the supernatant as trichloracetic acid insoluble molecules, after hyperthermia and hyperthermia plus 1 mM lanthanum (mean value ± SD of three incubations)

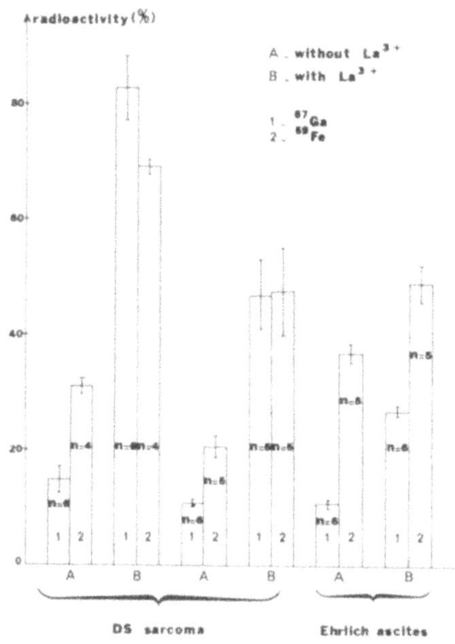

Fig. 10. Effects of pretreatment with lanthanum at 4° C on the uptake of ^{67}Ga- and ^{59}Fe-citrate by DS sarcoma and Ehrlich ascites tumor cells (mean value ± SD of each group of tubes)

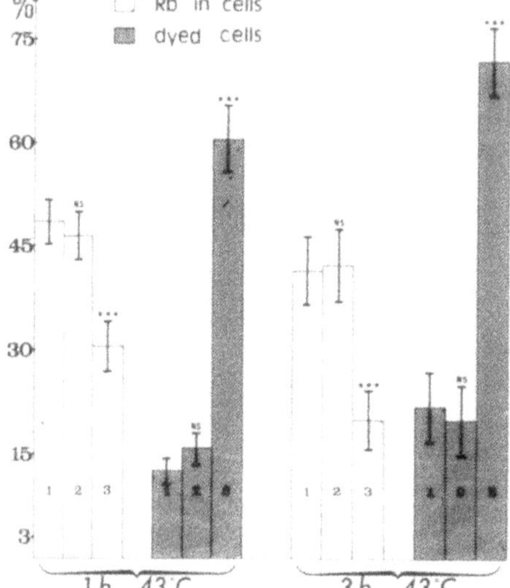

Fig. 11. Effects of lanthanum and procaine on trypan blue inclusion and release of ^{86}Rb. *1*, control cells; *2*, cells incubated in the presence of 1 mM procaine; *3*, cells incubated with 1 mM $LaCl_3$. (Mean value ± SD of ten incubation tubes; *** means $P < 0.0005$)

tracellular translocation of a calcium pool as well as cell membrane calcium ion transport mechanisms (Lehninger 1970). As calcium ion is displaced, cell membrane fluidity changes. A comparative study performed with equimolar concentrations of procaine and lanthanum ion has shown that the modifications due to lanthum ion are far more drastic than those induced by procaine (Fig. 11) (Anghileri et al. 1983b).

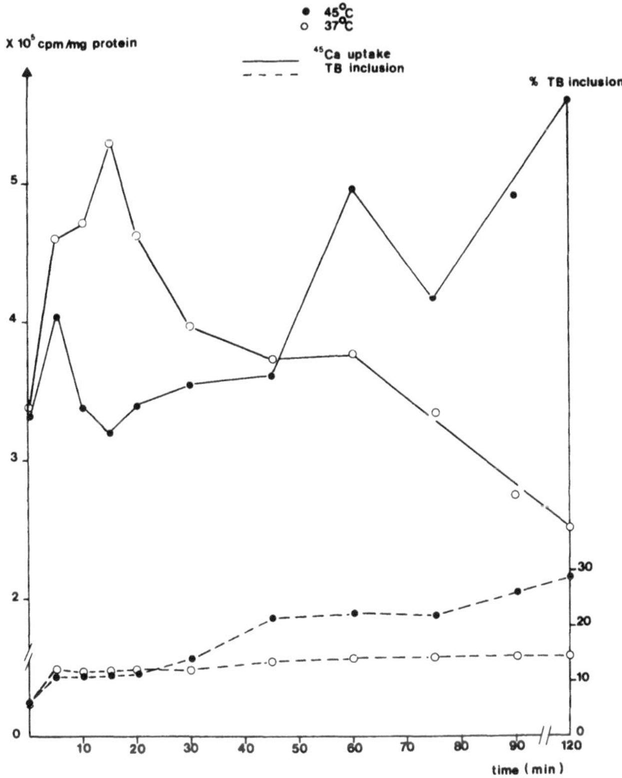

Fig. 12. Trypan blue inclusion and ^{45}Ca uptake by Ehrlich ascites tumor cells during incubation at 37° C and 45° C (mean values of three tubes)

Hyperthermic treatment of tumor cells is characterized by changes in the plasma membrane properties that provoke an increased in- and outflux of molecules. We have demonstrated this phenomenon for calcium ion, and its increased influx occurs concomitantly with an augmentation of trypan blue inclusion (plasma membrane alterations) (Fig. 12). From these observations we have inferred that uncontrolled calcium ion influx might be responsible for the toxic cell death provoked by an irreversible overlaoding of intracellular calcium (Schanne 1979). In the case of hyperthermia in combination with lanthanum ion administration, it is possible that the lethal effect is greatly increased by the effects of lanthanum ion on the calcium pump (Ca^{2+}-ATPase inhibition), permitting a massive calcium influx. Extracellular calcium ion concentration is 1000- to 10000-fold higher than the intracellular concentration, and the calcium pump (Ca^{2+}-ATPase) is responsible for keeping the intracellular calcium level at values compatible with cell life. A recent publication on sensitization of rat hepatocytes to hyperthermia by calcium (Malhotra et al. 1986) corroborates a similar phenomenon already reported by us for tumor cells (Anghileri et al. 1985b).

As a concluding remark on the use of lanthanum ions, I would like to point out the potential use of this cation to enhance interferon stability and binding to cells

(Sedmark and Grossberg 1981; Sedmark et al. 1986). Intravenous LD_{50} of lanthanum chloride for rabbit is 200-250 mg/kg (Haley 1965); because of this weak toxicity, concentrations of up to 2 mM and even higher can be used to enhance the stability and reactivity of interferon.

References

Agarwal N, Kalra VK (1983) Interaction of lanthanide cations and uranyl ion with calcium/proton antiport system in *Mycobacterium phlei.* Biochim Biophys Acta 727: 285-287

Anghileri LJ (1979) Effects of gallium and lanthanum on experimental tumor growth. Eur J Cancer 15: 1459-1462

Anghileri LJ, Marchal C, Crone MC, Robert J (1982) Enhancement of hyperthermia effects on cancer cells by cell membrane interaction with La^{3+}. Proceedings, 13th international cancer congress, 8-15 Sept, Seattle, Washington, p 514

Anghileri LJ, Marchal C, Crone MC, Robert J (1983a) Enhancement of hyperthermia lethality by lanthanum. Arch Geschwulstforsch 53: 335-339

Anghileri LJ, Crone MC, Marchal C, Robert J (1983b) Comparative enhancement of hyperthermia lethality on tumor cells by procaine and lanthanum. Neoplasma 30: 547-549

Anghileri LJ, Crone MC, Robert J (1985a) Intracellular ionic changes during hyperthermia of tumor cells in the presence of lanthanum. Neoplasma 32: 369-373

Anghileri LJ, Marchal C, Crone-Escanye MC, Robert J (1985b) Effects of extracellular calcium on calcium transport during hyperthermia of tumor cells. Eur J Cancer 21: 981-984

Djordjevic B, Szechter A (1981) Potentiation of radiation lethality in HeLa cells by mild hyperthermia and procaine. Radiology 141: 533-535

Durbin PW, Williams MH, Gee M, Newman RH, Hamilton JG (1956) Metabolism of the lanthanons in the rat. Proc Soc Exp Biol Med 91: 78-83

Evans CH (1983) Interesting and useful biochemical properties of lanthanides. TIBS 8: 445-449

Fahimi HD, Cotran RS (1971) Permeability studies in heat-induced injury of skeletal muscle using lanthanum as fine structural tracer. Am J Pathol 62: 143-152

Glick NB (1972) Inhibition of transport reactions. In: Holthers RM, Kates M, Quastel JH (eds) Metabolic inhibitors, vol 3. Academic, London, pp 1-44

Gordon LM, Dipple I, Sauerheber R, Esgate JA, Houslay MD (1980) The selective effects of charged local anesthetics on the glucagon- and fluoride-stimulated adenylate cyclase activity of rat liver plasma membranes. J Supramol Struct 14: 21-28

Haley TJ (1965) Pharmacology and toxicology of the rare earth elements. J Pharm Sci 54: 663-670

Hoffstein S, Gennaro DE, Fox AC, Hirsch J, Streuli F, Weissmann G (1975) Colloidal lanthanum as a marker for impaired plasma membrane permeability in ischemic dog myocardium. Am J Pathol 79: 207-214

Kass RS, Tsien RW (1975) Multiple effects of calcium antagonists on plateau currents in cardiac Purkinje fibers. J Gen Physiol 66: 169-173

Lehninger AL (1970) Mitochondria and calcium ion transport. Biochem J 119: 129-131

Levinson C, Mikiten TM, Smith TC (1972) Lanthanum-induced alterations in cellular electrolytes and membrane potential in Ehrlich ascited tumor cells. J Cell Physiol 79: 299-308

Luterbacher S, Schatzmann HJ (1983) The site of La^{3+} in the reaction cycle of the human red cell membrane Ca^{2+}-pump ATPase. Experientia 39: 311-312

Malhotra A, Kruuv J, Lepock JR (1986) Sensitization of rat hepatocytes to hyperthermia by calcium. J Cell Physiol 128: 279-284

Martinez-Palomo A, Benitez D, Alanis J (1973) Selective deposition of lanthanum in mammalian cardiac cell membranes. Ultrastructural and electrophysiological evidence. J Cell Biol 58: 1-10

Nayler WG (1976) The plasma membrane and sarcoplasmic reticulum of muscle. In: Jamieson GA, Hobinson DM (eds) Myocardial cell membranes. Butterworths, London, pp 45-65
Nayler WG, Harris JP (1976) Inhibition by lanthanum of the $Na^+ + K^+$ activated, ouabain sensitive adenosine triphosphatase enzyme. J Mol Cell Cardiol 8: 811-814
Padmanabhan M, Tuchweber B, Selye H (1963) Über direkt wirkende Verkalkungsstoffe. Arzneimittelforsch 13: 429-431
Pauling L (1960) The nature of the chemical bond. Cornell University Press, Ithaca, NY, p 3
Phillips CSG, Williams RJP (1966) Inorganic chemistry: II metals. Clarendon, Oxford, p 80
Schanne F, Kane AB, Young EE, Farber JL (1979) Calcium-dependence of toxic cell death: a final common pathway. Science 206: 700-702
Sedmark JJ, Grossberg SE (1981) Interferon stabilization and enhancement by rare earth salts. J Gen Virol 52: 195-198
Sedmark JJ, MacDonald HS, Kushnaryov VM (1986) Lanthanide ion enhancement of interferon binding to cells. Biochem Biophys Res Commun 137: 480-485
Seeman P (1972) The membrane actions of anesthetics and tranquilizers. Pharmacol Rev 24: 583-596
Skou JC (1965) Enzymatic basis for active transport of $Na^+ + K^+$ across the cell membrane. Physiol Rev 45: 596-606
von Breeman C, McNaughton E (1970) The separation of cell membrane calcium transport from extracellular calcium exchange in vascular smooth muscle. Biochem Biophys Res Commun 39: 567-569
Williams RJP (1971) Biochemistry of group IA and IIA cations. In: Gould RF (ed) Bioinorganic chemistry. Advances in chemistry series. American Chemical Society, Washington, DC, pp 155-173

Interactions of Hyperthermia with Hypoxic Cell Sensitisers

N. M. Bleehen, M.I. Walton, and P. Workman*

University Department of Clinical Oncology and Radiotherapeutics,
The Medical School, Hills Road, Cambridge CB2 2QH, Great Britain

Introduction

The role of hypoxic cell radiosensitisers has been extensively investigated for the past two decades. Efficacy in experimental models awaits validation in the clinic, but newer drugs currently entering clinical trial show considerable promise. Preferential hypoxic cell cytotoxicity by these electron-affinic agents was demonstrated about 10 years ago. Soon after the enhancement of this cytotoxity by hyperthermia was reported in cells in monolayer culture (Stratford and Adams 1977; Hall et al. 1977), multicellular tumour spheroids (Morgan and Bleehen 1981) and experimental tumours in vivo (Bleehen et al. 1977a; George et al. 1977). The purpose of this paper is briefly to review the topic of the interaction of heat with some hypoxic cell sensitisers. In addition we will also present some of our recent data on aspects of the pharmacology of this combination of treatment modalities. This updates reviews presented at the 2nd International Hyperthermia Symposium in Essen (Bleehen et al. 1978) and more recently by Adams et al. (1982).

The agents studied are all nitroheterocyclic compounds. There is a strong correlation between their electron affinity, hypoxic cell radiosensitisation and hypoxic cell cytotoxicity. However, there are differences in the mechanisms involved in radiosensitisation and cytotoxicity, and in particular their temperature dependence. The hypoxic radiosensitising effect of these drugs (and of O_2) is much less affected by temperature than is their cytotoxicity. This observation strongly suggests that metabolic activation is required for the cytotoxic effects, and this is generally thought to involve reduction of the nitro group (Rauth 1984).

The most frequently studied drug in the context of heat-sensitiser interaction has been misonidazole (MISO) because of its extensive clinical evaluation. We and other groups have also studied a range of other nitroheterocyclic compounds in attempts to understand the phenomenon more generally. In particular, we have studied the neutral 2-nitroimidazole MISO and two closely related analogues cur-

* We wish to thank our many colleagues who have contributed to this work, especially Ms. D.J. Honess. Part of this work was supported by a grant from the Cancer Research Campaign.

Recent Results in Cancer Research, Vol. 109

rently undergoing clinical trial: SR 2508, a hydrophilic compound with reduced neurotoxicity compared with MISO (Coleman et al. 1984), and Ro 03-8799, a more potent, basic analogue of MISO which concentrates in tissues (Williams et al. 1982; Roberts et al. 1986).

Review of Earlier Work

Cytotoxicity in Vitro

The majority of the work in vitro on mammalian cell cytotoxicity has been with MISO, a 2-nitroimidazole with a one-electron reduction potential (E_7^1) of −389 mV. The hyperthermic enhancement of MISO cytotoxicity was first demonstrated on cells grown in vitro and shown to be very much greater under conditions of hypoxia (Bleehen et al. 1977b, 1978; Hall et al. 1977; Stratford and Adams 1977). Stratford and Adams (1977) reported effects on V79 cells over the temperature range 25°-41° C and drug concentrations over the range 0.5-2 mM. An Arrhenius analysis of the data from hypoxic exposure shows a well defined breakpoint at a temperature of around 36° C. They suggested that this was evidence for two mechanisms of interaction. The first, predominant at the lower temperatures, was due to the reaction of MISO with a critical target in the cell, as also seen with oxic cells. The second reaction, predominant at the higher temperatures, was associated with the products of metabolic bioactivation.

Our own data using EMT6 cells confirm the above general observations and conclusions (Bleehen et al. 1977b). Other nitroheterocyclic compounds investigated in vitro include nifurpipone, nimorazole (Stratford et al. 1978), nitrofurantoin and metronidazole (Rajaratnam et al. 1982). The latter authors showed that the greatest heat activation was with the compound of the lowest electron affinity (metronidazole) and the least with nitrofurantoin, which has the highest electron affinity. This is to be expected if a redox reaction is involved, as the compound with the lowest electron affinity should have the largest activation energy and consequently the largest temperature effect. They also showed a pH relationship for the effect, with enhancement of cytotoxicity when the extracellular pH was dropped experimentally from 7.4 to 6.6. We did not observe any differences in the hyperthermic enhancement of MISO cytotoxicity in EMT6 cells treated in fresh or old medium in which the pH was reduced as a result of cellular metabolism (Bleehen et al. 1977b). The pH range, however, was not as extreme as in the work reported by Rajaratnam et al. (1982). Hall and his colleagues (1977) also reported on hyperthermic potentiation of MISO cytotoxicity using a technique of oxygen depletion brought about by incubation of V79 cells in sealed ampoules, a system in which a lowering of pH might be expected.

The role of chronic acidic pH in enhancing MISO cytotoxicity must therefore remain uncertain, but if confirmed would serve to increase the relevance of this combination in regions of tumour with poor nutrition and oxygenation. We have used EMT6 Ca/VJAc multicellular tumour spheroids (MTS) as models of this metabolic environment within tumours (Morgan and Bleehen 1981, 1982; Bleehen and Morgan 1982). Sutherland and his colleagues (1980) demonstrated cytotoxicity in large EMT6/Ro MTS with MISO, desmethylmisonidazole and SR 2508 at

37° C, and this was both drug concentration and exposure time dependent. Cytotoxicity was also enhanced when MTS were grown in 2.5% compared to 20% oxygen. They were able to relate the degree of cell kill to what appeared to be a sensitive subpopulation of cells which were demonstrated histologically to be located in the inner regions of the spheroids surrounding the necrotic zone.

We have used the MTS model to investigate the mechanism of the hyperthermic interaction with MISO. We demonstrated potentiation of hyperthermic cytotoxicity (1-1.5 h at 43° C) following hypoxic preincubation of 200 μm and 650 μm diameter MTS with 5 mM MISO at 37° C (Morgan and Bleehen 1981). This could be demonstrated both by clonogenic assay and growth delay end points. We chose conditions of normothermic pre-incubation with the drug to dissociate possible direct hyperthermic potentiation of the drug metabolism as suggested in the work of Stratford and Adams (1977) in which simultaneous treatment was used. Our studies indicate that hypoxia-dependent metabolic activation of MISO occurs at 37° C, with subsequent interaction with a temperature-sensitive cellular target.

This pre-treatment effect was reversed by a 6-h incubation in fresh medium at 37° before hyperthermic treatment (Morgan and Bleehen 1981). We suggested that one of two events occurred during the recovery interval: either metabolic recovery from sublethal MISO damage or diffusion of toxic products away from the MTS. In an attempt to distinguish between these two mechanisms we investigated the effect of holding the MTS at 0° C between the pre-incubation and hyperthermia treatments. Using large spheroids (650 μm) cell killing continued to increase during the holding period. This suggested an inhibition of repair processes. Smaller MTS (200 μm) also showed no recovery from the sensitisation induced in the pre-incubation period, upon similar holding at 0° C, before hyperthermia (1 h × 43° C).

We have interpreted these data to indicate that the heat sensitisation has a component of sublethal damage induced by hypoxic pre-incubation; this may be repaired during a recovery period at 37° C but this repair is inhibited at 0° C. If loss of toxic products by diffusion was solely responsible for this we should have expected to see some recovery after prolonged incubation at 0° C.

Further attempts to clarify the mechanisms involved have been reported by using cysteamine as a radical scavenger. Hall and colleagues (1977) reported that 5 mM cysteamine present during hypoxic incubation of V79 cells at 37.5° C was able to protect from the hypoxic cytotoxicity of 5 mM MISO. In our own work, addition of cysteamine to MISO in a pre-incubation period at 37° C increased cell kill during subsequent hyperthermia (Bleehen and Morgan 1982). Protection was only afforded if the cysteamine was added during the period of hyperthermia. We have no good explanation for the difference between these two reports other than differences in the experimental conditions. However, our own work does not rule out the explanation given by Hall and colleagues on the likely role of cysteamine as a scavenger of active species which are produced during nitroreduction.

Cytotoxicity in Vivo

Several groups have investigated the interaction of MISO and heat in vivo to see if effects comparable to those discussed in vitro can be demonstrated. Nitroimidazole cytotoxicity towards tumour cells at normal temperature in mice may be demonstrated when the sensitiser enhancement ratios are compared before or after a dose of radiation (Denekamp 1978). Using the EMT6 tumour heated in mice given 1 mg g^{-1} body weight of MISO, we were able to show marked enhancement of hyperthermic cytotoxicity without employing radiation. An in vitro clonogenic assay was used on cells disaggregated from the tumour immediately after heating (Bleehen et al. 1977a). A similar observation was reported for the Fib T tumour in WHT mice (George et al. 1977). In our work the magnitude of cell kill was considerably greater than that to be expected from the known hypoxic fraction of the tumour. This suggested that either diffusible toxic products were produced or other physiological factors associated with the hyperthermia treatment altered the overall interaction.

Experiments in which the effect of the combined treatment was monitored totally in vivo by tumour growth delay showed a much smaller effect than in vitro assays (Honess et al. 1978). We could not demonstrate an effect due to recovery of potentially lethal damage but other factors possibly related to the presence of temperature detectors and a lack of uniformity of heating may have contributed to the differences between the in vivo and in vitro assays. In studies with Ro 03-8799 we have only seen a very small growth delay in the KHT tumours after hyperthermia (Walton et al. unpublished).

Two other groups of workers have failed to demonstrate hyperthermia-enhanced MISO cytotoxicity in vivo using a growth delay assay. Overgaard (1980) found no change in the radiation TCD_{50} when hyperthermia was given to C3H mice with transplanted mammary carcinomas, with or without MISO after the irradiation. Under these conditions no heat-induced MISO tumour cytotoxicity could be seen. Likewise, Wondergem et al. (1982) could see no effect of MISO on the response of the M8013X murine mammary tumour to hyperthermia. There remains uncertainty, therefore, as to whether there is a significant enhancement of MISO tumour cytotoxicity in vivo by hyperthermia.

Recent Pharmacological Studies

Introduction

To date, there have been very few studies of the effects of either whole-body hyperthermia (WBH) or local hyperthermia on drug pharmacokinetics and metabolism. We have recently been investigating the effects of WBH on the pharmacokinetics of MISO, SR 2508 and Ro 03-8799 in mouse plasma and tumour tissue. We have also studied the effects of local hyperthermia, a clinically more manageable form of heating, on the pharmacokinetics of Ro 03-8799 in mice.

Methods

We have used male C3H/He mice bearing KHT leg tumours in the size range 0.3–0.8 g. Ro 03-8799 doses and concentrations are reported as the free base. Drugs were administered either i.p. or i.v. in Hanks' balanced salt solution, either

10 min before WBH or 5 min before local hyperthermia. WBH was induced in groups of three or four mice for a duration of 50 min as previously described (Honess and Bleehen 1982). This produced a steady-state rectal temperature of 41° ± 0.5° C for 35 min after an initial 15-min equilibration phase.

Local hyperthermia was administered to conscious mice contained in Perspex jigs using a novel waterbath and 13.56 MHz radiofrequency (RF) heating system, similar in design to that of Joiner and Vojnovic (1982). Central tumour temperatures were regulated to ± 0.2° C by a microcomputer controlled RF heating system (Sathiaseelan et al. 1983). Local hyperthermia treatments (43.5° C × 30 min) were administered to the whole tumour-bearing leg. Core temperatures were controlled to ⩽ 38.0° C.

Drug concentrations in mouse plasma and KHT tumours were assayed using reverse-phase isocratic HPLC as previously described (Workman et al. 1978; Malcolm et al. 1983). All samples were handled on ice and prepared as previously reported (Brown and Workman 1980; Workman 1980). Pharmacokinetic parameters were calculated as described in detail elsewhere (Workman and Brown 1981; White and Workman 1980). Significance levels were determined using Student's *t*-test. LD_{50} values were calculated as described before (Workman 1979). Mice were observed for 7 days after treatment.

Results

Acute Toxicity

Whole-body hyperthermia markedly increased the acute toxicity of MISO, SR 2508 and Ro 03-8799. The $LD_{50/7d}$ for MISO was decreased twofold from 1350 to 700 μg g^{-1}. SR 2508 $LD_{50/7d}$ was decreased fivefold from 5480 to 1080 μg g^{-1} and Ro 03-8799 $LD_{50/7d}$ was reduced threefold from 779 to 259 μg g^{-1} ($P < 0.01$ in all cases).

In contrast, local hyperthermia did not significantly alter Ro 03-8799 toxicity, the $LD_{50/7d}$ values being 710 and 776 μg g^{-1} for heat and sham treatments respectively ($P = 0.1$). Subsequent pharmacokinetic experiments were carried out at 60% $LD_{50/7d}$ of heated mice.

Effects of WBH on MISO Pharmacokinetics

Figure 1 a shows the effects of WBH in the plasma clearance of 420 μg g^{-1} MISO i.p. Plasma MISO concentrations were similar in both heated and unheated mice during WBH and up to 2 h after drug administration. At later times, WBH increased MISO plasma concentrations, prolonging the elimination $t_{1/2}$ by 18% from 1.33 to 1.6 h ($0.01 < P < 0.05$). This resulted in a 20% increase in plasma $AUC_{0-\infty}$ in heated animals, and a consequent 17% decrease in plasma clearance (P_{Cl}) from 0.409 to 0.491 ml g^{-1} h^{-1}.

Steady-state MISO tumour concentrations of 92% were reached after 20 min in both heated and control mice, indicating good tumour penetration. WBH in-

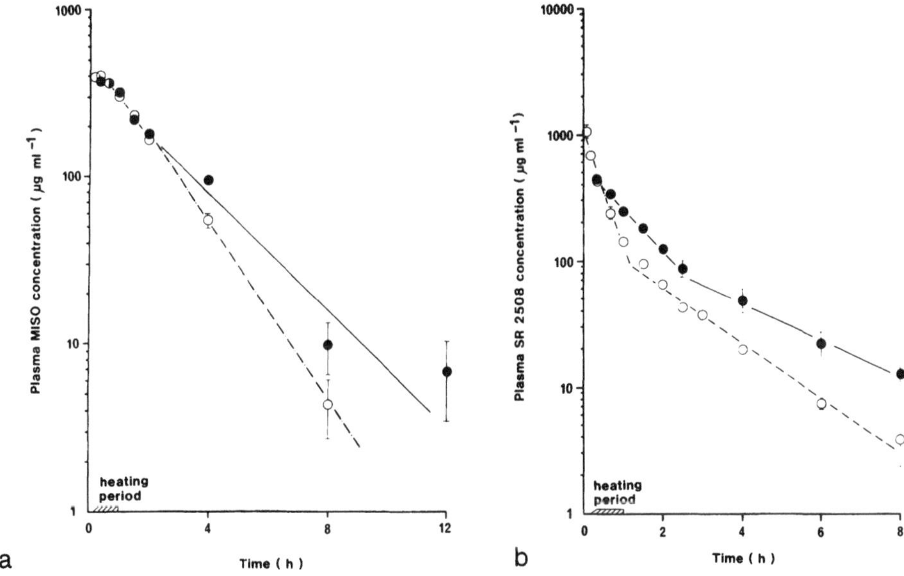

Fig. 1 a, b. Effects of WBH on the plasma pharmacokinetics of **a** 420 µg g^{-1} MISO i.p. and **b** 650 µg g^{-1} SR 2508 i.v. in C3H/He mice. *Symbols:* ● with WBH, and ○ without. Data from two or three independent experiments with 3-12 mice per point. Results are mean ± 2SE

Table 1. The effects of WBH on steady-state tumour/plasma ratios for MISO, SR 2508 and Ro 03-8799 in C3H/He mice

Drug	Steady-state period	Tumour/plasma (%)[a]	
		WBH	Control
MISO	40 min-8 h	89.3 ± 5.0 (n=40)	92.3 ± 6.6 (n=41)
SR 2508	40 min-4 h	97.1[b] ± 8.5 (n=32)	128 ± 6.7 (n=35)
Ro 03-8799	20 min-2 h	164[b] ±20 (n=31)	224 ±34 (n=23)

[a] Values are mean ± 2SE for n samples. Data derived from 2-3 independent experiments for each drug.
[b] $P < 0.01$ significantly different from control.

creased tumour and plasma MISO levels to a similar extent such that tumour/plasma ratios were very similar in both heated and control mice over this period (Table 1).

Effects of WBH on SR 2508 Pharmacokinetics

After i.v. administration SR 2508 plasma clearance was biphasic (Fig. 1 b) with a distribution phase $t_{1/2}\hat{\alpha}$ (with 95% confidence limits) of 14.6 (13.4-16.1) min and a terminal phase $t_{1/2}\hat{\beta}$ of 82.7 (77.4-88.2) min. WBH increased plasma SR 2508 concentrations over the whole time course and prolonged the $t_{1/2}\alpha$ in heated animals by 106% to 31.1 (24.6–42.1) min and the $t_{1/2}\beta$ by 45% to 121 (97.8–157) min ($P<0.01$). Plasma $AUC_{0-\infty}$ was elevated by 43% from 277 to 397 μg ml^{-1} h^{-1} and P_{Cl} reduced by 34% from 1.06 to 0.70 ml g^{-1} h^{-1}.

Table 1 shows that steady-state tumour penetration was very good in control mice, with tumour/plasma ratios over 100%. WBH increased tumour levels of SR 2508 but to a lesser extent than in plasma, resulting in significantly lower tumour/plasma ratios ($P<0.01$).

Effects of WBH on Ro 03-8799 Pharmacokinetics

Figure 2a shows the effects of WBH on the plasma clearance of 175 μg g^{-1} Ro 03-8799 i.v. Elimination was treated as monoexponential. WBH elevated plasma concentrations, particularly at later times, and significantly prolonged its elimination $t_{1/2}$ by 26% from 23.5 (21.8–25.4) min to 29.1 (27.5–31.0) min ($P<0.01$). Plasma $AUC_{0-\infty}$ was correspondingly increased by 22% from 44.9 to 54.8 μg ml^{-1} h^{-1}, resulting in a 36% reduction in P_{Cl} from 1.1 to 0.7 ml g^{-1} h^{-1}.

A feature of this basic radiosensitiser is its ability to concentrate in tissue, giving tumour/plasma ratios markedly in excess of 100%. In contrast to plasma, WBH did not alter steady-state tumour Ro 03-8799 concentrations. This resulted in reduced tumour/plasma ratios, and the difference became significant at times beyond 90 min ($P<0.01$).

Figure 2b shows the effect of WBH on the plasma concentrations of the N-oxide metabolite (Ro 31-0313) of Ro 03-8799. WBH greatly increased peak

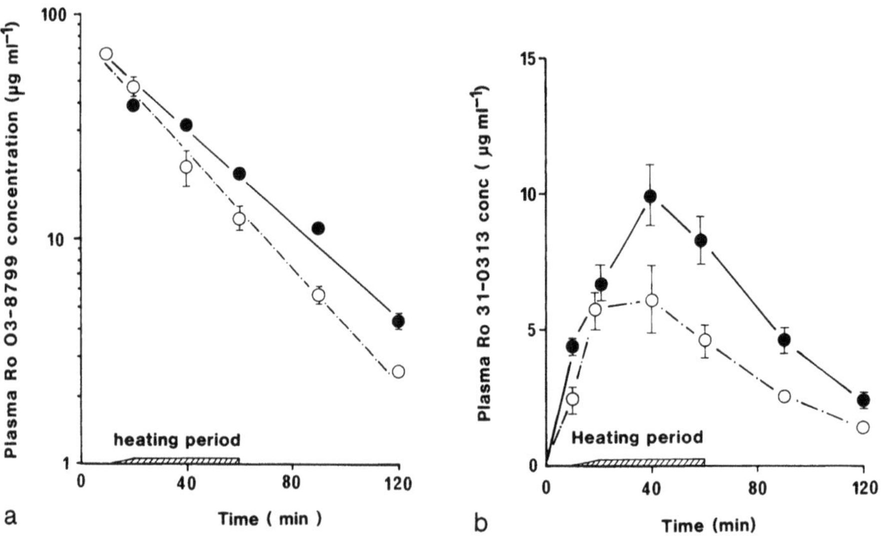

Fig. 2a, b. Effects of WBH on **a** the plasma pharmacokinetics of 175 μg g^{-1} Ro 03-8799 i.v. and **b** the plasma concentrations of the N-oxide metabolite, Ro 31-0313, after 175 μg g^{-1} Ro 03-8799 i.v. in C3H/H^e mice. *Symbols:* ● with WBH, and ○ without. Data from two independent experiments with three to seven mice per point. Results are mean ± 2SE

Ro 31-0313 plasma concentrations during the heating period, e.g. by 81% from 4.61 to 8.35 μg ml^{-1} at 60 min. Consequently the $AUC_{0-\infty}$ was increased by 57% from 65.6 to 103 μg ml^{-1} h^{-1}.

Effects of Local Hyperthermia on Ro 03-8799 Pharmacokinetics

Figure 3a shows the plasma clearance of Ro 03-8799 (437 μg g^{-1} i.v.) in mice given either local hyperthermia or sham treatment. There was no significant effect on clearance $t_{1/2}$, the values being 34.7 (32.3-37.5) min and 36.0 (32.9-39.8) min for heated mice and controls respectively. Plasma $AUC_{0-\infty}$ was also similar at 21.4 and 19.8 μg ml^{-1} h^{-1} respectively.

Tumour Ro 03-8799 concentrations equilibrated with plasma after 10 min in heated and 35 min in sham-treated mice. Local hyperthermia markedly lowered the tumour Ro 03-8799 concentration over the whole time course, and the $AUC_{0-\infty}$ was reduced by 31% from 191 to 132 μg g^{-1} h^{-1}. The average steady state tumour/plasma ratio was markedly reduced from 143%±21.8% to 87%±10.9% (mean±2SE) in heated tumours ($P<0.05$).

Peak plasma levels of the N-oxide metabolite, Ro 31-0313, were slightly increased in locally heated animals, e.g. by 15% from 12.5 to 14.4 μg ml^{-1} immediately after heating. However, the plasma $AUC_{0\text{-}180\,min}$ was increased by only 7% from 19.8 to 21.4 μg ml^{-1} h^{-1}.

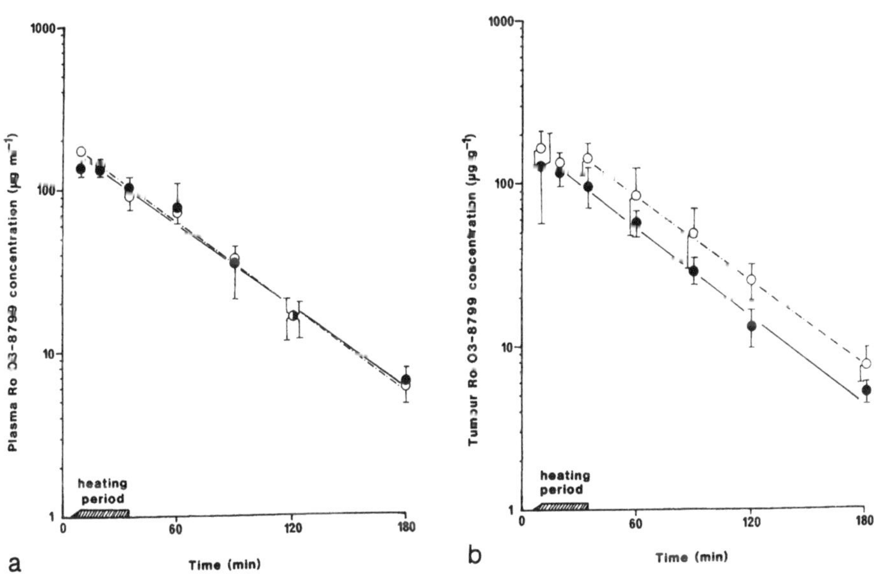

Fig. 3a, b. Effects of local hyperthermia on the pharmacokinetics of Ro 03-8799 (437 μg g^{-1} i.v.) in **a** plasma and **b** KHT tumours from C3H/He mice. *Symbols:* ● with local hyperthermia, and ○ without. Data from two independent experiments with four to six mice per point. Results are mean±2SE

Discussion

Our results show that WBH (41° C × 35 min) increased the acute lethality of MISO, SR 2508 and Ro 03-8799 by two-, seven- and threefold respectively. A similar twofold increase in MISO toxicity was noted by Gomer and Johnson (1979) when C3H mice core temperatures were maintained at 35°-37° C for 3 h after drug administration instead of becoming hypothermic. MISO toxicity was also reported to increase by 40% with local hyperthermia, where core temperatures approached 40° C towards the end of heating (Overgaard 1979). In contrast, when Ro 03-8799 was given with local hyperthermia but core temperatures were held at 35°-38° C, the drug was no more toxic than in unheated mice. These results suggest a need for careful core temperature control if 2-nitroimidazole acute toxicity is to be minimised during local hyperthermia.

Although hyperthermia, both whole body and local, is being evaluated in combination with various anticancer drugs (see Bleehen 1983) there have been few detailed studies of its effects on drug pharmacokinetics. Previous work with adriamycin and WBH (42.3° C × 60 min) showed no effect on adriamycin $t_{1/2}$ or plasma clearance in rabbits (Mimnaugh et al. 1978). Studies with methotrexate and WBH (43° C × 60 min) in dogs showed significantly higher methotrexate plasma concentrations at 24 and 48 h in heated animals compared to controls (Daly et al. 1984).

Our results with MISO, SR 2508 and Ro 03-8799 show a complex effect of WBH on the pharmacokinetics of each drug. WBH increased the plasma concentrations of all three drugs, particularly at later time points, and this was accompanied by a prolongation of their respective elimination $t_{1/2}$ values. This increase in plasma drug levels resulted in higher AUCs in heated mice and a reduced plasma clearance for all three radiosensitisers. This may result from WBH-impaired renal function. In support of this hypothesis we have shown that this heating technique almost completely inhibits glomerular filtration specifically during the heating period (Walton et al. 1987a). Other studies have also shown that mild heat stress can reduce glomerular filtration in man (Smith et al. 1952).

The precise effects of WBH on tumour drug concentrations were different for each radiosensitiser. MISO tumour concentrations were increased to the same extent as plasma by WBH and tumour/plasma ratios were unaltered, indicating good tissue-plasma equilibration. On the other hand SR 2508 tumour levels were increased by WBH but did not fully equilibrate with the higher plasma concentrations, resulting in lower tumour/plasma ratios for heated animals. Ro 03-8799 tumour levels were unaltered by WBH, resulting in decreased tumour/plasma ratios, particularly at later times. Reduced tumour/plasma ratios have also been noted at later time points for mice subjected to WBH and melphalan (Honess et al. 1985). These reduced ratios may be a result of several factors. WBH might decrease blood flow and hence tumour drug delivery and uptake. In the case of Ro 03-8799 subtle changes in the plasma/intracellular tumour pH ratios may limit drug accumulation during WBH (Dennis et al. 1985; Watts and Jones 1985). Alternatively the lower drug levels in heated tumours might reflect heat-stimulated reductive metabolism to non-UV-detectable metabolites. In support of the latter, we have shown that mild hyperthermia enhances the reductive metabolism of the lipophilic, neutral 2-nitroimidazole benznidazole in vitro (Walton et al. 1987b).

The marked increase in Ro 03-8799 N-oxide plasma concentrations during WBH may be a consequence of heat-stimulated hepatic N-oxidation and/or reduced plasma clearance of this metabolite. We have also shown that mild hyperthermia enhances MISO 0-demethylation in vitro (Walton et al., unpublished data), which further supports the former possibility.

In contrast to the results with WBH, local hyperthermia (43.5° C × 30 min) did not alter the plasma concentrations or elimination $t_{1/2}$ of Ro 03-8799, and plasma AUCs were similar in sham-treated and heated mice. Previous studies with local hyperthermia (44° C × 60 min) and MISO showed that the plasma elimination $t_{1/2}$ was also unaltered (Honess et al. 1980).

Tumour Ro 03-8799 concentrations were substantially decreased by local hyperthermia, as indicated by the 31% reduction in heated tumour AUC and the 39% decrease in tumour/plasma ratios. This finding is similar to that reported for MISO and local hyperthermia, where heated tumour $AUC_{0\text{-}8h}$ was decreased by 25% (Honess et al. 1980). This reduction in tumour drug levels with heating may arise through impaired drug delivery to the tumour or hyperthermia-stimulated reductive metabolism, as proposed earlier for WBH. Further support for the latter explanation is provided by studies combining local hyperthermia (43° C × 60 min) and adriamycin (Magin et al. 1980), where heated tumours were shown to have increased concentrations of reduced adriamycin metabolites (aglycones).

Local hyperthermia slightly increased plasma concentrations of Ro 31-0313. This may reflect a small increase in oxidative metabolism and/or decreased plasma clearance. Previous studies have shown that local hyperthermia decreases peak plasma concentrations of Ro 05-9963, the 0-demethylated metabolite of MISO, though the AUCs were comparable in heated and control mice (Honess et al. 1980). In contrast to WBH, local hyperthermia has minimal effects on the N-oxidation of Ro 03-8799 in mice.

In summary, WBH substantially increased the acute lethality of MISO, SR 2508 and Ro 03-8799. By contrast, local hyperthermia had no effect on Ro 03-8799 acute toxicity. WBH increased the plasma concentrations of all three radiosensitisers and decreased their plasma clearance, possibly in part through impaired renal function. WBH did not affect MISO tumour/plasma ratios but decreased these ratios for both SR 2508 and Ro 03-8799. WBH increased the plasma Ro 03-8799 N-oxide concentrations, possibly through enhanced oxidative metabolism. Local hyperthermia, on the other hand, did not alter Ro 03-8799 plasma pharmacokinetics, and only slightly increased plasma N-oxide concentrations. However, tumour Ro 03-8799 concentrations were markedly reduced by local hyperthermia, possibly through heat-stimulated nitroreductive bioactivation.

These results show that hyperthermia, both local and whole body, has a complex effect on the pharmacokinetics and metabolism of 2-nitroimidazoles. Further studies are required to elucidate the effects of hyperthermia on drug delivery and oxidative and reductive metabolism, particularly in view of the cytotoxic potential of the latter pathway and its possible stimulation in locally heated tumours.

Conclusions

The value of the hyperthermic potentiation of nitroimidazole cytotoxicity remains uncertain. A marked increase in cell kill is seen with hypoxic cells in monolayer and suspension cultures in vitro as well as in MTS. This may arise through a heat-induced increase in nitroreduction with the production of toxic intermediates.

The extent of heat-induced alterations of drug metabolism will depend not only on the temperature and the type of drug, but also on the physiological changes caused by the treatment. Changes in pH and oxygen tension consequent on changes in blood flow may be as important as the direct metabolic changes resulting from the raised temperature (see Bleehen et al. 1978). General systemic effects resulting in alterations in renal clearance will also affect the duration of tissue exposure to a drug. Hyperthermia may also increase the intracellular uptake of some 2-nitroimidazole hypoxic cell radiosensitisers in vitro (Brown et al. 1983). Should such changes occur in vivo they may influence the magnitude of radiosensitisation if hyperthermia is administered before radiotherapy.

The clinical relevance for a combined modality treatment strategy remains undefined. As a result of our early observations on in vivo tumours (Bleehen et al. 1977a), we proposed a potential therapeutic strategy. We postulated that it might be advantageous to use a regime in which a sensitiser was given before radiation to enhance the effect of the latter on the tumour hypoxic fraction. Subsequently hyperthermia could be employed so that it would enhance the cytotoxicity of both the radiation and the sensitiser (Bleehen et al. 1978). Although we have not investigated this triple treatment combination ourselves, two other groups have reported results for such combinations. Overgaard (1980) demonstrated MISO radiosensitisation and either hyperthermic radiosensitisation or independent hyperthermic cytotoxicity depending on whether the heat was given simultaneously with the radiation or delayed for 4 h. However, no MISO cytotoxicity was seen. In contrast and of great interest are the results reported by Wondergem et al. (1982). They were able to demonstrate a cytotoxic effect of MISO after radiation and hyperthermia which could not be seen in the nonirradiated tumour. A likely explanation for these differences is the increased population of hypoxic cells to be found in tumours immediately following irradiation, when tumour control end points are used. Under these conditions a greater cytotoxic effect of MISO would be seen than might otherwise occur with the smaller hypoxic fraction present in nonirradiated tumours.

On the basis of the experimental evidence presented in this paper there clearly remains both promise and uncertainty for a clinical combination of hypoxic cell sensitisers together with radiation and hyperthermia. Further investigation of optimal treatment conditions based on pharmacological studies of existing and new nitroheterocyclic compounds is required, together with in vivo assays of the antitumour effects of such combinations.

References

Adams GE, Stratford IJ, Rajaratnam S (1982) Interaction of the cytotoxic and sensitizing effects of electron-affinic drugs and hyperthermia. Natl Cancer Inst Monogr 61: 27-35

Bleehen NM (1983) Heat and drugs: current status of thermo-chemotherapy. In: Steel GG, Adams GE, Peckham MJ (eds) The biological basis of radiotherapy. Elsevier, Amsterdam, pp 321-332

Bleehen NM, Morgan JE (1982) Interaction between misonidazole, hyperthermia, and some cytotoxic drugs on multicellular tumour spheroids. In: Karcher KH et al. (eds) Progress in radio-oncology II, Raven, New York, pp 457-464

Bleehen NM, Honess DJ, Morgan JE (1977a) Interaction of hyperthermia and the hypoxic-cell sensitizer Ro 07-0582 on the EMT6 mouse tumour. Br J Cancer 35: 299-306

Bleehen NM, Honess DJ, Morgan JE (1977b) Interaction of the hypoxic cell sensitizer Ro 07-0582 and hyperthermia on EMT6 tumour cells in vitro and in vivo. In: Radiobiological research and radiotherapy, vol 1. International Atomic Energy Agency, Vienna, pp 211-220

Bleehen NM, Honess DJ, Morgan JE (1978) The combined effects of hyperthermia and hypoxic cell sensitizers. In: Streffer C (ed) Cancer therapy by hyperthermia and radiation. Urban und Schwarzenberg, Munich, pp 62-71

Brown DM, Cohen MS, Sagerman RH, Gonzales-Mendez R, Hahn GM, Brown JM (1983) Influence of heat on the intracellular uptake and radiosensitisation of 2-nitroimidazole hypoxic cell sensitisers in vitro. Cancer Res 43: 3138-3142

Brown JM, Workman P (1980) Partition coefficient as a guide to the development of radiosensitizers which are less toxic that misonidazole. Radiat Res 82: 171-190

Coleman CN, Urtasun RC, Wasserman TD, Hancock S, Harris JW, Halsey J, Hirst VK (1984) Initial report of the phase 1 trial of the hypoxic cell radiosensitizer SR 2508. Int J Radiat Oncol Biol Phys 10: 1749-1753

Daly JM, Wang YM, Kapelanski D, Howard-Frazier O (1984) Systemic thermochemotherapy, toxicity and plasma pharmacokinetics of methotrexate and doxorubicin. J Surg Res 37: 343-347

Denekamp J (1978) Cytotoxicity and radiosensitization in mouse and man. Br J Radiol 57: 636-637

Dennis MF, Stratford MRL, Wardman P, Watts ME (1985) Cellular uptake of misonidazole analogues with acidic or basic functions. Int J Radiat Biol 47: 629-643

George KC, Hirst DG, McNally NJ (1977) Effect of hyperthermia on the cytotoxicity of the radiosensitizer Ro 07-0582 in a solid mouse tumour. Br J Cancer 35: 372-375

Gomer CJ, Johnson RJ (1979) Relationship between misonidazole toxicity and core temperature in C3H mice. Radiat Res 78: 329-333

Hall EJ, Astor M, Geard C, Biaglow J (1977) Cytotoxicity of Ro 07-0582; enhancement by hyperthermia and protection by cyteamine. Br J Cancer 35: 809-815

Honess DJ, Bleehen NM (1982) Sensitivity of normal mouse marrow and RIF-1 tumour to hyperthermia combined with cyclophosphamide or BCNU: a lack of therapeutic gain. Br J Cancer 46: 236-248

Honess DJ, Morgan JE, Bleehen NM (1978) The hyperthermic potentiation of the cytotoxic effect of misonidazole on the EMT6 mouse tumour: relevance of in vitro measurement of in vivo effect. Br J Cancer 37 [Suppl III]: 173-177

Honess DJ, Workman P, Morgan JE, Bleehen NM (1980) Effects of local hyperthermia on the pharmacokinetics of misonidazole in the anaesthetized mouse. Br J Cancer 41: 529-540

Honess DJ, Donaldson J, Workman P, Bleehen NM (1985) The effects of systemic hyperthermia on melphalan pharmacokinetics in mice. Br J Cancer 51: 77-84

Joiner MC, Vojnovic B (1982) Radiofrequency diathermy for uniform heating of mouse tumours. Br J Cancer 45 [Suppl V]: 71-76

Magin RL, Cysyk RL, Litterst KL (1980) Distribution of adriamycin in mice under conditions of local hyperthermia which improve systemic drug therapy. Cancer Treat Rep 64 : 203-210

Malcolm SL, Lee A, Groves JK (1983) High-performance liquid chromatographic analysis of the new hypoxic-cell radiosensitizer Ro 03-8799, in biological samples. J Chromatogr 273: 327-333

Mimnaugh EG, Waring RW, Sikic BI, Magin RL, Drew R, Litterst CL, Gram TE, Guarino AM (1978) Effects of WBH on the disposition and metabolism of adriamycin in rabbits. Cancer Res 38: 1420-1425

Morgan JE, Bleehen NM (1981) Interactions between misonidazole and hyperthermia in EMT6 spheroids. Br J Cancer 44: 810-818

Morgan JE, Bleehen NM (1982) Heat sensitivity of EMT6 multicellular tumour spheroids following misonidazole pre-treatment. Natl Cancer Inst Monogr 61: 153-155

Overgaard J (1979) Effects of local hyperthermia on the acute toxicity of misonidazole in mice. Br J Cancer 39: 96-98

Overgaard J (1980) Effects of misonidazole and hyperthermia on the radiosensitivity of a C3H mouse mammary carcinoma and its surrounding normal tissue. Br J Cancer 41: 10-21

Rajaratnam S, Adams GE, Stratford IT, Clarke C (1982) Enhancement of the cytotoxicity of radiosensitizers by modest hyperthermia: the electron-affinity relationship. Br J Cancer 46: 912-917

Rauth AM (1984) Pharmacology and toxicology of sensitizers: mechanism studies. Int J Radiat Oncol Biol Phys 10: 1293-1300

Roberts JT, Bleehen NM, Walton MI, Workman P (1986) A clinical phase I toxicity study of Ro 03-8799: plasma, urine, tumour and normal brain pharmacokinetics. Br J Radiol 59: 107-116

Sathiaseelan V, Har-Kedar I, Howard GCW, Bleehen NM (1983) A microcomputer-controlled microwave hyperthermia system. J Microcomp Appl 6: 261-277

Smith JM, Robinson S, Pearcy M (1952) Renal responses to exercise, heat and dehydration. J Appl Physiol 4: 659-665

Stratford IJ, Adams GE (1977) Effect of hyperthermia on differential cytotoxicity of a hypoxic cell radiosensitizer, Ro 07-0582, on mammalian cells in vitro. Br J Cancer 35: 307-313

Stratford IJ, Watts ME, Adams GE (1978) The effect of hyperthermia on the differential cytotoxicity of some electron-affinic hypoxic cell radiosensitizers on mammalian cells in vitro. Streffer C (ed) Cancer therapy by hyperthermia and radiation. Urban and Schwarzenberg, Munich, pp 267-270

Sutherland RM, Bareham BJ, Reich KA (1980) Cytotoxicity of hypoxic cell sensitizers in multicell spheroids. Cancer Clin Trials 3: 73-83

Walton MI, Bleehen NM, Workman P (1987a) The effects of whole body hyperthermia on the pharmacokinetics and toxicity of the basic 2-nitroimidazole radiosensitizer Ro 03-8799 in mice. Br J Cancer 55: 469-476

Walton MI, Bleehen NM, Workman P (1987b) Heat stimmulated nitroreductive bioactivation of the 2-introimidazole benzoidazole in vitro. Biochem Pharmacol 36: 2627-2632

Watts ME, Jones NR (1985) The effect of extracellular pH on radiosensitization by misonidazole and acidic and basic analogues. Int J Radiat Biol 47, 6: 645-653

White RAS, Workman P (1980) Pharmacokinetic and tumour penetration properties of the hypoxic-cell radiosensitizer desmethylmisonidazole (Ro 05-9963) in dogs. Br J Cancer 41: 268-276

Williams MV, Denekamp J, Minchinton AL, Stratford MRL (1982) In vivo assessment of basic 2-nitroimidazole radiosensitizers. Br J Cancer 46: 127-137

Wondergem J, Haveman J, van der Schueren E, van der Hoeven H, Breur K (1982) Effect of hyperthermia and misonidazole on the radiosensitivity of a transplantable murine tumour: influence of factors modifying the fraction of hypoxic cells. Int J Radiat Oncol Biol Phys 8: 1323-1331

Workman P (1979) Effects of pretreatment with phenobarbitone and phenytoin on the pharmacokinetics and toxicity of misonidazole in mice. Br J Cancer 40: 335-353

Workman P (1980) Dose-dependence and related studies on the pharmacokinetics of misonidazole in mice. Cancer Chemother Pharmacol 5: 27-37

Workman P, Brown JM (1981) Structure-pharmacokinetic relationships for misonidazole analogues in mice. Cancer Chemother Pharmacol 6: 39-49

Workman P, Little CJ, Marten TR, Dale AD, Ruane RJ, Flockhart IR, Bleehen NM (1978) Estimation of the hypoxic cell sensitizer misonidazole and its 0-demethylated metabolite in biological materials by reverse-phase high-performance liquid chromatography. J Chromatogr 145: 507-512

*Thermal Enhancement of the Cell Killing Effect of X-Irradiation in Mammalian Cells in Vitro and in a Transplantable Mouse Tumor: Influence of pH, Thermotolerance, Hypoxia, or Misonidazole**

J. Haveman and J. Wondergem**

Radiotherapy Department, University of Amsterdam, Medical Center (AMC), Meibergdreef 9, 1105 AZ Amsterdam, The Netherlands

Introduction

Many experimental results indicate that the lethal effects of X-irradiation on mammalian cells are the result of damage to DNA. Radiosensitization by hyperthermia, i.e., treatment at temperatures in the range of 42°-47° C, is caused by inhibition of the repair of radiation-induced damage (Bronk 1976). Most of the lethal effects induced by hyperthermia alone are presumably due to damage to other cellular targets, including the plasma membrane and other membrane structures of the cell (Hahn 1982). Both the direct cell-killing effect of hyperthermia and radiosensitization might be exploited in the clinical application of hyperthermia.

Solid tumors are often poorly vascularized. This is thought to be one of the factors that plays an important role in the presumed selective effect of hyperthermia on tumor tissue. The poor vascularization is partly the result of the relatively rapid proliferation of tumor cells, which leads to a retardation of the required increase in vascular endothelial cells. This inadequate blood vessel structure in its turn leads to necrotic areas in (solid) tumors. In the regions between healthy tumor tissue and necrotic areas many cells suffer from hypoxia, lack of nutrients, lack of cellular energy, and a relatively low intercellular pH. Many data concerning the influence of hypoxia, pH, and lack of nutrients or cellular energy on radiation and heat sensitivity and on heat radiosensitization come from work with mammalian cells cultured in vitro. In view of the clinical interest, many studies on the enhancement of radiation effects by hyperthermia have been done with transplantable tumors, and with normal tissues, in experimental animals. In several of these studies some differential effect was observed, indicating a therapeutic gain (Haveman 1986).

* Part of the research described here was supported by grants from the KWF (Koningin Wilhelmina Fonds) and from the IRS (Interuniversitair Instituut voor Radiopathologie en Stralenbescherming).
** We thank Mrs. H. Erkelens for the careful typing of the manuscript.

When radiation is applied in fractions it appears that part of the radiation-induced damage to cells may be repaired in the intervals between fractions. However, the intrinsic sensitivity of the cells to a subsequent radiation fraction will not have been changed (Elkind and Whitmore 1967). When hyperthermia is applied in fractions, the effect of a fraction after the first one may be greatly reduced and much less than would be expected from recovery of sublethal heat damage alone. This change in intrinsic sensitivity to hyperthermia has been called thermotolerance.

Thermotolerance is a transient phenomenon: it decays when the interval between two fractions of heat is long enough. It has been observed with cells cultured in vitro (Henle and Dethlefsen 1978) and with normal tissues (Field and Anderson 1982) and tumors (Kamura et al. 1982) in experimental animals. Thermotolerance can also be induced by continuous heating at temperatures below 42.5° C (or other temperatures, depending on the cell line or tissue under investigation, cf. Field and Morris 1983; Nielsen 1986).

Thermotolerance for heat radiosensitization has been observed with several cell lines cultured in vitro. In vivo, the effect has been observed in tumors (Nielsen et al. 1983), in skin (Law et al. 1979; Wondergem and Haveman 1984), and in intestine (Hume and Marigold 1985) after a priming heat treatment and in intestine also after continuous heating (Marigold and Hume 1983). Conflicting results in this respect were obtained by Nielsen (1983), using cultured murine L1A2 cells. Nielsen did not observe any influence of thermotolerance on heat radiosensitization. The conclusion from the other results is often that the influence of thermotolerance on heat radiosensitization is relatively small compared to its influence on direct heat-induced cell lethality. This is related to the fact that different cellular targets are involved in heat-induced cell killing and heat radiosensitization.

The radiosensitizer misonidazole has been used extensively in experimental studies and in clinical trials as a drug which sensitizes hypoxic cells in tumors to irradiation (Brown 1975; Denekamp et al. 1980; Fowler et al. 1976). Misonidazole may also exhibit a direct cytotoxic effect on hypoxic cells (Brown 1977). The hypoxic cell toxicity is related to the electron affinic properties of the drug. Several studies have shown that hyperthermia and low pH are able to enhance the direct cytotoxicity of misonidazole (Bleehen et al. 1978; Hall et al. 1977; Rajaratnam et al. 1982; Stratford and Adams 1977).

The following sections will be used to describe a selection of experimental results concerning the influence of pH, thermotolerance, and hypoxia and misonidazole on thermal enhancement of radiation effects. The experimental work on normal tissues in this respect will be mentioned only briefly as it is treated elsewhere (Hume, this volume); in this chapter mainly work on cultured cells and on thermal enhancement of radiation effects in transplantable tumors will be discussed.

pH

The results in Fig. 1 (Haveman 1983b) show the influence of pH in the range from 6.5 to 8.5 on the enhancement by heat of the effects of 3.5-Gy X-rays. It is clear from the data in this figure that M8013 cells resist combined treatment best be-

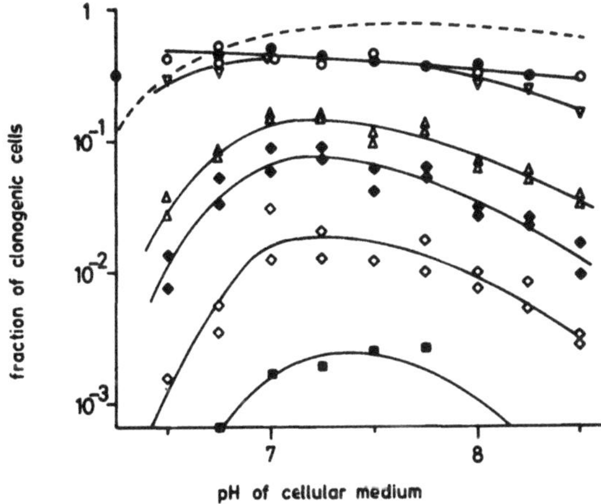

Fig. 1. Influence of the pH of the cellular medium on the effectiveness of irradiation and heat treatment. The M8013 cells were kept for 60 min in buffered Hanks' balanced salt solution and irradiated halfway during this period as described by Haveman (1983b); radiation dose: 3.5 Gy. ○, without heat treatment; ●, irradiated at 37° C in buffered Hanks' balanced salt solution 4 h and 15 min after a prior 30-min 42° C treatment in culture medium; ▽, irradiated halfway during heat treatment, 30 min at 41° C; △, irradiated during heat treatment, 30 min at 42° C; ◇, irradiated during heat treatment, 30 min at 43° C; ◆, irradiated during heat treatment, 30 min at 43° C 4 h after prior treatment as above; ■, irradiated during heat treatment, 30 min at 44° C 4 h after prior treatment as above. The *dashed curve* is redrawn from survival data after 30 min at 43° C without irradiation. After 30 min at 41° C or 42° C survival of the cells was not significantly different from control cells in the pH rage 6.5-8.5

tween pH 7.0 and 7.5. Radiosensitization is relatively strong below pH 7.0 and above pH 7.8.

Generally in the literature only two or few pH values are compared. Freeman and Malcolm (1985), for instance, showed that thermal radiosensitization was increased when Chinese hamster ovary (CHO) cells were treated at pH 6.8 compared to pH 7.2, independent of the media used (either McCoy's medium containing fetal bovine serum or glucose-free Hanks' balanced salt solution).

Holahan et al. (1984) correlated the thermal enhancement ratios (TERs) (calculated from the final slope data of the radiation survival curves, $1/D_0$) with the cell-killing effects of heat alone (Fig. 2). They observed that TER increased continuously with increasing cell-killing effect of the 45.5° C heat treatment alone in G1 phase CHO cells. Moreover, data on TER (D_0) obtained from experiments performed at pH 6.75 and 7.4 as a function of cell killing after heat only could be approximated by the same curve. This latter observation indicates that the degree of cell killing induced by heating, whatever the pH, may predict the degree of radiosensitization to be provoked by the same heat treatment. pH apparently modifies heat-induced cell killing and TER equally.

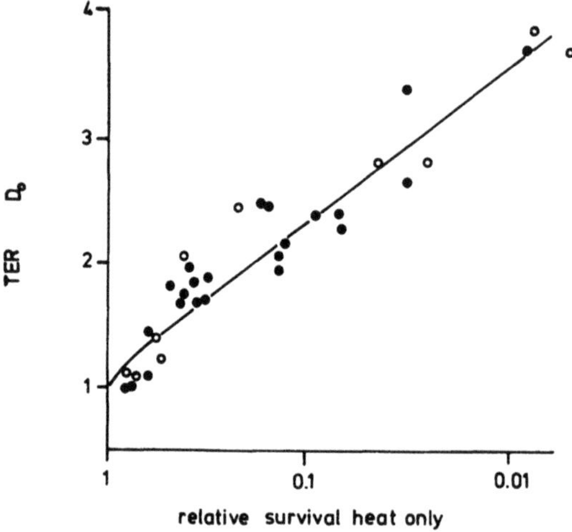

Fig. 2. Thermal enhancement ratios (ratio of D_os of heated G1 phase CHO cells as a function of heat-induced damage expressed as survival after heat treatment alone (redrawn from Holahan et al. 1984). The cells were heated at 45.5° C for various durations at pH 7.4 *(closed symbols)* or 6.75 *(open symbols)* and then incubated, without changing the pH, at 37° C for 10 min before irradiation. The cellular medium during heating (modified McCoy's medium) contained fetal calf serum. Changing the pH to a lower value was done by flushing the cell medium with an air mixture with enhanced CO_2 pressure

Thermotolerance

A decreased radiosensitization by heat, leading to lower TER values, as a result of thermotolerance has been reported in several in vitro studies with different cell lines, using both continuous heating at a relatively low temperature (Holahan et al. 1984; Raaphorst and Azzam 1983) and a priming heat treatment (Hartson-Eaton et al. 1984; Henle et al. 1979; Haveman 1983 (a, b); van Rijn et al. 1984; Holahan et al. 1986; Haveman et al. 1986). The influence of thermotolerance on radiosensitization is well illustrated in Fig. 3: The effectiveness of the heat treatment in thermotolerant cells is equivalent to a treatment at a 1° C lower temperature in nontolerant cells. When TER (D_o) was considered as a function of the cell-killing effects of heat treatment alone, thermotolerance did not seem to have any influence in either the data of Haveman et al. (1986) on asynchronous M8013 cells or those of Holahan et al. (1986) on G1 phase Chinese hamster ovary cells (Figs. 4, 5). These latter observations suggest that thermotolerance modifies the effectiveness of hyperthermia for direct cell killing and radiosensitization equally in both cell lines. The TER values calculated from the 45.5° C data on CHO cells of Holahan et al. (1984, 1986) are lower than those obtained with M8013 cells by Haveman et al. (1986). Holahan et al. did not irradiate during heat treatment but they used a 10-min interval at 37° C between heat and irradiation. Whether this explains the lower TER values is not certain: in M8013 cells a 10-min interval would not lead to much lower TER values when radiation is applied shortly after heating (cf. Figs. 6, 7), while in CHO cells it might be important (see the discussion by Hahn

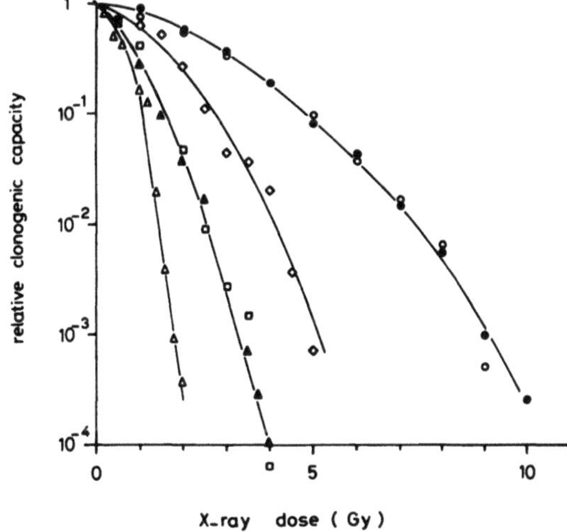

Fig. 3. Radiation survival curves of M8013 cells treated in culture medium, pH 7.3. ○, ●: irradiated at 37° C. △, □, ◇, ▲: irradiated halfway during a 30-min heat treatment at 45° C, 44° C, 43° C, and 45° C respectively. *Open symbols:* nontolerant cells; *closed symbols:* thermotolerant cells, heated for 30 min at 43° C, 5½ h prior to irradiation. The datum points are all based on the average of data from two or three dishes. The data are corrected for the effect of heat only, so that all curves start at unity. After 30-min heat treatment alone at 43°, 44°, and 45° C, relative clonogenic capacity was 0.90, 0.47, and 0.14 respectively with nontolerant cells; after similar heat treatment at 45° C it was 0.74 with thermotolerant cells. Note that there is no difference in radiosensitivity between nontolerant and thermotolerant cells at 37° C

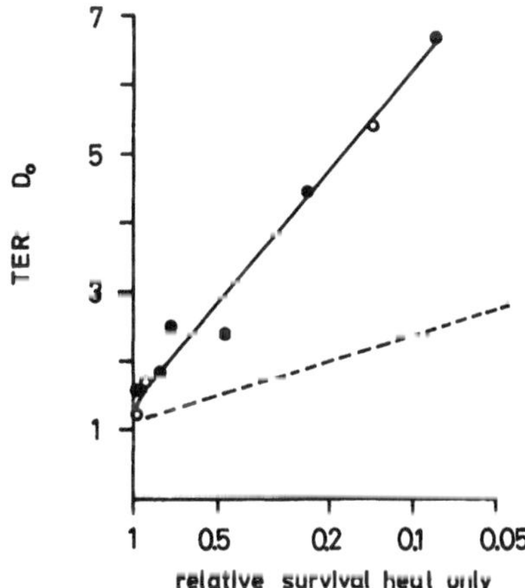

Fig. 4. Thermal enhancement ratios as a function of the cell-killing effect of heat treatment alone. The cells were irradiated halfway through a 30-min hyperthermic treatment at various temperatures as described by Haveman et al. (1986). The cells were kept in Eagle's minimum essential medium with fetal calf serum during treatment. *Open symbols,* nontolerant asynchronous M8013 cells; *closed symbols,* thermotolerant cells. Thermotolerance was induced by a priming heat treatment, 5 h before combined treatment. The *dashed curve* in this figure is redrawn from Fig. 2. (This figure is reproduced with kind permission from the editors of the International Journal of Radiation Biology)

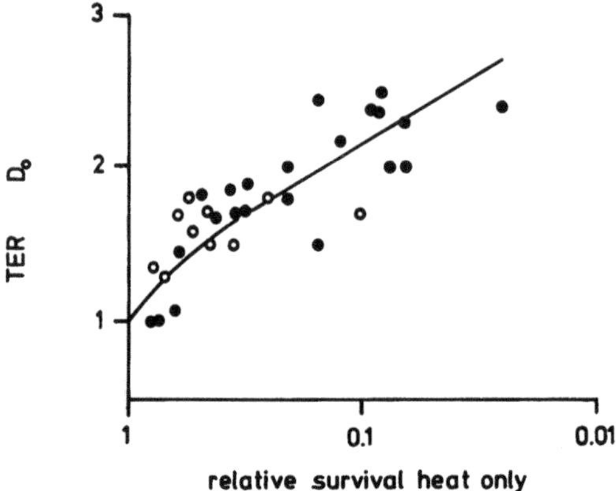

Fig. 5. Thermal enhancement ratios plotted as a function of the cell-killing effect of a 45.5° C heat treatment for various durations (redrawn from data by Holahan et al. 1986). TER values were calculated from D_0. *Open symbols:* thermotolerant cells, thermotolerance was induced by a priming heat treatment to G1 phase cells 12 or 24 h before the final heat treatment at 45.5° C. *Closed symbols,* nontolerant G1 phase CHO cells. The interval between heat treatment at 45.5° C and X-irradiation was 10 min

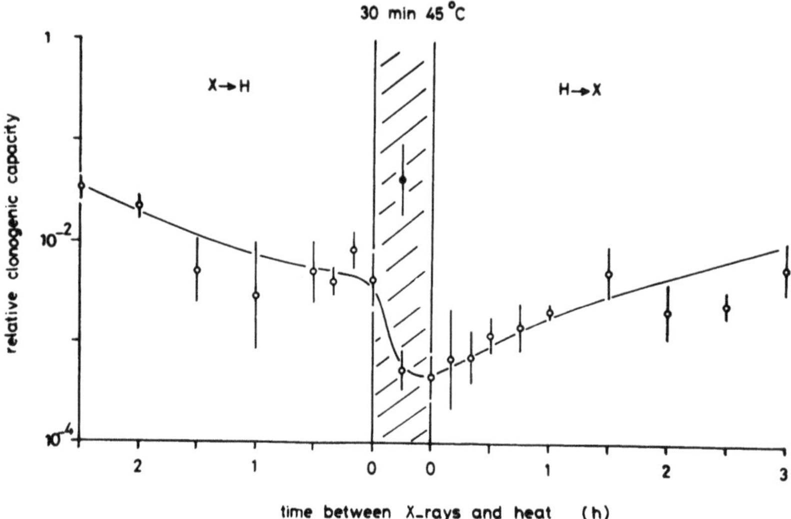

Fig. 6. Influence of the interval between heat treatment (30 min at 45° C) and X-irradiation (1.50 Gy). The M8013 cells were treated in culture medium containing fetal calf serum, pH approximately 7.3, as described by Haveman et al. (1986). *Open symbols,* survival of cells after heat *plus* X-rays; *closed symbol,* survival after only the heat treatment. Irradiation with 1.50 Gy alone would reduce the fraction of clonogenic cells to approximately 0.65

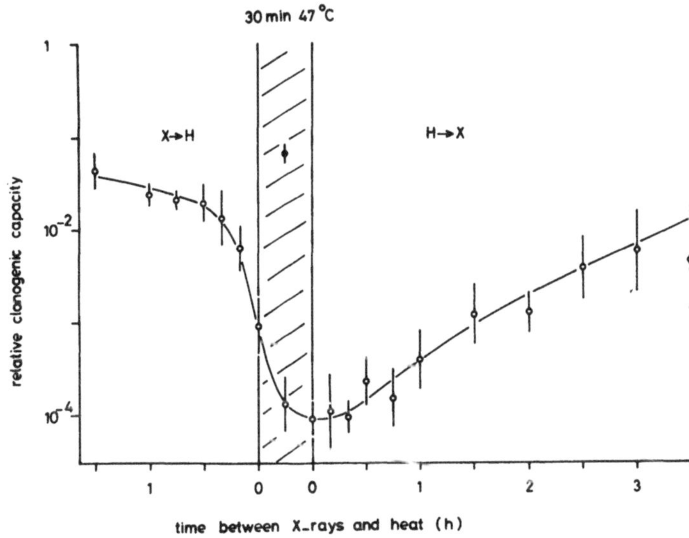

Fig. 7. Influence of the interval between heat treatment (30 min at 47° C) and X-irradiation (1.00 Gy) in thermotolerant M8013 cells. Thermotolerance was induced by 30-min treatment at 43° C, always exactly 5 h prior to the treatment at 47° C. *Open symbols*, survival of cells after heat *plus* X-rays; *closed symbol*, survival after only heat treatment. Irradiation with 1.00 Gy alone would reduce the fraction of clonogenic cells to approximately 0.8

1982). Apart from the differences in cell lines, the fact that Holahan et al. used G1 phase cells might also play a role.

The data on TER in Figs. 2, 4, and 5 do not show a maximum in TER below some level of cell survival. In both cell lines TER increases continuously with increased cell killing by hyperthermia alone, in M8013 cells even up to TER values of approximately 7.

Based on the in vitro observations mentioned above, Haveman et al. (1983) suggested that several in vivo results could also be explained by equal modification by thermotolerance of the direct effects of heat and the effects of heat radiosensitization. The influence of thermotolerance on direct heat effects and on TER in studies on mouse foot deformity was equivalent to a reduction in the effective temperature of about 1° C in both cases (cf Haveman et al. 1986; Wondergem and Haveman 1985). Hume and Marigold (1980, 1985), using another priming heat treatment to induce thermotolerance, observed a reduction in the effective temperature of 0.5° C as a result of thermotolerance for direct heat effects and for thermal enhancement of radiation effects in mouse intestine. As the effects of hyperthermia on tissues in animal experiments may interfere with those of irradiation, it is often not easy to obtain TER values which reflect merely radiosensitization. Therefore it is difficult to correlate TER with the effectiveness of only the heat treatment, as is done in Figs. 4 and 5. Moreover, in animal experiments on TER often a heat dose is employed which would not lead to "visible" damage at the end point used when applied alone. Still, in our opinion the observations on normal tissues mentioned above indicate that thermotolerance modifies the effects of heat

(i. e., its direct effects and its effect on radiosensitization) in the same way in vitro and in vivo.

Hypoxia and Misonidazole

In this section we switch from cells in vitro to transplantable mouse tumors. Several studies have shown that mouse tumors become progressively more resistant to X-irradiation with increasing tumor volume (Haveman et al. 1981; Shipley et al. 1975; Stanley et al. 1977; Wondergem et al. 1981). Moreover, pentobarbitone sodium, an anesthetic which is frequently used in animal experiments, influences the radiation response of large solid tumors by rendering them more radioresistant (Denekamp et al. 1979; Sheldon and Chu 1979; Sheldon et al. 1977). The radioresistance that developed with the increase in volume and with the anesthetic disappeared after administration of the hypoxic cell radiosensitizer misonidazole. This indicates that the influence of volume on radiosensitivity is mainly a result of a large fraction of hypoxic cells in larger tumors. The hypoxic cells in question are presumably mainly "chronically" hypoxic. Pentobarbital anesthesia affects radiosensitivity apparently by further increasing the fraction of hypoxic cells. The increase in the number of hypoxic cells resulting from anesthesia involves "acutely" hypoxic cells. The hypoxic cell fraction may be more than 50% (Wondergem et al. 1981) in large M8013 tumors (murine mammary carcinoma) in anesthetized animals.

The results shown in Fig. 8 nicely illustrate the consequences of an increase in the fraction of hypoxic cells with regard to sensitivity to irradiation, to hyperthermia, or to combined treatment with X-rays and heat. These experiments show that there is no change in sensitivity to hyperthermia with increasing tumor volume. Although hypoxic cells presumably are more sensitive to heat treatment compared with well oxygenated cells, we could not demonstrate that increased sensitivity to heat alone resulted from the larger number of hypoxic cells with increasing tumor volume. Probably the regrowth of a tumor after single heat treatment is mainly determined by the size of the heat-resistant cell fraction. As mentioned above, the large hypoxic cell fraction in tumors in anesthetized animals mainly involves acutely hypoxic cells: the chronically hypoxic cell fraction does not increase to more than about 5%–11% in large (~300 mm^3) tumors. The fact that the very large increase in the fraction of acutely hypoxic cells does not enhance the effect of a hyperthermic treatment indicates that acutely hypoxic cells do not show an enhanced sensitivity to heat.

When hyperthermia is combined with radiation a large percentage of the well oxygenated cells are killed by the X-rays. This will lead to a relatively greater contribution of the increase in chronically hypoxic cell fraction with regard to the effects of heat treatment (Fig. 8 a, top curve).

Results on TCD^{50} (radiation dose required to control 50% of the treated tumors) are given in Table 1. TERs in these data never exceed a corresponding sensitizer enhancement ratio. This indicates that in these experiments all thermal enhancement may be explained by effects of heat on the chronically hypoxic cell fraction. The effects of heat in this respect resemble those of the radiosensitizer misonida-

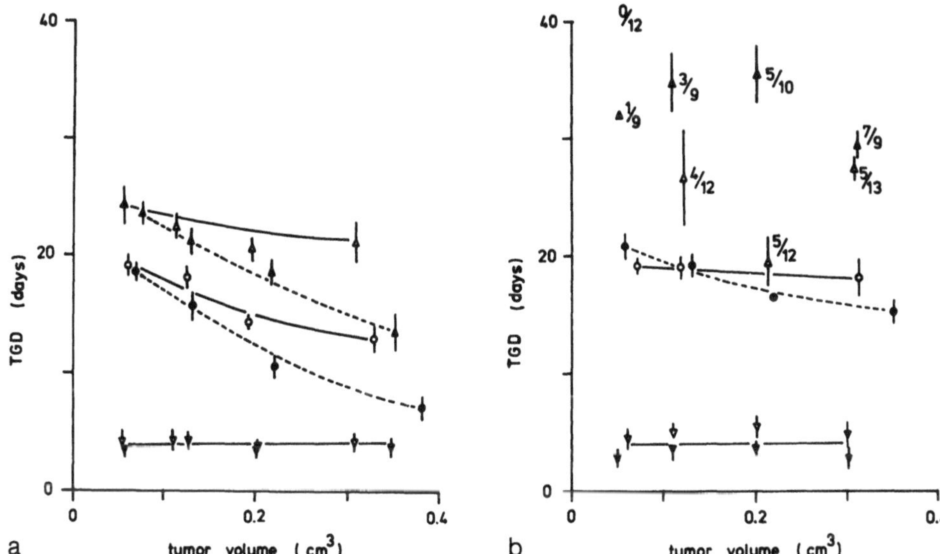

Fig. 8a, b. Tumor growth delay *(TGD)* as a result of treatment of transplantable M8013 tumors in D_2B mice with irradiation at 15 Gy (O, ●), with hyperthermia for 1 h at 43° C (▽, ▼), or with irradiation immediately followed by hyperthermia for 1 h at 43° C (△, ▲). The mice were treated without *(open symbols)* or with *(closed symbols)* anesthesia (50 mg/kg body weight pentobarbital sodium). Results are shown for mice treated **a** without and **b** with misonidazole (0.5 g/kg body weight, 30 min before irradiation). The *error bars* represent ± SEM (8-12 mice per treatment group). If tumor cures were observed in a treatment group, the fraction of animals that were not cured is given next to the datum point; the fraction 0/12 in one case indicates that no animal could contribute to data on TGD. The data in this figure are redrawn from Wondergem et al. (1982)

zole. A contribution of more radiosensitization by heat could not be observed in these data (cf Wondergem et al. 1982). It must be kept in mind that neither of the end points studied, TGD and TCD^{50}, is able to discriminate between direct heat effects and thermal radiosensitization. Nevertheless, thermal radiosensitization has been observed in tumor experiments where the sequence and interval between heat and X-rays was changed. These experiments will not be discussed here (cf Hahn 1982).

Misonidazole strikingly enhances the effects of heat + X-rays (cf. Fig. 8 and Table 1) when all three modalities are combined. The "extra" effect of the "sensitizer" may presumably be explained by an enhanced cytotoxicity of misonidazole toward hypoxic cells in tumors under hyperthermic conditions. The enhanced cytotoxicity was not observed after hyperthermia alone as the changes in hypoxic cell fraction in the tumor volume range 50-350 mm³ are relatively small. Killing of a fixed proportion of well oxygenated cells by X-rays makes the contribution of the changes in the fraction of chronically hypoxic cells more important, also in this respect. The large increase in the hypoxic cell fraction as a result of anesthesia does not further enhance the cytotoxic effects of misonidazole; this indicates that it is not hypoxia as such which leads to the enhanced cytotoxicity and that factors

Table 1. TCD^{50} (Gy) values, calculated thermal enhancement ratios (*TER* = TCD^{50} radiation alone/TCD^{50} radiation with heat), and sensitizer enhancement ratios (*SER* = TCD^{50} treatment without/with sensitizer) for 100 mm^3 and 300 mm^3 M8013 tumors in mice. Treatment with irradiation was immediately followed by heating for 60 min at 43° C. Mice were treated with or without anesthesia (50 mg/kg pentobarbital sodium). Misonidazole was administered at a dose of 0.5 g/kg body weight 30 min before irradiation. The 95% confidence intervals were determined using the Litchfield-Wilcoxon Method (Litchfield and Wilcoxon 1949). In each TCD^{50} experiment 40-50 mice were used. Data in this table are from Wondergem et al. (1982)

Treatment	TCD^{50} (Gy) with 95% confidence intervals		TER	SER (X)	SER (X+H)
	X alone	X + heat			
100 m^3 tumors					
Without anesthesia	35.0 (32.7-37.4)	21.5 (20.3-22.7)	1.6		
With anesthesia	35.0 (33.3-36.8)	29.5 (27.5-31.6)	1.2		
Misonidazole (without anesthesia)	21.5 (19.4-23.8)	15.0 (12.8-17.5)	1.4	1.6	1.4
Misonidazole (with anesthesia)	22.5 (21.2-23.8)	15.0 (13.8-16.3)	1.5	1.6	1.4
300 m^3 tumors					
Without anesthesia	45.2 (42.6-47.9)	23.0 (21.1-25.1)	2.0		
With anesthesia	50.0 (47.2-53.0)	32.5 (30.5-34.7)	1.6		
Misonidazole (without anesthesia)	22.5 (20.7-24.5)	15.0 (12.4-18.1)	1.5	2.0	1.5
Misonidazole (with anesthesia)	22.5 (20.8-24.4)	15.0 (12.6-17.9)	1.5	2.0	1.5

like the pH and nutritional state also play a role. In vitro results of Stratford and Adams (1977) indeed showed enhanced cytotoxicity of misonidazole at low pH. Perhaps the increased acidity in the tumor as a result of chronic hypoxia causes the enhanced sensitivity toward misonidazole during hyperthermia which emerges in the experiments where heat, X-rays, and the drug are combined.

Conclusion

Both pH and thermotolerance influenced heat-induced cell killing and thermal radiosensitization equally. In other words: the degree of radiosensitization could be predicted from the direct effects of heat, regardless of pH or thermotolerance. Although this conclusion was reached from experiments on cells in vitro, it presumably also applies to the situation in vivo. Some results from experiments on normal tissues, indeed, may clearly be explained in this way.

Experiments by us on combined treatment of a murine tumor (M8013) with radiation and heat did not show radiosensitization in spite of the fact that the heat treatment immediately followed X-irradiation. All "thermal" enhancement could be explained by effects of heat on chronically hypoxic cells.

In experiments with misonidazole it appeared that, apart from the radiosensitizing effect on both chronically and acutely hypoxic cells, misonidazole greatly enhanced the effect of heat combined with irradiation. This latter effect of misonidazole is explained by enhanced cytotoxicity of the drug toward chronically hypoxic tumor cells under hyperthermic conditions.

References

Bleehen NM, Honess DJ, Morgan JE (1978) The combined effects of hyperthermia and hypoxic cell sensitizers. In: Streffer C et al. (eds) Cancer therapy by hyperthermia and radiation. Urban and Schwarzenberg, Baltimore, pp 62-71

Bronk BV (1976) Thermal potentiation of mammalian cell killing: clues for understanding and potential for tumor therapy. Adv Radiat Biol 6: 276-324

Brown JM (1975) Selective radiosensitization of the hypoxic cells of mouse tumors with the nitroimidazoles metronidazole and RO-07-0582. Radiat Res 64: 633-647

Brown JM (1977) Cytotoxic effects of the hypoxic cell radiosensitizer RO-07-0582 to tumor cells in vivo. Radiat Res 72: 469-486

Denekamp J, Terry NHA, Sheldon PW, Chu AM (1979) The effect of pentobarbital anesthesia on the radiosensitivity of four mouse tumours. Int J Radiat Biol 35: 277-280

Denekamp J, Hirst DG, Stewart FA, Terry NHA (1980) Is tumour radiosensitization by misonidazole a general phenomenon? Br J Cancer 41: 1-9

Elkind MM, Whitmore GF (1967) The radiobiology of cultured mammalian cells. Gordon and Breach, New York

Field SB, Anderson RL (1982) Thermotolerance: a review of observations and possible mechanisms. Nat Cancer Inst Monogr 61: 193-199

Field SB, Morris CC (1983) The relationship between heating time and temperature: its relevance to clinical hyperthermia. Radiother Oncol 1: 179-186

Fowler JF, Adams GE, Denekamp J (1976) Radiosensitizers of hypoxic cells in solid tumours. Cancer Treat Rev 3: 227-256

Freeman ML, Malcolm A (1985) Acid modification of thermal damage and its relationship to nutrient availability. Int J Radiat Oncol Biol Phys 11: 1823-1826

Hahn GM (1982) Hyperthermia and cancer. Plenum, New York

Hall EJ, Astor M, Geard C, Biaglow J (1977) Cytotoxicity of RO-07-0582; enhancement by hyperthermia and protection by cysteamine. Br J Cancer 35: 809-815

Hartson-Eaton M, Malcolm AW, Hahn GM (1984) Radiosensitivity and thermosensitization of thermotolerant Chinese hamster cells and RIF-1 tumors. Radiat Res 99: 175-184

Haveman J (1983a) Influence of a prior heat treatment on the enhancement by hyperthermia of X-ray induced inactivation of cultured mammalian cells. Int J Radiat Biol 43: 267-280

Haveman J (1983b) Influence of pH and thermotolerance on the enhancement of X-ray induced inactivation of cultured mammalian cells by hyperthermia. Int J Radiat Biol 43: 281-289

Haveman J (1986) Enhancement of radiation effects by hyperthermia. In: Anghileri LJ, Robert J (eds) Hyperthermia in cancer treatment, vol I. CRC, Boca Raton, Florida, pp 169-181

Haveman J, Jansen W, van der Schueren E, Breur K (1981) Radiosensitivity of microscopic tumours of a transplantable mammary adenocarcinoma in mice. Br J Cancer 43: 864-870

Haveman J, Hart AAM, Wondergem J (1987) Thermal radiosensitization and thermotolerance in cultured cells from a murine mammary carcinoma. Int J Radiat Biol 51: 71-80

Henle KJ, Dethlefsen LA (1978) Heat fractionation and thermotolerance: a review. Cancer Res 38: 1843-1851

Henle KJ, Tomasovic SP, Dethlefsen LA (1979) Fractionation of combined heat and radiation in asynchronous CHO cells. 1. Effects on radiation sensitivity. Radiat Res 80: 369-377

Holahan EV, Highfield DP, Holahan PK, Dewey WC (1984) Hyperthermic killing and hyperthermic radiosensitization in Chinese hamster ovary cells: effects of pH and thermal tolerance. Radiat Res 97: 108-131

Holahan PK, Wong RSL, Thompson LL, Dewey WC (1986) Hyperthermic radiosensitization of thermotolerant Chinese hamster ovary cells. Radiat Res 107: 332-343

Hume SP, Marigold JCL (1980) Transient heat-induced thermal resistance in the small intestine of mouse. Radiat Res 82: 526-535

Hume SP, Marigold JCL (1985) Time-temperature relationships for hyperthermal radiosensitization in mouse intestine: influence of thermotolerance. Radiother Oncol 3: 165-171

Kamura T, Nielsen OS, Overgaard J, Andersen AM (1982) Development of thermotolerance during fractionated hyperthermia in a solid tumor in vivo. Cancer Res 42: 1744-1748

Law MP, Ahier RG, Field SB (1979) The effect of prior heat treatment on the thermal enhancement of radiation damage in the mouse ear. Br J Radiol 52: 315-321

Litchfield JF, Wilcoxon F (1949) A simplified method of evaluating dose effect experiments. J Pharmacol Exp Ther 96: 99-113

Marigold JCL, Hume SP (1983) Effect of prolonged heating on the thermal enhancement ratio in X-irradiated murine intestine. Int J Radiat Biol 44: 285-291

Nielsen OS (1983) Influence of thermotolerance on the interaction between hyperthermia and radiation in L1A2 cells in vitro. Int J Radiat Biol 43: 665-673

Nielsen OS (1986) Evidence for an upper temperature limit for thermotolerance development in L1A2 tumour cells in vitro. Int J Hyperthermia 2: 299-309

Nielsen OS, Overgaard J, Kamura J (1983) Influence of thermotolerance on the interaction between hyperthermia and radiation in a solid tumour in vivo. Br J Radiol 56: 267-273

Raaphorst GP, Azzam EI (1983) Thermal radiosensitization in Chinese hamster (V79) and mouse C3H 10T½ cells. The thermotolerance effect. Br J Cancer 48: 45-54

Rajaratnam S, Adams GE, Stratford IJ, Clarke C (1982) Enhancement of the cytotoxicity of radiosensitizers by modest hyperthermia: the electron affinity relationship. Br J Cancer 46: 912-917

Sheldon PW, Chu AM (1979) The effects of anesthetics on the radiosensitivity of a murine tumor. Radiat Res 79: 568-578

Sheldon PW, Hill SA, Moulder JE (1977) Radioprotection by pentobarbitone sodium of a murine tumour in vivo. Int J Radiat Biol 32: 571-575

Shipley WU, Stanley JA, Steel GG (1975) Tumor size dependency in the radiation response of the Lewis lung carcinoma. Cancer Res 35: 2488-2493

Stanley JA, Shipley WA, Steel GG (1977) Influence of tumour size on hypoxic fraction and therapeutic sensitivity of Lewis' tumour. Br J Cancer 36: 105-113

Stratford IJ, Adams GE (1977) Effect of hyperthermia on differential toxicity of a hypoxic cell sensitizer RO-07-0582, on mammalian cells in vitro. Br J Cancer 35: 307-313

Van Rijn J, van der Berg J, Schamhart DHJ, Van Wijk R (1984) Effect of thermotolerance on thermal radiosensitization in hepatoma cells. Radiat Res 97: 318-328

Wondergem J, Haveman J (1984) A study on the effects of prior heat treatment on the skin reaction of mouse feet after heat alone or combined with X-rays: influence of misonidazole. Radioth Oncol 2: 159-170

Wondergem J, Haveman J (1985) Thermal enhancement of the radiation damage in the mouse foot at different heat and radiation dose: influence of thermotolerance. Int J Radiat Biol 48: 337-348

Wondergem J, Haveman J, van der Schueren E, van der Hoeven H, Breur K (1981) The influence of misonidazole on the radiation response of murine tumors of different size: possible artifacts caused by pentobarbital sodium anesthesia. Int J Radiat Oncol Biol Phys 7: 755-760

Wondergem J, Haveman J, van der Schueren E, van der Hoeven H, Breur K (1982) Effect of hyperthermia and misonidazole on the radiosensitivity of a transplantable murine tumor: influence of factors modifying the fraction of hypoxic cells. Int J Radiat Oncol Biol Phys 8: 1323-1331

Thermal Enhancement of Drug Cytotoxicity in Vivo and in Vitro

D. J. Honess and N. M. Bleehen*

Medical Research Council Clinical Oncology and Radiotherapeutics Unit, MRC Centre, Hills Road, Cambridge CB2 2QH, Great Britain

Introduction

Hyperthermia as an adjunct to conventional radiotherapy is currently being extensively tested throughout the world, but interest in its use as a potentiator of conventional chemotherapy is less widespread. Nonetheless, its efficacy in enhancing the cytotoxicity of a variety of commonly used antitumour agents, particularly the alkylating agents, is now well established. The possibility of treating a patient with a systemically administered drug and dramatically potentiating its activity exclusively at the site of a tumour by means of locally applied hyperthermia is an attractive one. It is especially so because significant potentiation can be achieved with relatively modest temperature increases. In view of the difficulties being encountered in many clinics in heating some tumours to the desired minimum temperature, usually around 43° C, the potential benefits of thermo-chemotherapy must be increasingly recognised.

This paper reviews some of our previous work and presents some new data to illustrate the value of thermal enhancement of common anticancer agents, with particular emphasis on melphalan.

Initial in Vivo Studies with Anticancer Drugs in Tumour and Skin

Initial studies were carried out with the EMT6 tumour using a waterbath heating technique, with mice under pentabarbitone anaesthesia but with minimal restraint. Using leg tumours, with response assayed by regrowth delay, thermal potentiation was demonstrated for the toxicity of 133 mg kg^{-1} cyclophosphamide (CTX) given intraperitoneally (Table 1). Drug-induced growth delay was 6.5 days in heated mice compared with about 1 day in unheated animals. In contrast, no potentiation was found for 15 mg kg^{-1} intravenous bleomycin (BLM), which produced only 1 day's delay in both heated and unheated animals (Table 1). Twentyman et al.

* We wish to thank J. J. Shaw for carrying out the experiments with RIF-1 suspension culture.

Table 1. Effect of heat (60 min at a waterbath temperature of 43.5° C) immediately after 133 mg kg^{-1} CTX or 15 mg kg^{-1} BLM on EMT6 leg tumours in Balb/C mice[a]

Treatment	n[b]	Time to reach 4 × treatment volume (days)	Drug-induced growth delay (days)
Unheated control	10	10.7 (10.0–11.3)[c]	–
CTX i.p. unheated	9	11.6 (10.9–12.3)	0.97
BLM i.v. unheated	11	11.9 (11.2–12.7)	1.3
Heat alone control	10	12.0 (10.3–13.7)	–
CTX i.p. heated	10	18.5 (15.8–21.2)	6.5
BLM i.v. heated	7	12.5 (11.2–13.8)	0.6

[a] All animals underwent pentobarbitone anaesthesia.
[b] n, number of animals per group.
[c] Figures in parentheses are 95% confidence limits.

(1978), using a waterbath temperature of 43° C, demonstrated potentiation of activity of BCNU at 20 mg kg^{-1} using both regrowth delay and clonogenic cell survival assays.

We also conducted a normal tissue study on mouse foot skin in anaesthetised Balb/C mice, using the same heating method. Since the response of skin to drugs is not readily assayed, a different approach was taken and drug enhancement of heat damage caused by 1 h at a waterbath temperature of 44° C was measured. Significant ($P<0.05$) enhancement by CTX at 133 mg kg^{-1} and BCNU at 20 mg kg^{-1} was found with dose modification factors of 1.3 and 1.2 respectively (Honess and Bleehen 1980). However, although single doses of BLM up to 25 mg kg^{-1} were ineffective, three fractions of 8.3 mg kg^{-1} BLM, each combined with 45 min × 44° C, caused significant potentiation of heat damage. Thus substantial interactions were found in normal tissue, which raised the question of whether there was a therapeutic gain for tumour over isothermal normal tissue, and prompted a more extensive programme of study.

Comparative Studies on Tumour and Normal Marrow

Measurement of Therapeutic Ratio

The normal tissue selected for comparison with tumour was bone marrow, being the dose-limiting target for the majority of alkylating agents tested. Experiments were carried out in C3H mice, with the KHT and RIF-1 tumours, without the use

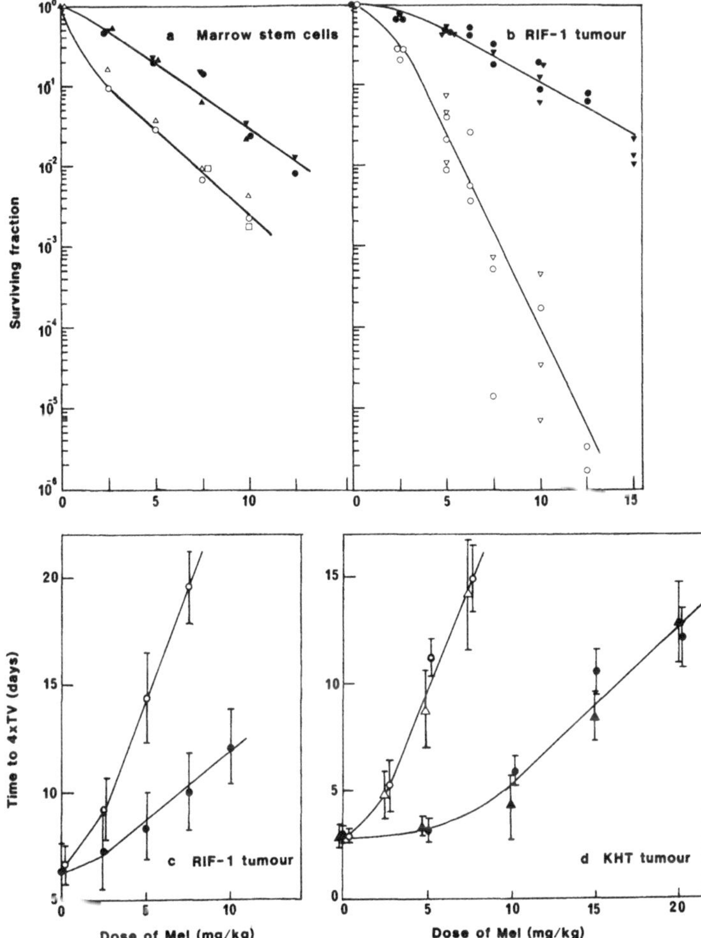

Fig. 1. The effect of 45 min systemic hyperthermia at 41° C on the response to melphalan of normal marrow stem cells assayed 24 h after treatment *(panel a)*, RIF-1 tumour assayed by clonogenic cell survival 24 h after treatment *(panel b)* and RIF-1 and KHT tumour assayed by regrowth delay *(panels c and d* respectively*)*. *Closed symbols* show data for unheated animals, *open symbols* for heated ones. Different symbols show data from different experiments. Lines were fitted by regression analysis in panels a and b and by eye in panels c and d. In panel a, each *point* is derived from the mean colony count for a group of 7-12 spleens. In panel b, each *point* shows the response of a single tumour from one animal. In panels c and d *error bars* show ± 2SE for groups of 7-11 animals. 4 × TV = 4 times treatment volume. (Reproduced from Honess and Bleehen 1985a, with permission)

of anaesthesia or restraint. Systemic hyperthermia (41° C) was used in order to guarantee isothermal treatment of both femoral marrow and tumour, which was grown intramuscularly in the leg. Full dose response curves were constructed for marrow and tumour in unheated and heated animals for a variety of agents; CTX, BCNU, CCNU, cis-platinum, chlorambucil and melphalan. Drugs were injected intraperitoneally at the start of heating (45 min at 41° C). Heat was found to potentiate drug toxicity equally in tumour and marrow for all agents except mephalan. For this one drug, potentiation was greater in tumour, and there was therapeutic gain (Honess and Bleehen 1982, 1985a, b). The magnitude of the effect is illustrated in Fig. 1. Therapeutic ratios (TRs) were calculated for a series of doses of drug in unheated animals by taking, for each dose, the ratio of the isoeffect dose with heat in marrow to that in tumour. TR values of up to 2.0 were calculated for melphalan in KHT tumour and rather less for RIF-1, up to 1.6 (Honess and Bleehen 1985a), demonstrating substantial therapeutic gain for the combination.

Scheduling

Using melphalan, the timing of drug administration was found to be very critical. Maximum potentiation in both the KHT tumour and marrow was obtained when drug was given at the start of heating, although some potentiation was found in KHT when the start of heat was delayed for 30 min (Honess and Bleehen 1985a). Subsequent pharmacokinetic studies using the RIF-1 tumour (Honess et al 1985) provide a reason for this. The melphalan concentration peak was fairly broad, from 10-20 min after i.p. injection, and at times later than 20 min, melphalan concentrations were higher in heated animals in both plasma and tumour. However, by 40 min after injection (at almost the end of heating) drug concentrations had dropped substantially, the plasma half-life being about 25 min. Hence the greater the delay between drug injection and the start of heating, the smaller the drug concentrations available for potentiation. This short duration of relatively high drug concentrations in the tumour explains why heat and drug must be given simultaneously for maximum potentiation. This observation has also been made in other model systems (Dahl and Mella 1983).

Effect of Cell Environment

Leg tumours used in the studies summarised above were grown intramuscularly and were treated at 300-600 mm^3 in size. It is thought probable that a large proportion of cells in tumours of this size are likely to be subject to conditions which may increase drug potentiation by heat. Low pH, for example, has been shown to enhance the degree of thermal potentiation of another alkylating agent, BCNU (Hahn and Shiu 1983). Hypoxia and general nutritional deprivation existing in tumours of this size would also be expected to increase thermally potentiated drug damage. The possibility that therapeutic gain for melphalan could be attributed to the relatively poor nutritional milieu of the tumour cells compared with those in marrow was investigated by measuring melphalan heat potentiation in tumour cell microcolonies in the lung. These microcolonies, comprising two to eight cells at the time of treatment, were assayed by their ability to survive to form macrocolonies by 17 (for KHT) or 24 (for RIF-1) days after initiation. Melphalan potentiation proved to be greater in microtumours than in marrow, again resulting in therapeutic gain, but this was somewhat smaller for microtumours than leg tumours (TR up to 1.6) (Honess and Bleehen 1985b). This difference was due to heat ap-

Table 2. Comparison of slopes of melphalan dose-response curves in unheated and heated animals. (Data taken from Honess and Bleehen 1985a, b)

Tissue	Treatment details	Slope (mg^{-1} kg)		Heated: unheated
		Unheated	Heated	
KHT tumour	Lung microtumour treated 3 days after initiation	0.16 (0.09-0.24)[a]	0.37 (0.28-0.46)	2.3 (1.1-3.5)
	Lung microtumour treated 4 days after initiation	0.12 (0.09-0.15)	0.34 (0.16-0.52)	2.9 (1.3-4.5)
	Leg tumour treated at 300-600 mm^3 (growth delay assay)	0.76[b]	1.9[b]	2.5
RIF-1 tumour	Lung microtumour treated 4 days after initiation	0.23 (0.17-0.29)	0.90 (0.39-1.41)	4.0 (2.6-5.4)
	Leg tumour treated at 300-600 mm^3 (clonogenic assay)	0.31 (0.26-0.35)	1.26 (1.04-1.49)	4.1 (3.1-5.0)
	Leg tumour treated at 300-600 mm^3 (growth delay assay)	0.54[b]	2.1[b]	3.9
Marrow	Femoral marrow CFUs assay	0.36 (0.34-0.39)	0.51 (0.46-0.57)	1.41 (1.22-1.59)

[a] Figures in parentheses are 95% confidence limits.
[b] Units are day mg^{-1} kg.

parently eliminating more of the shoulder of the dose-response curves in the leg tumours than in microtumours, these differences in the shoulder region affecting the estimate of TR. However, comparison of the heat-induced changes in the slope of the melphalan dose-response curves in both systems shows that the changes are remarkably consistent for each tumour (Table 2). The increase for KHT is from 2.3 to 2.9, and for RIF-1 from 3.9 to 4.0. The conclusions from the study were two-fold: firstly, that cell environmental differences between microtumours and 300-600 mm^3 tumours apparently can influence the size of the shoulder of the response curve; secondly, that each tumour type has an inherent capacity for potentiation of melphalan damage at this heat dose, and that this is greater than that of marrow, where the factor is only 1.4 (Table 2). This difference in change of slope is the major determinant of therapeutic gain.

Blood Flow Considerations

Blood flow is of great importance in local hyperthermia in determining the temperatures achieved in areas of differing blood flow, or where heat can variously modify that flow. It is of crucial importance in thermo-chemotherapy for the delivery of the drug to be potentiated. In our systemic hyperthermia system, with isothermal tissue and blood, vascular cooling was not a problem. However, the well recognised apparent predisposition of tumour vasculature to occlusion by lower temperatures and/or thermal doses than are deleterious to normal tissue (e.g. Dewhirst et al. 1984; Dudar and Jain 1984) can be a disadvantage in thermo-chemotherapy if temperatures achieved are sufficient to block drug access. In our study, 41° C for 45 min is apparently below the threshold for tumour vascular compromise as reported by others (Dewhirst et al. 1984; Dudar and Jain 1984). We have not actually measured blood flow in heated leg tumours, but some of the pharmacokinetic data imply that some obstruction may have occurred. Plasma melphalan concentrations were elevated in heated animals by a factor of 2.5 to 4, whereas the factor in tumours was smaller, 1.5 to 2. There was no evidence for a difference in half-life of the drug in plasma and tumour; hence this observation may reflect some reduction in drug delivery. The large potentiation in tumour, however, far outweighed this difference. This observation illustrates the value of relatively low temperatures in thermo-chemotherapy, and emphasises the need to use thermal doses below the threshold for severe vascular occlusion, at least until the majority of the drug has reached its target. This requirement has obvious implications for scheduling.

Comparative Studies with Different Types of RIF-1 Cells in Vitro

One of several aims of studies on thermal potentiation of melphalan toxicity to RIF-1 in vitro was to measure the thermopotentiation attributable to heat alone under defined conditions. Hence the magnitude of the effect of physiological factors contributing to thermopotentiation in vivo might be inferred from any difference between in vitro and in vivo data. We have used RIF-1 cells grown and treated in suspension culture (avoiding trypsinisation) and also a melphalan-sensitive and a melphalan-resistant clone of RIF-1 cells, which were grown and treated in monolayer (which necessitated trypsinisation).

For suspension culture, cells were propagated in 500 ml microcarrier stirring flasks in Eagle's MEM with low serum concentration (5%) and treated as 15-ml samples in universal containers, each equipped with a stirring bar. After treatment, cells were plated into medium with the full 20% of serum for cell survival assay. Melphalan-sensitive (L16) and -resistant (L20) clones of RIF-1 were derived by others in this laboratory (Reeve and Twentyman 1983; Reeve et al. 1983) and were grown and treated in conventional monolayer, using medium with 20% serum at all times. Dose-response curves at 37° C and 41° C were obtained and are presented in Fig. 2. Slopes of the exponential parts of the curves are given in Table 3. Figure 2 shows clearly the difference in sensitivity to melphalan of L20 and L16, the doses to reduce survival to 0.1 ($dose_{0.1}$) being 6.9 and 1.6 mg kg^{-1} respectively at 37° C. RIF-1 suspension culture has intermediate sensitivity, the $dose_{0.1}$ being 2.4 mg kg^{-1} for a 60-min treatment (data not shown) and 3.8 mg kg^{-1} for a 45-min treatment. Melphalan sensitivity data have also been obtained at 37° for a single cell suspension of RIF-1 tumour cells obtained from 300-600 mm^3 leg tumours by enzymatic digestion with neutral protease and treated for 45 min under exactly the same conditions as the RIF-1 suspension cultures. The slope of the curve was very similar to that for RIF-1 suspension (see Table 3) although the $dose_{0.1}$ was some-

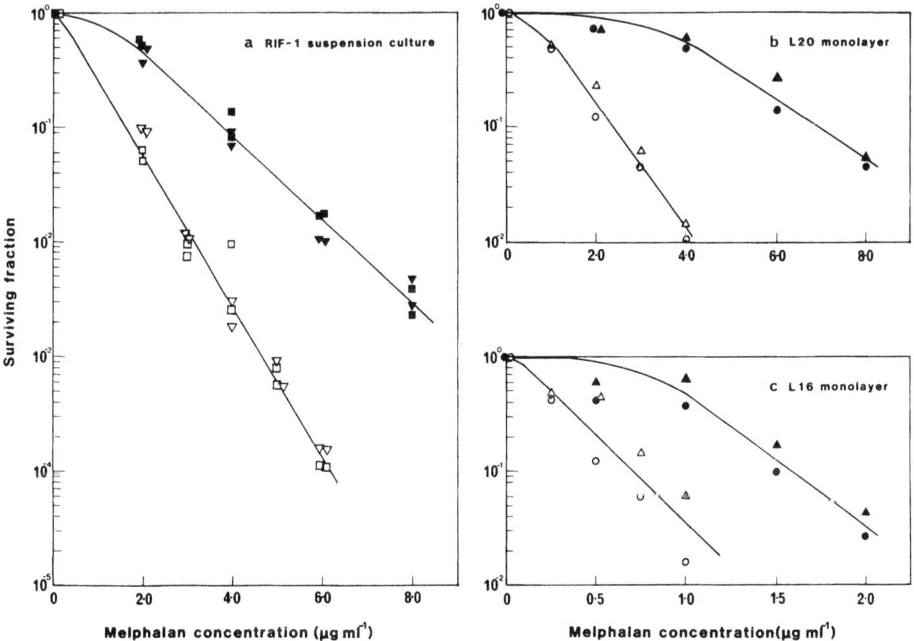

Fig. 2. The effect of hyperthermia at 41° C on the response to melphalan of various types of RIF-1 cells in vitro. *Closed symbols* show the response at 37° C, *open symbols* at 41° C. Different symbols indicate data from different experiments. Lines were drawn by regression analysis. For RIF-1 suspension culture *(panel a)* treatment time was 45 min; for L20 and L16 (*panels b and c* respectively) it was 60 min. Note difference in scale of x axis

Table 3. Slopes for melphalan response curves in vitro at 37° C and 41° C

Cell type	Treatment time	Slope (mg^{-1} kg) 37° C	Slope (mg^{-1} kg) 41° C	Slope 41° C/slope 37° C
RIF-1 suspension culture[a]	45 min	0.84 (0.78–0.90)[c]	1.52 (1.40–1.64)	1.8 (1.6–2.0)
RIF-1 suspension culture[b]	60 min	1.14 (0.98–1.31)	2.08 (1.93–2.23)	1.8 (1.5–2.1)
L20 monolayer (resistant clone)[a]	60 min	0.60 (0.46–0.73)	1.23 (1.07–1.39)	2.1 (1.5–2.6)
L16 monolayer (sensitive clone)[a]	60 min	2.66 (2.00–3.32)	3.12 (0.77–5.47)	1.35 (0.68–2.0)
RIF-1 suspension from tumour, treated in vitro[b]	45 min	0.91 (0.78–1.09)		

[a] Data shown in Fig. 2.
[b] Data not shown in Fig. 2.
[c] Numbers in brackets are 95% confidence limits.

what smaller (2.0 mg kg^{-1}) because the curve had a smaller shoulder. This suggested that the melphalan response of RIF-1 suspension culture was very similar to that of RIF-1 cells from in vivo tumours.

For the present comparison, the important feature of the data in Fig. 2 and Table 3 is that the heat-induced change in slope of the melphalan dose-response curve is only about a factor of 2 for RIF-1 suspension and L20, and rather less, 1.35, for the more sensitive L16. It is very striking that the largest difference found in vitro is only half of that found in vivo, where heat-induced changes in slope were by factors of 3.9 to 4.1 for this tumour (Table 2). This difference cannot be directly attributed to any differences in drug concentration between medium and plasma at 37° C. In vitro dose-response curves at 37° C are exponential between doses of 5 and 15 or 20 mg kg^{-1} in both leg tumours and lung microtumours. A dose of 7.5 mg kg^{-1} of melphalan gives a peak plasma concentration of 3–4 μg ml^{-1}, and one of 15 mg kg^{-1} a peak of 6–8 μg ml^{-1} (Honess et al. 1985), so the peak plasma concentration range is very similar to that in medium over which slopes of dose-response curves at 37° C have been measured in vitro. However, part of the explanation may lie in the different pharmacokinetics at 41° C for drug in vivo and in vitro. The half-life of melphalan in vivo at 37° C (20–25 min) is shorter than in vitro (80–90 min), since in vivo the drug is subject to elimination as well as spontaneous hydrolysis, which is the mechanism for depletion in medium. We have previously shown (Honess et al. 1985) that in vivo the plasma half-life is not shortened in heated animals, whereas in vitro the half-life is reduced to 50–60 min at 41° C. Thus for treatment at 41° C in vitro the total melphalan exposure is less than at 37° C, which would result in a smaller heat-induced change in slope than if the half-life were the same at both temperatures. This might partially explain why the in vitro data fail to predict the magnitude of the effect found in vivo. The discrepancy presented here, whatever its cause, emphasises the fact that in vitro experiments, however carefully modelled on in vivo conditions, cannot always predict the size of an effect in vivo.

Conclusions

The data presented above show that substantial potentiation of anticancer drugs, particularly alkylating agents, can be achieved at the relatively low hyperthermic temperature of 41° C. The data show a therapeutic gain for thermopotentiation of melphalan with systemic hyperthermia, and suggest much greater advantage for its combination with local heating. The necessity to apply heat at the time of maximum tumour drug concentration and to avoid thermally induced vascular occlusion in the tumour are highlighted. Finally, the in vitro studies with a variety of types of the same tumour line clearly demonstrate that thermopotentiation of cytotoxicity is an area where larger effects can be found in vivo than in vitro.

References

Dahl O, Mella O (1983) Effect of timing and sequence of hyperthermia and cyclophosphamide on a neurogenic rat tumour (BT_4 A) in vivo. Cancer 52: 983-987

Dewhirst MW, Sim DA, Gross J, Kundrat MA (1984) Effect of heating rate on tumour and normal tissue microcirculatory function. In: Overgaard J (ed) Hyperthermic oncology 1984, vol 1, summary papers. Taylor and Francis, London, pp 177-180

Dudar TE, Jain RK (1984) Differential response of normal and tumour microcirculation to hyperthermia. Cancer Res 44: 605-612

Hahn GM, Shiu EC (1983) Effect of pH and elevated temperatures on the cytotoxicity of some chemotherapeutic agents on Chinese hamster cells in vitro. Cancer Res 43: 5789-5791

Honess DJ, Bleehen NM (1980) Effects of the combination of hyperthermia and cytotoxic drugs on the skin of the mouse foot. In: Arcangeli G, Mauro F (eds) Proceedings, 1st meeting European Group of Hyperthermia and Radiation Oncology. Masson, New York, pp 151-155

Honess DJ, Bleehen NM (1982) Sensitivity of normal mouse marrow and RIF-1 tumour to hyperthermia combined with cyclophosphamide or BCNU: a lack of therapeutic gain. Br J Cancer 46: 236-248

Honess DJ, Bleehen NM (1985a) Thermochemotherapy with cis-platinum, CCNU, BCNU, chlorambucil and melphalan on murine marrow and 2 tumours: therapeutic gain for melphalan only. Br J Radiol 58: 63-72

Honess DJ, Bleehen NM (1985b) Potentiation of melphalan by systemic hyperthermia in mice: therapeutic gain for mouse lung microtumours. Int J Hyperthermia 1: 57-68

Honess DJ, Donaldson J, Workman P, Bleehen NM (1985) The effect of systemic hyperthermia on melphalan pharmacokinetics in mice. Br J Cancer 57: 77-84

Reeve JG, Twentyman PR (1983) Clonal variation in the arrest, survival and growth of RIF-1 mouse sarcoma cells in the lungs of C3H mice. Br J Cancer 47: 833-840

Reeve JG, Wright KA, Twentyman PR (1983) Response to X-radiation and cytotoxic drugs of clonal subpopulations of different ploidy and metastatic potential isolated from RIF-1 mouse sarcoma. Br J Cancer 47: 841-848

Twentyman PR, Morgan JE, Donaldson J (1978) Enhancement by hyperthermia of the effect of BCNU against the EMT6 mouse tumour. Cancer Treat Rep 62: 439-443

Effect of Heat and Combined Treatments on Human Tumors

Preclinical Hyperthermia in Human Tumors: Introductory Remarks

R. Engelhardt

Medizinische Klinik, Albert-Ludwigs-Universität, Hugstetter Straße 55, 7800 Freiburg, FRG

Chairman's Introduction

Hyperthermia is on the way to becoming a tool for the clinical treatment of cancer. For several reasons, discussed elsewhere (Engelhardt 1985, 1987; Hahn 1982), hyperthermia is going to be used preferentially in combination with radiation and cytotoxic chemotherapy. In developing the clinical approach one has to be aware of a huge number of complex interactions between the patient, the tumor, the heat, the irradiation, and the drugs. From the basic research data about heat effects and from our experience in clinical oncology we can predict a long list of circumstances that will modify the effect of heat applied alone or as part of a combined modality:

Patient
- Performance status
- Age
- Sex
- Other disease
- Supportive care

Tumor
- Type/histology/grading
- Burden/stage
- Size of lesions
- Site of lesion(s)
- Sensitivity
- Heterogeneity
  - clonal
  - cell cycle
  - environmental

Recent Results in Cancer Research, Vol. 109

Heat
- Heating rate
- Maximum level
- Duration
- Timing
- Fractionation
- Thermotolerance
- Application technique

Radiation
- Type
- Dosage
- Fractionation

Drug
- Type of action
- Dosage
- Pharmacokinetic
- Combinations
- Schedule of administration
- Route of administration

Most of our knowledge about heat effects stems from laboratory work done in cell lines of murine (or other mammalian) origin. Further experience has been gained with animal tumors "treated" after transplantation or, more seldom, in situ, i.e., at the site of origin.

It seems likely that the physical and biological phenomena which have been described in these experiments will also be found in human tumours. But due to biological differences between human and nonhuman tumors and between seemingly the same tumors in different individuals, profound differences in heat effects seem to occur. In addition, tumors are heterogeneous in respect of quite a number of phenotypic characteristics (Leith and Dexter 1986a), including radiation sensitivity, drug sensitivity, and heat sensitivity (Leith and Dexter 1986b), each alone as well as in combination. Therefore, it seems mandatory and reasonable to investigate to what degree heat effects, i.e., heat toxicity and heat sensitization, can be demonstrated in human tumors, and to ascertain the conditions for the induction of these effects. Although all the preclinical testing assays mimic the clinical situation in an arbitrary manner, they all have their value in providing the clinician with information to the design of clinical trials. Beyond this, the preclinical investigation of tumors from individual patients may be able to select those cases with a high probability of response or, vice versa, those unlikely to respond to heat alone or to combined heat and irradiation or heat and drug therapy. The investigations presented in the following section deal mainly with two problems: (1) The development of so-called predictive assays. The clonogenic assay, xenotransplants, morphological changes of tumor cells, and biochemical assays (dansyl lysine) are used. (2) The characterization of inter- and intraindividual tumor heterogeneity.

From what we know - and are learning - about the different types of heterogeneity and keeping in mind the long list of factors that influence the therapeutic effect, the predictive value of any of the assays mentioned above will be limited. But by way of encouragement it should be mentioned that in spite of these limitations, in "normothermic chemotherapy" high in vitro/in vivo correlations have been found: Using the clonogenic assay in a broad variety of tumors, sensitivity could be predicted in an average of 70% of the cases tested, the figure varying according to the tumor type, from 42% in multiple myeloma to 92% in ovarian cancer. Resistance prediction was reported to be possible at as high an average as 92%, ranging from 83% in multiple myeloma to 100% in ovarian cancer (DeVita 1985).

The clinical relevance of the data concerning the prediction of sensitivity or resistance to heat alone or in combination therapy must be confirmed by ongoing clinical trials.

References

DeVita VT (1985) Principles of chemotherapy. In: DeVita VT, Hellmann S, Rosenberg SA (eds) Cancer, principles and practice of oncology. 2nd edn. Lippincott, Philadelphia, pp 257-285

Engelhardt R (1985) Whole-body hyperthermia. Methods and results. Proceedings, 4th international symposium on hyperthermic oncology, 2-6 July 1984, Aarhus, Denmark. In: Overgaard J (ed) Hyperthermic oncology 1984, vol 2. Taylor and Francis, London, pp 263-276

Engelhardt R (1987) Hyperthermia and drugs. In: Streffer C (ed) Recent Results in Cancer Research, vol 104. Springer, Berlin Heidelberg New York Tokyo, pp 136-203

Hahn GM (1982) Hyperthermia and cancer. Plenum, New York

Leith JT, Dexter DL (1986a) Mammalian tumor cell heterogeneity. CRC, Boca Ranton, Florida, pp 11-22

Leith JT, Dexter DL (1986b) Mammalian tumor cell heterogeneity. CRC, Boca Raton, Florida, pp 97-120

*Microcirculatory and pH Alterations in Isotransplanted Rat and Xenotransplanted Human Tumors Associated with Hyperthermia**

P. Vaupel[1], F. Kallinowski[1], M. Kluge[1], E. Egelhof[1], and H. P. Fortmeyer[2]

[1] Abteilung für Angewandte Physiologie, Johannes-Gutenberg-Universität, Saarstraße 21, 6500 Mainz, FRG
[2] Tierversuchsanlage, Universitätsklinikum Frankfurt, Theodor-Stern-Kai 7, 6000 Frankfurt/M., FRG

Introduction

The rationale for considering the use of hyperthermia as an antitumor agent is based on three different mechanisms of action depending on the hyperthermia levels chosen: At moderate hyperthermia levels (40°-42.5° C) heat can increase the radiosensitivity and/or the chemosensitivity. At higher tissue temperatures (> 42.5° C) hyperthermia acts as a cytotoxic agent since mammalian cells die after heating in a temperature-, time-, and cell cycle-dependent manner. Besides direct effects on the cell membranes, on the cytoskeleton, on metabolic processes, on DNA replication, and on RNA and protein synthesis, *indirect effects* distinctly modulating the anticancer action of heat have to be considered. These indirect effects are mostly mediated through the cellular microenvironment, both for in vitro and for in vivo conditions. In most solid tumors, this microenvironment is characterized by hypoxia and even anoxia, acidosis, and energy deprivation, which are known to enhance the heat effect even under in vitro conditions. These characteristic features of the cellular microenvironment are mostly determined by tumor microcirculation. It is generally accepted that nutritive blood flow in most tumors is heterogeneously distributed and on the average insufficient at larger tumor sizes. This flow pattern in solid tumors has two relevant consequences:

1. It induces the hostile microenvironment described, thus rendering the tumor cells in vivo more heat sensitive as compared with normal tissues.
2. It limits the heat dissipation from the tumor tissue and thus the energy input required to reach a therapeutic tissue temperature level. The latter fact often implies the possibility of a relatively selective heating of the tumor tissue.

Considering the relative sensitivity of tumors to heat based on the hostile micromilieu, changes in the microenvironment upon heating are of interest, since an additional deterioration of the nutritive flow would further sensitize the cells to heat (for recent reviews see Song 1984; Reinhold and Endrich 1986; Vaupel and Kallinowski 1987), making a positive feedback mechanism feasible.

* This work was supported by the Bundesministerium für Forschung und Technologie (grant 01 VF 034).

Experiments on Isotransplanted Rat Tumors

Experiments performed using isotransplanted rat tumors have shown that changes in the micromilieu consistent with the above postulated feedback mechanism are frequently observed. As an example, in Fig. 1 the time-dependent drop in the mean local *tumor blood flow* (TBF) is depicted for Yoshida sarcomas transplanted subcutaneously into the dorsum of the left hind foot of Sprague-Dawley rats. Local hyperthermia was induced using an ultrasound feedback control system (1.7 MHz). Tissue temperature in the center of 1- to 2 g tumors was monitored with a miniaturized thermocouple, and mean arterial blood pressure (MABP) through a catheter in the thoracic aorta. Tumors were heated up to either 40.5° or 44° C for 60 min. During this period, the power to the ultrasound transducer was shut off every 20 min of heating and the subsequent thermal washout was recorded. In the control series, the tumor temperature was elevated to 38.5° C for 60 s and the thermal washout curves were recorded thereafter. This short-time temperature increase had no significant effect on TBF as shown with the ^{85}krypton-clearance technique.

Before heating, the average local TBF was 0.31 ± 0.05 ml g^{-1} min^{-1}. Whereas in the unheated control tumors there was only a slight decrease in TBF with time, during hyperthermia at 44° C a significant drop in flow occurred as a function of heating time. Tumors heated up to 40.5° C also showed a time-dependent decrease in flow. However, this decrease in TBF was not significantly different from that observed in the control group. This was mostly due to pronounced intertumor variability in the flow pattern during heating, as shown in Fig. 2. As a further consequence of this pronounced intertumor variability, it has to be stated that the temperature- and time-dependent flow changes cannot be predicted for the individual tumor. The individual flow patterns for hyperthermia at 44° C are shown in Fig. 3. Here again, anisotropic flow behavior is obvious.

Considering time- and temperature-dependent changes in TBF and in MABP under these conditions, tumor vascular functions can best be characterized by the *tumor vascular conductance* (TVC = TBF/MABP). In the unheated tumors (mean

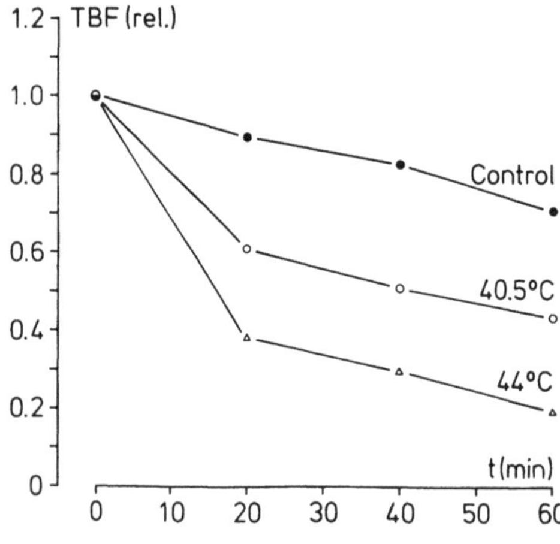

Fig. 1. Relative changes in TBF of subcutaneous Yoshida sarcomas as a function of exposure time and tissue hyperthermia level (40.5° C, 44° C, localized ultrasound heating). Sham-heated rat tumors served as controls

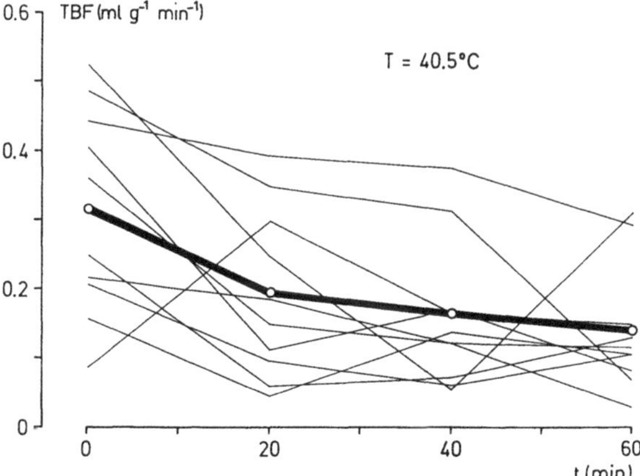

Fig. 2. Changes in TBF as a function of exposure time at 40.5° C in ten individual rat tumors *(thin lines)*. During heating pronounced intertumor variability is apparent. For comparison, the average flow change is also given *(thick line)*

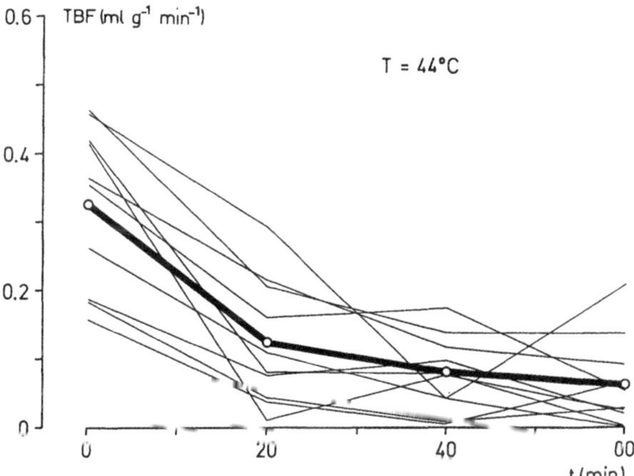

Fig. 3. Changes in TBF as a function of heating time at 44° C in ten individual rat tumors *(thin lines)*. The *thick line* indicates the mean flow change under these conditions

tumor tissue temperature: 34°–35° C) the average TVC was 3.5 ± 0.5 µl min^{-1} mmHg^{-1}. Upon heating at 40.5° C and 44° C, TVC decreased significantly in a time- and temperature-dependent manner, whereas in the unheated tumors it remained almost constant (Fig. 4). Here again, pronounced interindividual differences occurred.

On average, the *tissue oxygenation* of isotransplanted rat tumors parallels the heat-induced flow changes (Vaupel et al. 1982). The same holds true for the nutrient supply and the removal of acidic waste products. This indicates that nutritive blood flow is the main parameter determining the micromilieu surrounding the tumor cells (Vaupel et al. 1983).

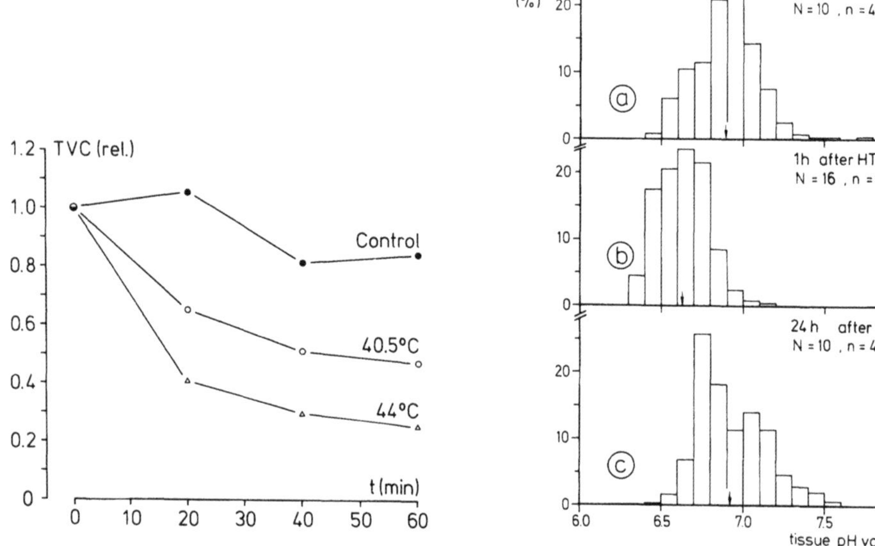

Fig. 4 *(left)*. Relative changes in tumor vascular conductance (TVC = TBF/MABP) of subcutaneous Yoshida sarcomas as a function of exposure time (20-60 min) and tissue hyperthermia level (40.5° C and 44° C). Sham-heated isotransplants served as controls

Fig. 5 a-c *(right)*. Frequency distributions of measured tumor tissue pH values (pH histograms) in Yoshida sarcomas (tumor wet weight: 2-3 g) **a** before, **b** 1 h after, and **c** 1 day after localized ultrasound hyperthermia at 44° C for 60 min (heating-up rate > 1.5° C/min). *Arrows* indicate the respective mean pH value. *N*, number of tumors investigated; *n*, number of pH measurements

When measuring the *tissue pH distribution* in subcutaneously growing Yoshida sarcomas with wet weights between 2 and 3 g, the results showed that under control conditions the tissue pH ranged from 6.40 to 7.80 with an average of 6.89 (upper panel in Fig. 5). At 1 h after heating (44° C for 60 min) the pH distribution significantly shifted to lower values, with an average pH of 6.63 (central panel in Fig. 5), i.e., upon hyperthermia employing thermal doses of ca. 540° C · min the mean tumor pH drops by about 0.25 pH units. From these results it can be concluded that the tissue pH is usually lower in rat tumors than in normal tissues (mean pH in muscle and subcutis: approx. 7.35) and that hyperthermia further decreases tumor pH if appropriate thermal doses are applied. At 24 h after heating the tumor pH distribution has returned to values obtained during preheating conditions.

The average tissue pH 1 day after heating is 6.92 (lower panel in Fig. 5); pH values higher than 7.2 are more frequent as compared with control conditions. Probably this is due to enlarged areas with necrotic debris following heat application (Vaupel 1982).

Different heating-up rates of the tumor tissue seem to induce different pH changes during hyperthermia at 44° C sustained for 60 min (see Fig. 6). Whereas

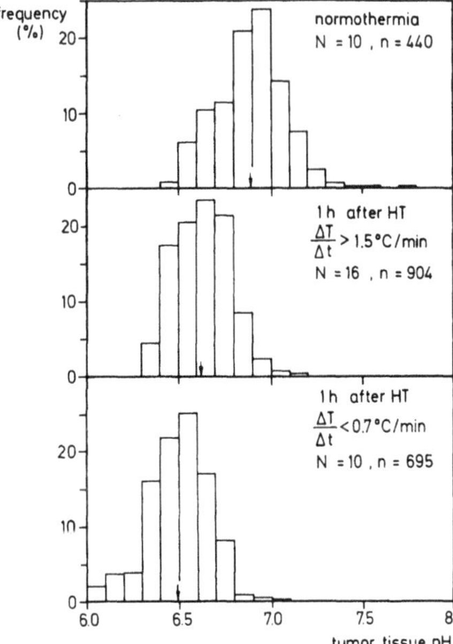

Fig. 6. pH histograms of Yoshida sarcomas (tumor wet weight: 2–3 g) before *(upper panel)* and 1 h after localized ultrasound hyperthermia at 44° C for 60 min using different heating-up rates ($\Delta T/\Delta t$). *Arrows* indicate the mean values. *N*, number of tumors; *n*, number of pH measurements

heating-up rates $<0.7°$ C/min are followed by a mean pH drop of approximately 0.4 pH units, after rapid heating ($\Delta T/\Delta t > 1.5°$ C/min^{-1}) the average fall in pH is only 0.25 pH units. Up to now there have been no convincing experimental hints that this difference is caused by the somewhat greater heat dose applied during hyperthermia at 44° C for 60 min and heating-up rates $<0.7°$ C/min as compared with rapidly heated tumors.

Experiments on Human Tumor Xenografts

For human tumors, only scarce data concerning these relevant parameters are available. In order to bridge the gap between rodent tumors and primary human tumors, human tumor xenografts in nude rats were systematically studied. In a first approach, breast cancers were investigated due to their frequency and problematic prognosis.

Following the experimental protocol used for isotransplanted rat tumors, local TBF was measured in human breast cancers xenotransplanted subcutaneously into rnu/rnu rats. Throughout all experiments xenografts with wet weights of approximately 3 g were studied. Here again, local TBF was evaluated using thermal washout curves and considering only convective and excluding conductive heat transfer.

Whereas in the subcutis a time- and temperature-dependent increase in flow (increase in the laser Doppler flow, unpublished results) occurred during the treatment period, a thermal dose related drop in flow was observed during hyperthermia in the human breast cancer xenografts. In a control series, no significant

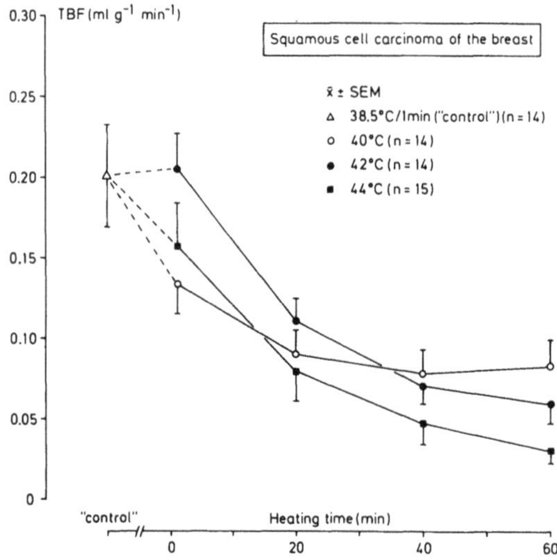

Fig. 7. Changes in TBF in human breast cancer xenografts (squamous cell carcinomas) in rnu/rnu rats as a function of exposure time and tissue hyperthermia level (40° C, 42° C, and 44° C, ultrasound heating). "Control" flow was measured using thermal washout curves after a 60 s heating period up to 38.5° C. Values are means ± standard error of the mean ($\bar{x} \pm$ SEM). *n*, number of tumors investigated

changes in blood flow were obvious in subcutaneous tumors with mean tissue temperatures of 34°-35° C during the observation period.

The blood flow pattern of *human squamous cell breast cancer xenografts* after 1, 20, 40, and 60 min of hyperthermia at 40° C, 42° C, and 44° C is presented in Fig. 7. The triangle indicates the local flow under "control" conditions (tissue temperature 38.5° C for 60 s). During treatment, a time- and temperature-dependent decrease in flow was again observed. Compared with the control values, after 60 min of hyperthermia significant reductions in TBF were obtained at all hyperthermia levels, the reduction being most pronounced at the highest tissue temperature. A total flow stop occurred in approximately 10% of the tumors heated to 40° C, in 20% of the tumors heated to 42° C, and in 50% of the tumors heated to 44° C.

Blood flow changes upon hyperthermia in *human medullary breast cancer xenografts* are shown in Fig. 8. Here, an initial TBF increase is obvious after 1 min at 44° C. Subsequently, a time- and temperature-dependent decrease in flow again occurred during treatment. However, the reduction in flow was somewhat less pronounced than that observed in the squamous cell carcinomas. After 60 min of treatment, significant reductions were seen for 42° and 44° C but not for 40° C. At that time, a total flow stop was obvious in 10% of the tumors heated to 40° C, 20% of the tumors with tissue temperatures of 42° C, and 30% of the xenografts heated to 44° C.

Considering individual xenografts, pronounced intertumor variability in the flow changes upon heat treatment was detectable, so that the biological behavior of the individual tumor at elevated tumor tissue temperature levels cannot be pre-

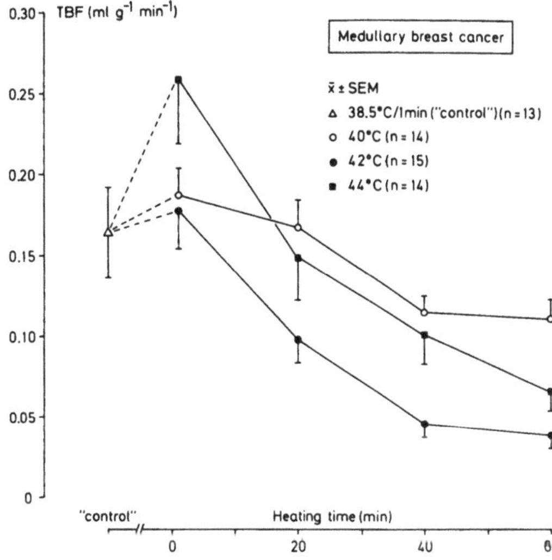

Fig. 8. Changes in TBF in human breast cancer xenografts (medullary breast cancers) in rnu/rnu rats as a function of exposure time and tissue hyperthermia level. For further details see legend to Fig. 7

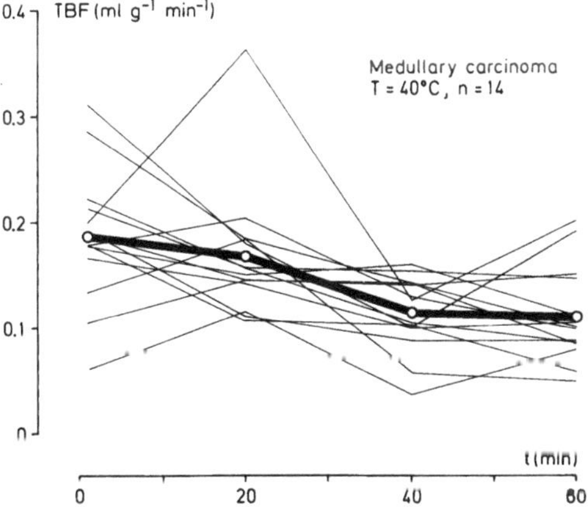

Fig. 9. Changes in TBF as a function of exposure time at 40° C in 14 individual human breast cancer xenografts *(thin lines)*. For comparison, the mean flow change is also given *(thick line)*

dicted. As was the case in rat tumors, the TBF changes of some individual tumors did not follow the average flow changes at a certain temperature level although comparable tumor sizes were considered (see Figs. 9-11).

When TBF in the squamous cell breast cancer xenografts is considered as a function of various thermal doses (TD = integral of the tissue temperature elevation above the starting temperature during the treatment period), it is seen to decrease continuously with increasing thermal dose (Fig. 12). TBF in medullary tu-

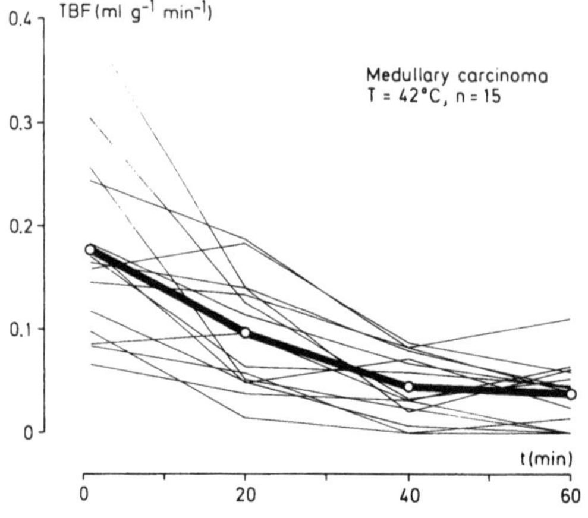

Fig. 10. Changes in TBF as a function of exposure time at 42° C in 15 individual human breast cancer xenografts *(thin lines)*. The mean flow change is indicated by the *thick line*

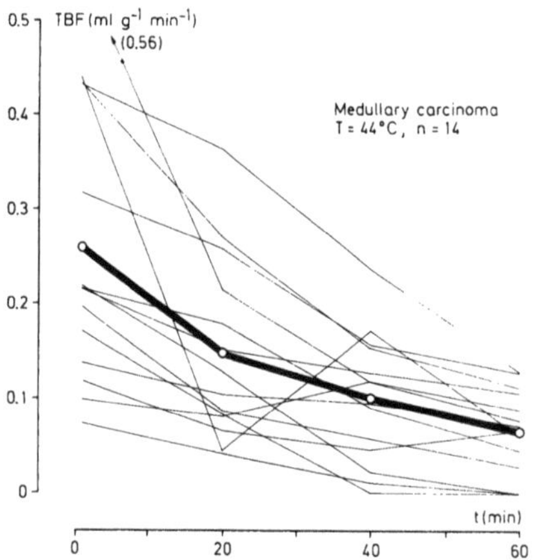

Fig. 11. Changes in TBF as a function of exposure time at 44° C in 14 individual human breast cancer xenografts *(thin lines)*. The average flow change is indicated by the *thick line*

mor xenografts as a function of the thermal dose is shown in Fig. 13; similarly, a continuous, but less pronounced reduction in flow was found with increasing thermal dose.

Whereas no pH changes upon hyperthermia are observed in the subcutis, in xenografts of the squamous cell carcinomas of the breast heat treatment was followed by a significant shift of the pH frequency distribution (pH histogram) to lower pH values, from 7.07 at control conditions to 6.91 after hyperthermia at 44° C for 60 min (see Fig. 14). Comparable shifts were also observed after hyperthermia at 44° C for 30 min and at 42° C for 60 min.

In xenografts of medullary breast carcinomas no significant pH shifts to lower values were found upon comparable thermal doses. However, there was a trend towards more acidic values with increasing thermal dose. The mean pH value was 6.82 under control conditions and 6.72 after tissue temperatures of 44° C for 60 min. This slight pH shift to more acidic values in the medullary tumors coincides with a less pronounced reduction in flow in this tumor type.

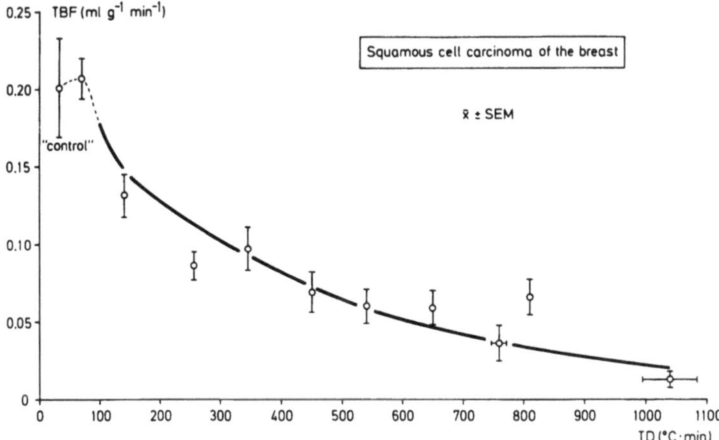

Fig. 12. TBF in human breast cancer xenografts (squamous cell carcinomas) as a function of various thermal doses *(TD)*. Values are means ± standard error of the mean ($\overline{x} \pm$ SEM). The *solid line* was fitted using a least squares method. The *broken line* indicates the trend at low thermal doses

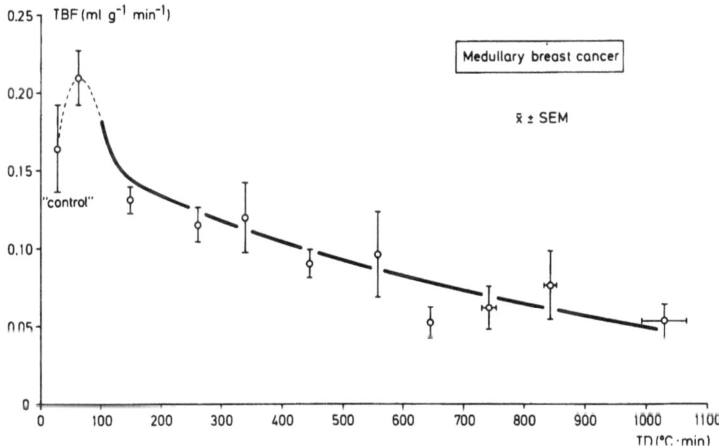

Fig. 13. TBF in human breast cancer xenografts (medullary breast cancers) as a function of various thermal doses *(TD)*. Values are means ± standard error of the mean ($\overline{x} \pm$ SEM). The *solid line* was fitted using a least squares method. The *broken line* indicates the trend at low thermal doses

Conclusions

The hostile tumor microenvironment as a consequence of an inadequate tumor microcirculation sensitizes tumor cells to heat. During heat treatment, a positive feedback mechanism is postulated, since adequate thermal doses further reduce tumor blood flow and further intensify the hostile micromilieu. This pattern can

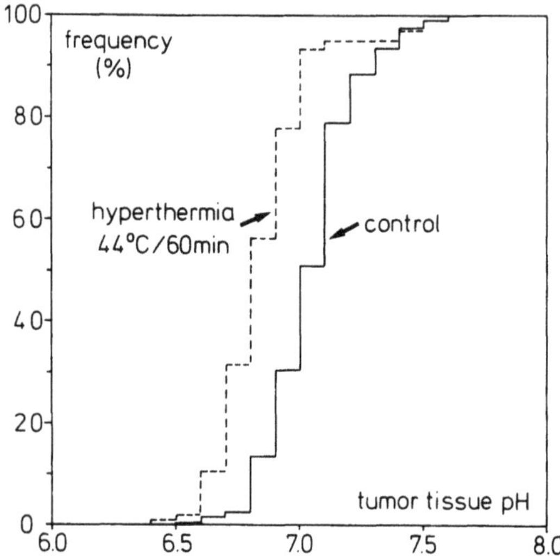

Fig. 14. Cumulative frequency distributions of measured tumor tissue pH values before (control, *solid line*) and 1 h after localized ultrasound heating of human breast cancer xenografts (squamous cell carcinomas) at 44° C for 60 min *(broken line)*

be observed both in isotransplanted rat tumors and in xenotransplanted human breast cancers. At comparable thermal doses, the changes in the latter tumors, however, are somewhat less pronounced.

References

Reinhold HS, Endrich B (1986) Tumour microcirculation as a target for hyperthermia. Int J Hyperthermia 2: 111-137

Song CW (1984) Effect of local hyperthermia on blood flow and microenvironment. Cancer Res (Suppl) 44: 4721s-4730 s

Vaupel P (1982) Einfluß einer lokalisierten Mikrowellenhyperthermie auf die pH-Verteilung in bösartigen Tumoren. Strahlentherapie 158: 168-173

Vaupel P, Kallinowski F (1987) Physiological effects of hyperthermia. In: Streffer C (ed) Hyperthermia and the therapy of malignant tumors. Springer, Berlin Heidelberg New York, pp 71-109 (Recent results in cancer research vol 104)

Vaupel P, Otte J, Manz R (1982) Oxygenation of malignant tumors after localized microwave hyperthermia. Radiat Environ Biophys 20: 289-300

Vaupel P, Mueller-Klieser W, Otte J, Manz R, Kallinowski F (1983) Blood flow, tissue oxygenation, and pH distribution in malignant tumors upon localized hyperthermia. Strahlentherapie 159: 73-81

*Effects of Heat Treatment in Vitro and in Vivo on Human Melanoma Xenografts**

T. Brustad and E. K. Rofstad

Institute for Cancer Research, The Norwegian Cancer Society,
The Norwegian Radium Hospital, Montebello, 0310 Oslo 3, Norway

Introduction and Methods

In the present paper inactivation of human melanoma xenografts will be discussed. Five different human melanomas, propagated in athymic mice, were used as a test system. The tumors were derived from metastases of patients at The Norwegian Radium Hospital and transplanted directly to nude mice without adaptation to in vitro culture conditions. The tumors were grown serially in nude mice by implanting small tumor fragments into the flanks of recipient mice. When the present work was carried out, the tumors had been grown for at least 20 passages in nude mice. The tumors used in hyperthermia experiments were implanted in the legs of the mice and had grown to a diameter of 8-12 mm when the experiments were carried out. Light microscopic and electron microscopic examination of the xenografts showed that they very nearly retained the morphology of the parent tumors.

The cells of the melanomas have the ability to form colonies when seeded in soft agar. The colony forming ability of the cells was thus used as an end point in the in vitro studies and in some of the in vivo studies. Single cell suspensions were prepared from the tumors by mechanical dispersion without the use of enzymes. The soft agar assay was similar to that developed by Courtenay and Mills (1978), applying Bacto agar, Ham's F12 medium, red blood cells from August rats, and an atmosphere of 5% O_2, 5% CO_2, and 90% N_2.

Heterogeneous Heat Sensitivity of Melanomas

An interesting discovery was that the heat sensitivity of cells isolated from the five melanomas differed quite dramatically. This is illustrated in Fig. 1, which shows survival curves for cells heated in vitro at 42.5° C. About 80% of the cells from the

* Financial support from The Norwegian Cancer Society, The Norwegian Research Council for Science and the Humanities, and The Nansen Scientific Fund is gratefully acknowledged.

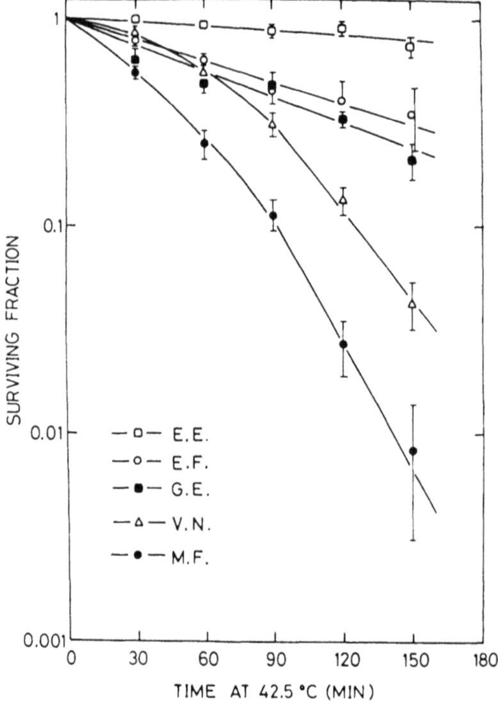

Fig. 1. Survival curves of cells from human melanoma xenografts heated at 42.5° C suspended in culture medium. Each *point* represents the mean surviving fraction of three to five independent experiments. Standard errors are indicated by *vertical bars*. The surviving fraction from each individual experiment was calculated from the mean number of colonies in five tubes with heated and five tubes with unheated cells

E. E. melanoma survived a heat treatment of 42.5° C for 150 min, whereas the same treatment resulted in a cell survival of about 1% for the M. F. melanoma, the most sensitive xenograft. Another interesting observation was that the melanomas were more heat sensitive when heated as solid tumors in vivo than when heated as single cells in vitro. This is illustrated in Fig. 2 for the E. E. and V. N. melanomas. When heated in vivo, the tumors were excised and assayed in vitro immediately after the heat treatment. It is likely that these differences in heat sensitivity are related to differences in the physiological conditions in vivo and in vitro.

In order to test whether the heat sensitivity of human melanomas in vivo could be enhanced by inducing extremely unfavorable physiological conditions as first shown for experimental animal tumors by Hill and Denekamp (1978), the melanomas were heated while the blood supply was occluded. A tourniquet was applied on the leg above the tumors 15 min before the start of the heat treatment and removed immediately after the treatment was completed. The tumors were excised and assayed in vitro immediately after the heat treatment. The results are shown in Fig. 3.

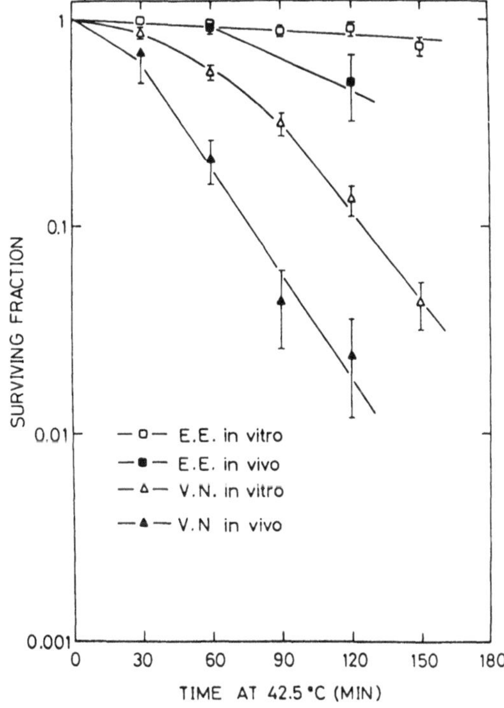

Fig. 2. Survival curves of cells from human melanoma xenografts heated at 42.5° C as solid tumors in nude mice. Each *point* represents the mean surviving fraction calculated from four tumors. Standard errors are indicated by *vertical bars*. The surviving fraction from each tumor was calculated from the mean number of colonies in five tubes with cells from the heated tumor and five tubes with cells from an unheated tumor. The survival curves in Fig. 1 of cells from the same melanomas heated in vitro are included for comparison

The data presented for the E. E. and V. N. melanomas demonstrate clearly that clamping results in a considerable enhancement of the heat sensitivity of human melanomas. This is the very opposite to the situation for treatment with ionizing radiation, where clamped tumors, due to hypoxia, are more resistant than unclamped tumors.

Heat Inactivation Caused by Direct and Indirect Processes

On the basis of results such as those described above, it was found relevant to shed more light on the possible effects of heat treatment on the microvasculature of the human melanoma xenografts, and the consequences of such treatments for cell survival. Microangiograms for unheated and heated tumors were thus established and studied. The vascular system of the tumors was filled with an X-ray contrast medium, and 720 μm thick freeze sections were irradiated by use of an X-ray unit.

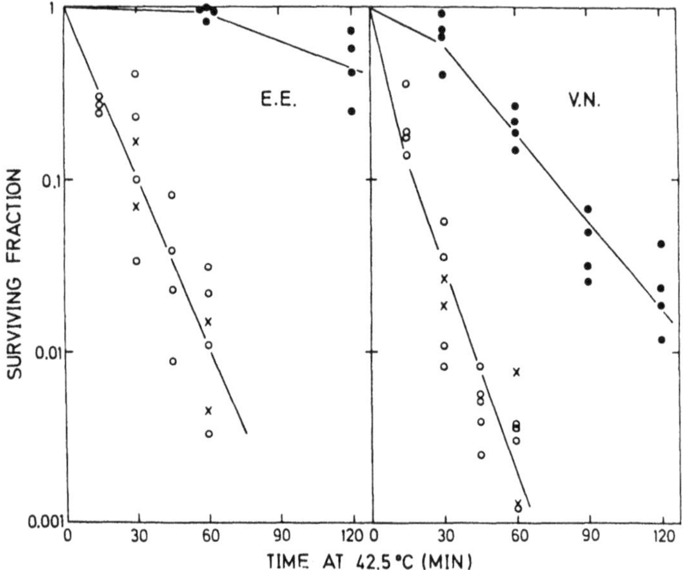

Fig. 3. Survival curves of cells from human melanoma xenografts heated (42.5° C) in vivo as solid tumors. The tumors were heated either in dead mice (x) or in air-breathing mice while clamped (O) or unclamped (●). Each *point* represents the surviving fraction of cells from one treated tumor, calculated from the mean number of colonies in five tubes with cells from this tumor and five tubes with cells from an untreated tumor. Exponential curves were fitted to the data by the method of least squares. The curves from the origin to the first set of data points were drawn by hand

Figure 4 illustrates changes in the vascular density induced by a heat treatment of 60 min at 42.5° C. Figure 4a demonstrates an untreated tumor in which the density of vascular structures is high except in a small central area, where the tumor was confirmed to be necrotic. The vascular density was considerably reduced at 24 h after treatment (Fig. 4b). The vascularized area increased in size by 3 days after treatment (Fig. 4c), and by 9 days the tumors were well vascularized (Fig. 4d). Consequences of this heat-induced vascular damage for cell survival are shown in Fig. 5.

Figure 5a shows relative tumor cell yield and Fig. 5b relative plating efficiency of the tumor cells as a function of time after treatment: 42.5° C for 60 min. The relative cell yield and the relative plating efficiency were multiplied to obtain the fraction of clonogenic cells (Fig. 5c), i.e., the number of clonogenic cells per unit tumor volume relative to that for untreated tumors. The fraction of clonogenic cells was already reduced to 60%–70% immediately after treatment, owing to the direct cytotoxic effect of the heat. Moreover, the fraction of clonogenic cells decreased with time after treatment toward a minimum of about 5×10^{-3} at 3 days, and then increased again. This reduction indicates that a considerable fraction of the tumor cells was killed *after* the heat treatment, probably because of the heat-induced vascular damage. Beyond the third day after treatment, at the time when the tumors, as shown above, became revascularized, the total number of repopu-

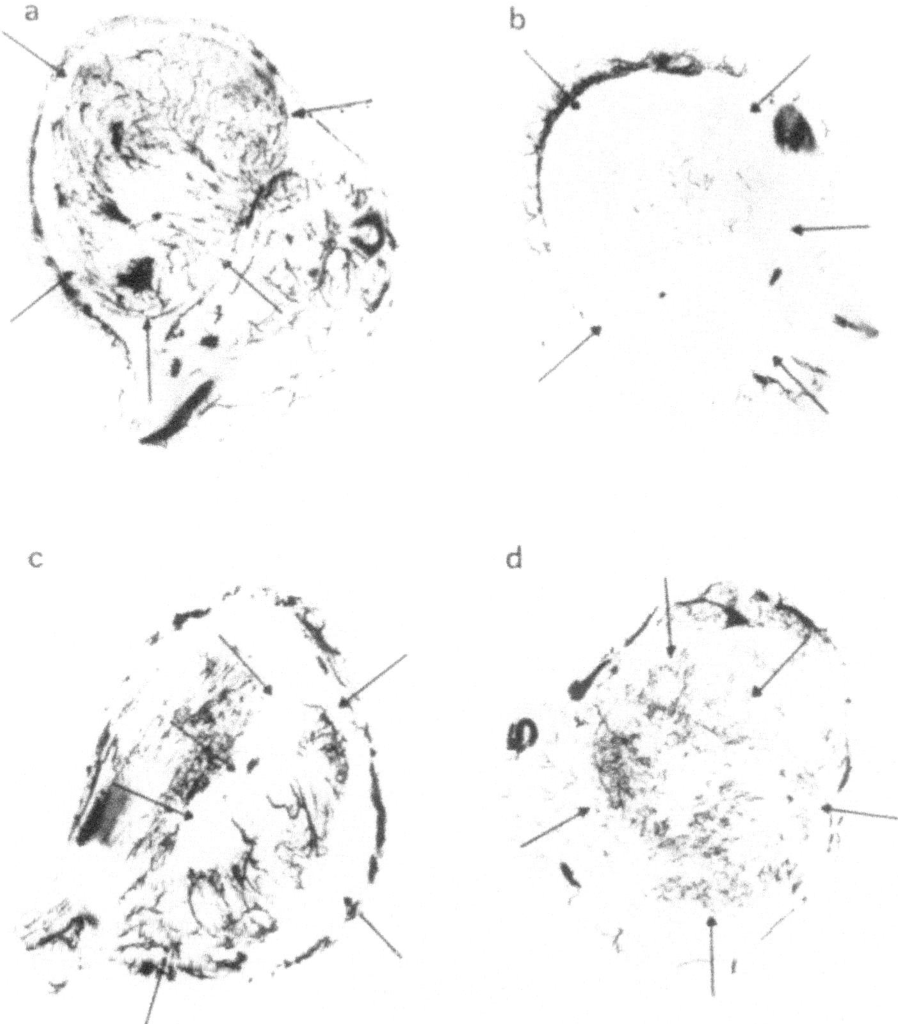

Fig. 4a–d. Microangiograms of 720 μm thick tumor sections from a human melanoma xenograft heated at 42.5° C for 60 min. An unheated tumor (**a**) and tumors fixed 24 h (**b**), 3 days (**c**), and 9 days (**d**) after treatment. All four sections were cut from the deeper third of a tumor, i.e., the third closest to the muscle tissue. The areas circumscribed by the *arrowheads* are tumor tissue, whereas the areas outside are normal tissue

lating cells was larger than the total number of dying cells, and the fraction of clonogenic cells increased.

At least two mechanisms are involved in heat-induced cell inactivation in vivo in our xenografts. Firstly, cells are inactivated due to the direct cytotoxic effect of high temperature per se. Secondly, delayed secondary cell death occurs, probably as a result of heat-induced vascular damage which gives rise to a variety of phe-

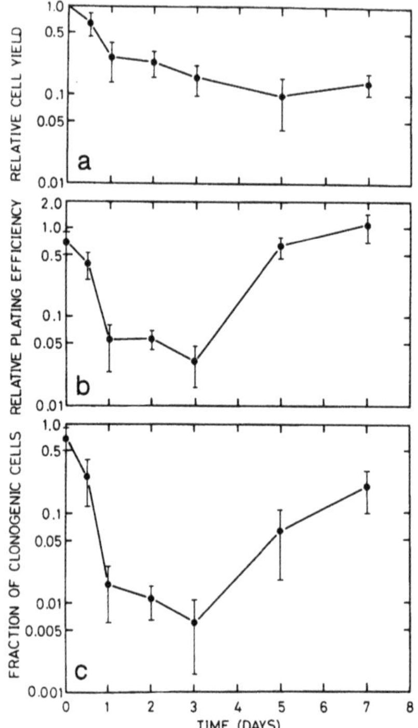

Fig. 5a–c. Cell yield per unit tumor volume (**a**), plating efficiency (**b**), and fraction of clonogenic cells (**c**) for a human melanoma xenograft heated at 42.5° C for 60 min as a function of the time elapsed after treatment. Tumor volumes were measured immediately before treatment. All values are expressed as fractions of the values for unheated control tumors. The fraction of clonogenic cells was obtained by multiplying the relative cell yield and the relative plating efficiency for each tumor. The *points* and the *vertical bars* represent mean values and standard errors, based on four to six individual tumors. The relative plating efficiency for each tumor was calculated from the number of morphologically intact cells seeded and the mean number of colonies in four or five tubes with cells from heated tumors and four or five tubes with cells from unheated tumors

nomena, such as protracted hypoxia, increased acidity, nutrient deficiency, and/or accumulation of toxic, metabolic products.

Recent studies have shown that the magnitude of the secondary cell death differs significantly among the different melanomas, as does the primary cell death. The secondary cell death is least pronounced in the melanomas in which most of the large vessels are embedded in broad bands of connective tissue.

Heat Response in Relation to Heating Time and Heating Temperature

Above we demonstrated that the heat response in vivo is partly governed by physiological and microvascular conditions. In the following the relationship between the heat response of the melanomas and the corresponding heating time/temperature will be discussed, first in vitro, then in vivo.

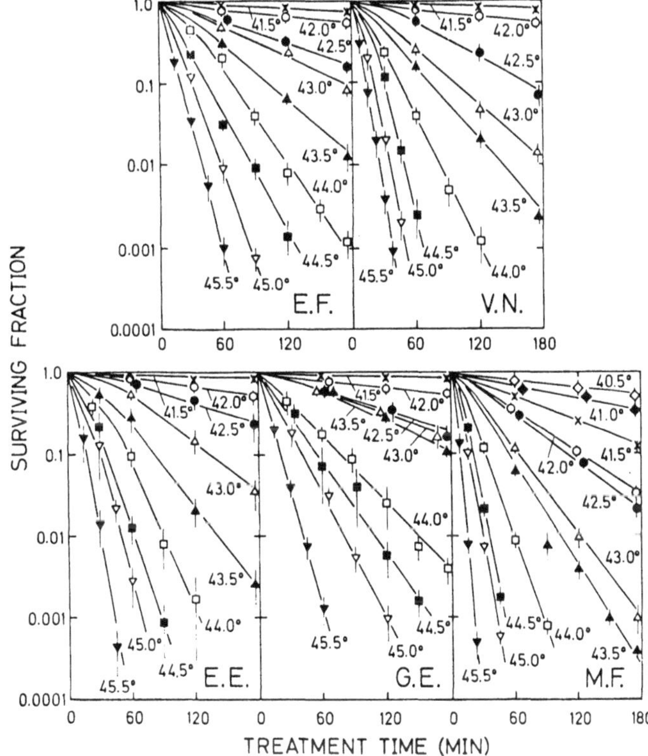

Fig. 6. Survival curves for cells from each of the five human melanoma xenografts heated at 40.5°-45.5° C in soft agar. Each *point* represents the mean surviving fraction from three to seven independent experiments. The *vertical bars* represent SE. The surviving fraction from each individual experiment was calculated from the mean number of colonies in four tubes with heated and four tubes with unheated cells

Heating Under in Vitro Conditions

Survival curves for cells from the melanomas heated in vitro are shown in Fig. 6, reflecting that the heat sensitivity differs among the melanomas at all temperatures within the range 41.5°-45.5° C.

Arrhenius curves (Field and Morris 1983) are derived from these survival curves by plotting the slopes of the survival curves versus the reciprocal value of the heating temperature. Such Arrhenius curves are shown in Fig. 7. The M. F. melanoma showed an inflection point at 41.5° C and the other melanomas inflection points at 42.5° C.

Heating Under in Vivo Conditions

Specific growth delay data for the melanomas heated in vivo are shown in Fig. 8 as a function of heating time. The heating temperature was varied from 40.5° to 44.0° C for the M. F. melanoma and from 41.5° to 44.0° C for the other melano-

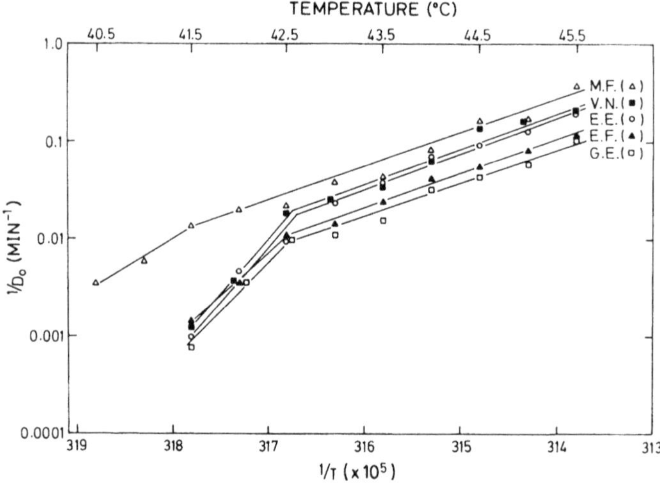

Fig. 7. Arrhenius curves for cells from human melanoma xenografts heated in vitro in soft agar at 40.5°-45.5° C. The data were derived from the slopes of the curves presented in Fig. 6

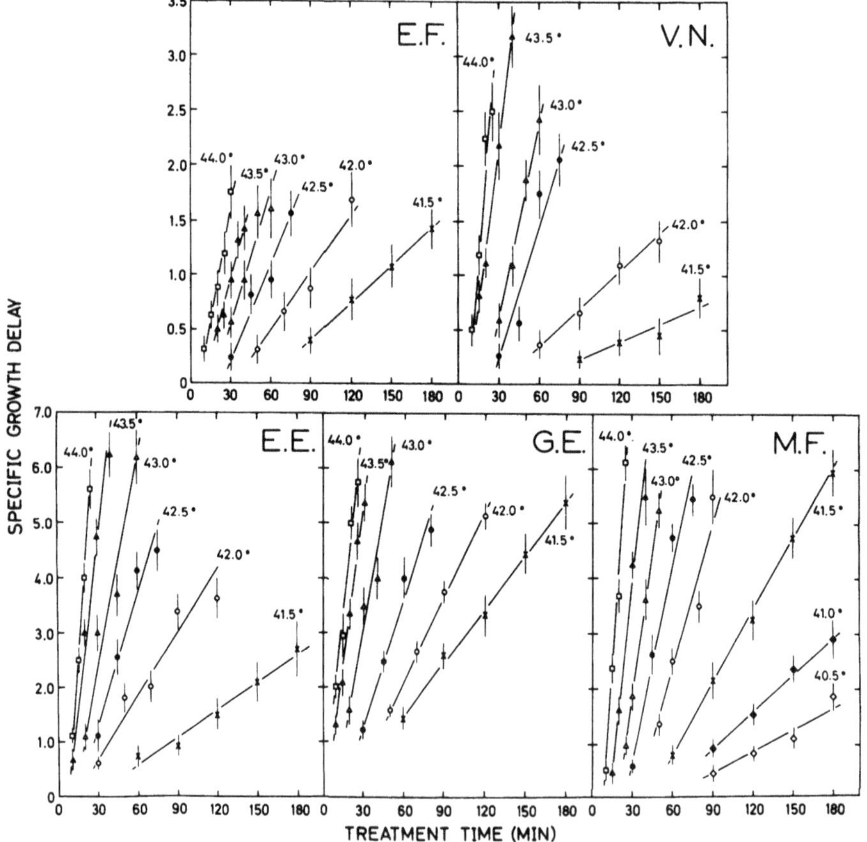

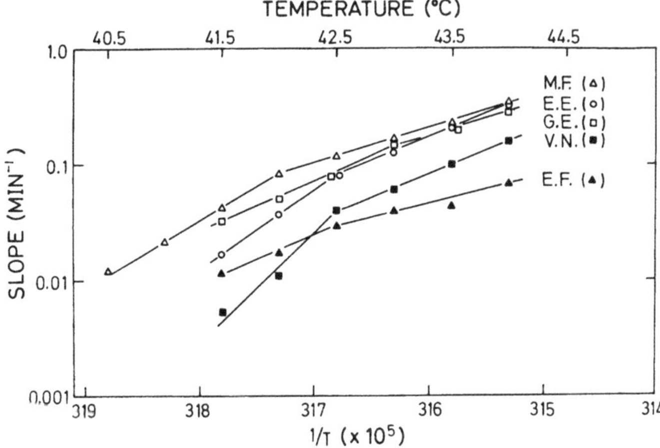

Fig. 9. Arrhenius curves for human melanoma xenografts heated in vivo at 40.5°-44.0° C. The data were derived from the slopes of the curves presented in Fig. 8

mas. The corresponding Arrhenius curves, based on the slopes of the specific growth delay dose-response curves, are presented in Fig. 9. Such curves are quite demanding to determine accurately. Nevertheless, it appears that all the Arrhenius curves have inflection points within a temperature range of 42.5° C ± 0.5° C.

Various parameters derived from the Arrhenius curves (Figs. 7 and 9) are summarized in Table 1. From this table certain conclusions may be drawn: The inflection point occurred at almost the same temperature in vivo and in vitro. The activation energies at temperatures above the inflection points were not significantly

Table 1. Activation energies[a] calculated from Arrhenius curves

Melanoma	In vivo			In vitro		
	Inflection point t(° C)[b]	μ (kJ/mole) T<t[c]	μ (kJ/mole) T>t[c]	Inflection point t (° C)[b]	μ (kJ/mole) T<t[c]	μ (kJ/mole) T>t[c]
E. F.	42.5	774 ± 67	426 ± 79	42.5	1691 ± 129	676 ± 37
V. N.	42.5	1661 ± 261	771 ± 76	42.5	2190 ± 281	739 ± 65
E. E.	42.5	1296 ± 84	760 ± 68	42.5	1839 ± 414	685 ± 39
G. E.	43.0	841 ± 75	507 ± 34	42.5	2134 ± 267	693 ± 57
M. F.	42.0	1072 ± 69	554 ± 39	41.5	1118 ± 135	678 ± 51

[a] Mean values ± SE.
[b] Inflection points were determined to the nearest 0.5° C.
[c] Activation energies at temperatures below (T<t) and above (T>t) the inflection point.

◀ **Fig. 8.** Specific growth delay for human melanoma xenografts heated at 40.5°-44.0° C as a function of treatment time. Note that the scale along the ordinate is different for the upper two and the lower three panels. Each *point* represents mean values based on 10-25 tumors. The *vertical bars* represent SE

different in vivo and in vitro for any of the melanomas. These activation energies do not seem to be significantly different from those reported for cells in culture (Henle and Dethlefsen 1980), murine tumors, and murine normal tissues (Overgaard and Suit 1979). Below the inflection point, the activation energies were found generally to be lower in vivo than in vitro. The observed activation energies in vitro in this temperature range were similar to those reported for established cell lines and murine normal tissues (Field and Morris 1983; Morris and Field 1985). Studies of cells in culture have indicated that the activation energy is reduced below, but remains unchanged above the inflection point when cells are heated at acid pH (Gerweck 1977; Henle and Dethlefsen 1980). These results support the assumption that the differences between the activation energies in vivo and in vitro at lower temperatures for our melanomas may probably be attributed to differences in the physiological conditions in vivo and in vitro. This may lead to the working hypothesis that hyperthermic treatments at temperatures below 42.5° C may be of particular interest in clinical situations where heat-induced normal tissue damage is a limiting factor.

Are Heat Responsiveness and Radiation Responsiveness Correlated?

Hyperthermia seems to have a particularly significant potential in the treatment of cancer when used as a cytotoxic agent in combination with radiation (Perez and Meyer 1985). A major concern, however, is that radioresistant tumors also may be resistant to heat, and that just radiosensitive tumors may be heat sensitive. Indeed, a study by Suit (1977) of experimental animal tumors indicated that tumor cure by heat alone can be achieved with particularly radiosensitive tumors only. In order to clarify whether there is any correlation between heat and radiation responsiveness of the human melanomas, we also carried out a study of their X-ray responsiveness.

Figure 10 shows specific growth delay after two different heat treatments, one at a low (41.5° C) and the other at a high (44.0° C) temperature, as a function of specific growth delay after a given radiation treatment (15 Gy). From these data it follows that there is no correlation between the heat and the radiation responses of the melanomas. This indicates that the heat responsiveness of melanomas in vivo is independent of the radioresponsiveness.

On the basis of these results it seems appropriate to stress that it is not justified to conclude that a radioresistant tumor is necessarily also heat resistant. Other criteria must be found to decide whether a tumor is likely to respond well to heat, and thus provide a guideline for the clinicians as to whether hyperthermic treatment should be prescribed.

Induced Thermotolerance in Human Melanomas

Hyperthermic treatments are known to induce a transient resistance to subsequent heat exposure, a phenomenon called thermotolerance. In the following the kinet-

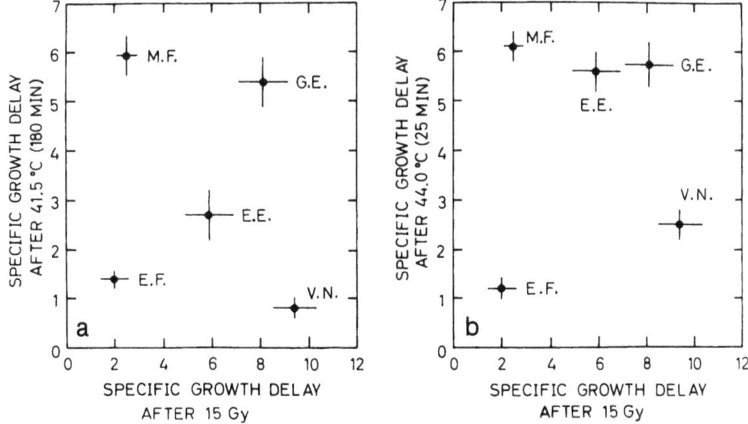

Fig. 10. **a** Specific growth delay in vivo after 41.5° C (180 min) and **b** specific growth delay in vivo after 44.0° C (25 min) versus specific growth delay in vivo after a single radiation dose of 15 Gy for human melanoma xenografts. The *points* and the *bars* represent mean values ± SE

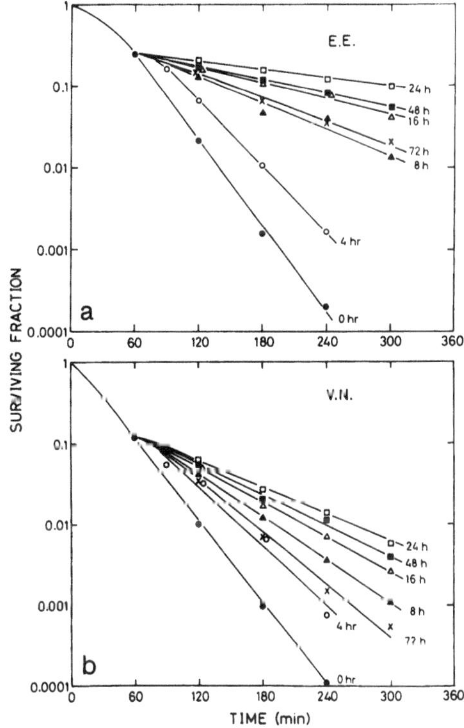

Fig. 11a, b. Survival curves for cells from human melanoma xenografts given two heat treatments at 43.5° C. The first treatment lasted 60 min, and the second 30, 60, 120, 180, or 240 min. The fractionation intervals were 0, 4, 8, 16, 24, 48, and 72 h, as indicated. The surviving fractions were calculated from the mean number of colonies in four tubes with heated and four tubes with unheated cells

ics of induced thermotolerance in vitro and in vivo of the melanoma xenografts will be discussed and certain possible implications of these results for fractionated clinical hyperthermia derived.

Kinetics of Induction of Thermotolerance in Vitro

Split-dose survival curves for cells from two of the melanomas (E. E. and V. N.) heated in vitro are shown in Fig. 11. The priming treatment was 43.5° C for 60 min. Second graded treatments at 43.5° C were given after fractionation intervals up to 72 h. From these curves thermotolerance ratios (TTRS) were calculated as the ratio of the slopes for preheated and single heated cells, the results of which are shown in Fig. 12. It can be seen that maximum TTR was reached 24 h after the priming treatment for all, but the maxima varied significantly among the melanomas, and that for the E. E. was about 3.5 times higher than that for the V. N. melanoma.

Kinetics of Induction of Thermotolerance in Vivo

Dose-response curves for the E. E. melanoma following split heat treatments in vivo are shown in Fig. 13. Tumor volumetric tripling time, i. e., the time from the day the first treatment was given to the day the tumor volumes had reached three times the initial volumes, was used as the measure of response. The priming treatment was 42.5° C for 30 min. Second graded treatments at 42.5° C were given after fractionation intervals up to 168 h (1 week). TTR was calculated as the ratio of the slopes for preheated and single heated tumors. TTR versus fractionation interval for the E. E. melanoma in vivo is shown in Fig. 14.

It follows from this figure that TTR reached a maximum of 4.9 at about 16 h and then decayed slowly toward unity at 1 week. This melanoma was the one

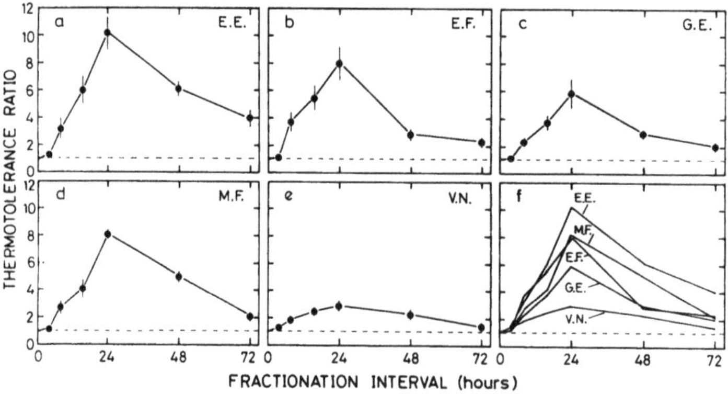

Fig. 12a–f. TTR as a function of fractionation interval for cells from human melanoma xenografts. *Curves*, kinetics of thermotolerance induced by heating at 43.5° C for 60 min; *bars*, SE; ----, TTR = 1.0. The curves are redrawn without experimental points for comparison

showing the highest degree of thermotolerance under in vitro conditions. Consequently, if there is a relationship between the thermotolerance induced under in vitro and in vivo conditions, a time interval of 1 week between heat fractions of 42.5° C for 30 min appears required to ensure complete decay of thermotolerance for the majority of melanomas.

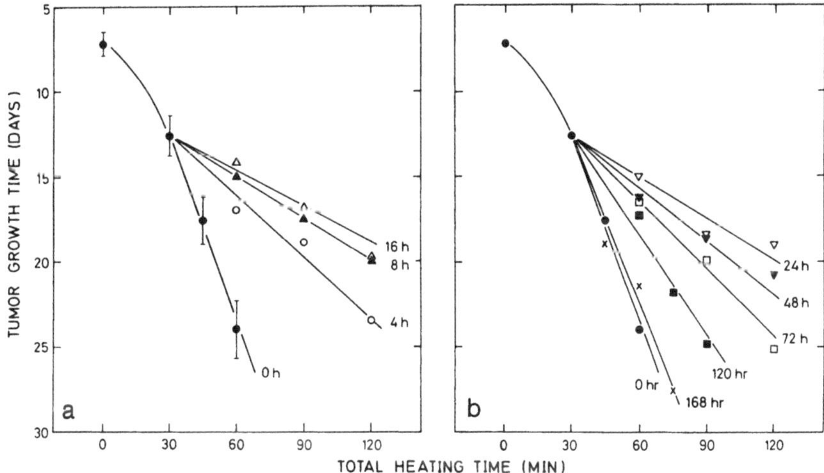

Fig. 13a, b. Tumor volumetric tripling time as a function of total heating time for a human melanoma xenograft given two treatments at 42.5° C. The first treatment lasted 30 min, and the second lasted 15, 30, 45, 60, or 90 min. The fractionation intervals were 0, 4, 8, and 16 h (**a**), and 24, 48, 72, 120, and 168 h (**b**). Each *point* is based on 15-20 tumors and represents mean values

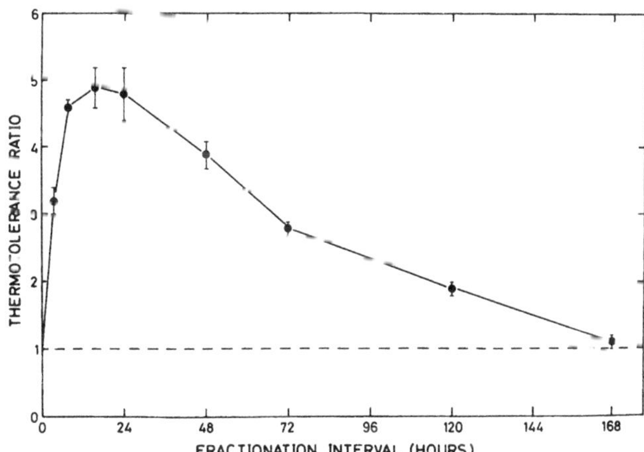

Fig. 14. TTR as a function of fractionation interval for a human melanoma xenograft. The *curve* illustrates the kinetics of thermotolerance induced by heating at 42.5° C for 30 min. The TTR values were calculated from the slopes of the curves in Fig. 13. *Bars*, SE; ----, TTR = 1.0

Possible Implications for Design of Clinical Hyperthermia Regimens

These results may have some implications for the choice of fractionation regimens in clinical treatment of cancer with hyperthermia. It will be of paramount importance to utilize the differences in thermotolerance between the tumor tissue and the limiting normal tissue when clinical hyperthermia regimens are to be designed. It may, however, be extremely difficult to predict the thermotolerance in a given tumor and in the limiting normal tissue in clinical practice (Overgaard 1985). Some of the reasons are:

1. The magnitude and kinetics of thermotolerance induced by equal treatments appear to vary considerably among different normal tissues and different tumors.
2. The tumor heating is usually heterogeneous due to vascular cooling or inadequate heating techniques.
3. Tumors may contain cell subpopulations with different heat sensitivities.

The problems related to the development of thermotolerance may be considerably reduced by using treatment regimens with fractionation intervals sufficiently long to ensure complete decay of thermotolerance. A therapeutic gain is then to be expected on the basis of differences between the tumor and the normal tissues in temperature and physiology.

The question then arises: How long should the interval between two fractions be? The thermotolerance induced in the E. E. melanoma xenograft by a heat dose of 42.5° C for 30 min decayed completely within 7 days after treatment. If temperatures above 42.5° C are maintained for 30 min or longer, complete decay of thermotolerance will probably require more than 7 days. Consequently, the present results indicate that treatment protocols probably should not prescribe more than one hyperthermic treatment per week.

Summary

The heat response in vitro and in vivo of five human melanoma xenografts grown in athymic nude mice was studied. The melanomas differed significantly in terms of heat sensitivity both in vitro and in vivo. At least two different mechanisms governed the overall heat response of the melanomas in vivo: the primary cell death, induced during treatment, was due to direct cytotoxic effects of the heat; the secondary cell death, induced after completion of treatment, was due to heat-induced vascular damage. The activation energies for the melanomas were not significantly different in vitro and in vivo at temperatures above the inflection point of the Arrhenius curves. Below the inflection point, on the other hand, the activation energies were higher in vitro than in vivo, probably as a consequence of differences in the physiological conditions in vitro and in vivo. The heat responsiveness of the melanomas in vivo was not related to the radioresponsiveness, whether the heat treatment was given at a low or a high temperature. All melanomas developed thermotolerance after a priming heat treatment. The thermotolerance differed significantly in magnitude among the five melanomas. It was concluded from the thermotolerance data that clinical treatment protocols probably should not prescribe more than one hyperthermic treatment per week.

References

Courtenay VD, Mills J (1978) An in vitro colony assay for human tumours grown in immune-suppressed mice and treated in vivo with cytotoxic agents. Br J Cancer 37: 261-268

Field SB, Morris CC (1983) The relationship between heating time and temperature: its relevance to clinical hyperthermia. Radiother Oncol 1: 179-186

Gerweck LE (1977) Modifications of cell lethality at elevated temperatures. The pH effect. Radiat Res 70: 224-235

Henle KJ, Dethlefsen LA (1980) Time-temperature relationships for heat-induced killing of mammalian cells. Ann NY Acad Sci 335: 234-253

Hill SA, Denekamp J (1978) The effect of vascular occlusion on the thermal sensitization of a mouse tumour. Br J Radiol 51: 997-1002

Morris CC, Field SB (1985) The relationship between heating time and temperature for rat tail necrosis with and without occlusion of the blood supply. Int J Radiat Biol 47: 41-48

Overgaard J (ed) (1985) Hyperthermic oncology 1984, vol 2. Review lectures, symposium summaries and workshop summaries. Taylor and Francis, London

Overgaard J, Suit HD (1979) Time-temperature relationship in hyperthermic treatment of malignant and normal tissue in vivo. Cancer Res 39: 3248-3253

Perez CA, Meyer JL (1985) Clinical experience with localized hyperthermia and irradiation. In: Overgaard J (ed) Hyperthermic oncology, vol 2. Review lectures, symposium summaries and workshop summaries. Taylor and Francis, London, pp 181-198

Suit HD (1977) Hyperthermic effects on animal tissues. Radiology 123: 483-487

*Intrinsic Thermosensitivity of Various Human Tumors**, **

W. Hinkelbein, G. Bruggmoser, A. Würdinger, and H. H. Fiebig

Abteilung Strahlentherapie, Radiologische Klinik, Albert-Ludwigs-Universität, Hugstetter Straße 55, 7800 Freiburg, FRG

Introduction

Hyperthermia is currently being tested clinically in combination with radiotherapy or chemotherapy. Often local or regional hyperthermia is combined with irradiation in the treatment of superficial tumors, this modality showing improved response rates over radiotherapy alone (Overgaard 1985). There is a wide range of response to hyperthermia, perhaps owing to the different intrinsic thermosensitivity of human tumors. Other reasons may be related to microcirculation (Reinhold and Endrich 1986), variations in pH or in nutrient concentration, immunological factors, and the development of thermotolerance (Meyer et al. 1986). If the intrinsic heat sensitivity could be predicted by an in vitro assay, this would permit the clinician to determine whether the patient might benefit from combining irradiation with hyperthermia.

In this paper, we report the heat sensitivity of various human tumor xenografts in a clonogenic stem cell assay (Hamburger and Salmon 1977; Salmon 1984). We have used human tumors growing in serial passages in nude mice to obtain a higher plating efficiency and to be able to reproduce the experiments (Henss et al. 1984).

Material and Methods

Tumors

Untreated human tumors established in serial passage in NMRI nu/nu mice were used (Fiebig et al. 1984, 1985). The animals were housed in Macrolon cages set in laminar flow shelves. In only 20% of the xenografts did the histological appearance of the mouse-grown tumors show some variation in degree of differentiation

* Dedicated to Professor Dr. med., Dr. h. c. G. W. Löhr on his 65th birthday.

** This work was supported by the DFG (grant Hi 368/1-1).

Recent Results in Cancer Research, Vol. 109

as compared with the original human tumors. The human origin of the tumors was demonstrated by isoenzyme technique. The tumors were studied in vitro after one to ten passages in nude mice.

Preparation of Single Cell Suspension

A single cell suspension was obtained by mechanical disaggregation and subsequent incubation with 0.04% collagenase, 0.07% DNAse, and 0.1% hyaluronidase at 37° C for 30 min. Afterwards, the cells were washed and passed through sieves (200- and 50-μm mesh size) to remove any remaining clumps. The cells were counted in a hemocytometer and the viable cells were determined by trypan blue exclusion.

Culture Methods and Heat Treatment

A modification of the double-layer soft agar culture system introduced by Hamburger and Salmon (1977) was used. The base layer consisted of 1 ml Iscove's modified Dulbeccos medium with L-glutamine containing 10% fetal calf serum and 0.5% agar, which was plated in 35-mm Petri dishes. Between 2 and 5×10^5 viable human tumor cells were added in a volume of 1 ml (0.3% agar, 30% fetal calf serum, and medium over the base layer). The top agar layer was covered by 1 ml medium containing 30% fetal calf serum (Fig. 1). Cultures were incubated at 37° C (control group), 40.5° C, 42° C, 43.5° C, or 45° C for 90 min, followed by incubation at 37° C in a humidified atmosphere containing 7% CO_2. Each treatment group had three dishes, the control groups six dishes. The growth of the control groups was monitored every other day using an inverted microscope. At the time of maximum colony formation (7–21 days after plating) the colonies (60–80 μm) were counted by an automatic image analysis system (Bausch and Lomb, OMNICON, FAS III) 24 h after vital staining with 1 ml tetrazolium chloride as negative controls (Alley et al. 1982). For the purpose of quality control, cultures were stained with tetrazolium chloride on day 0 and 2 and frozen at −20° C 1 day after addition of 1 ml glycerin until final evaluation.

Careful selection of viable tumor cells and passaging the tumors in nude mice was able to increase the growth rate to 86% with a median plating efficiency of 0.07% (Table 1).

Figure 2a shows the colony formation of a rapidly growing thyroid cancer (XF 117), and Fig. 2b shows the growth curve of a slowly growing malignant melanoma (MEXF 276).

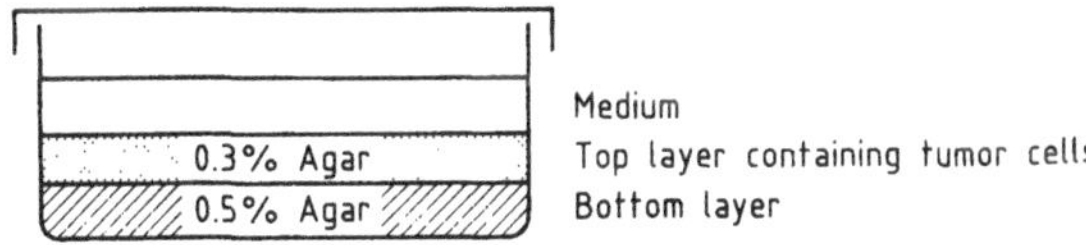

Fig. 1. Schematic illustration of a culture dish in the clonogenic tumor stem cell assay (semisolid double layer agar system)

Table 1. Plating efficiency of the human tumor stem cell assay

Seeded cells (× 1000)	200-500
Average number of colonies	100-800
Plating efficiency (%), median	0.07
Range	0.01-0.40
Tumor growth (%) (minimum of 30 colonies in untreated control plates)	86

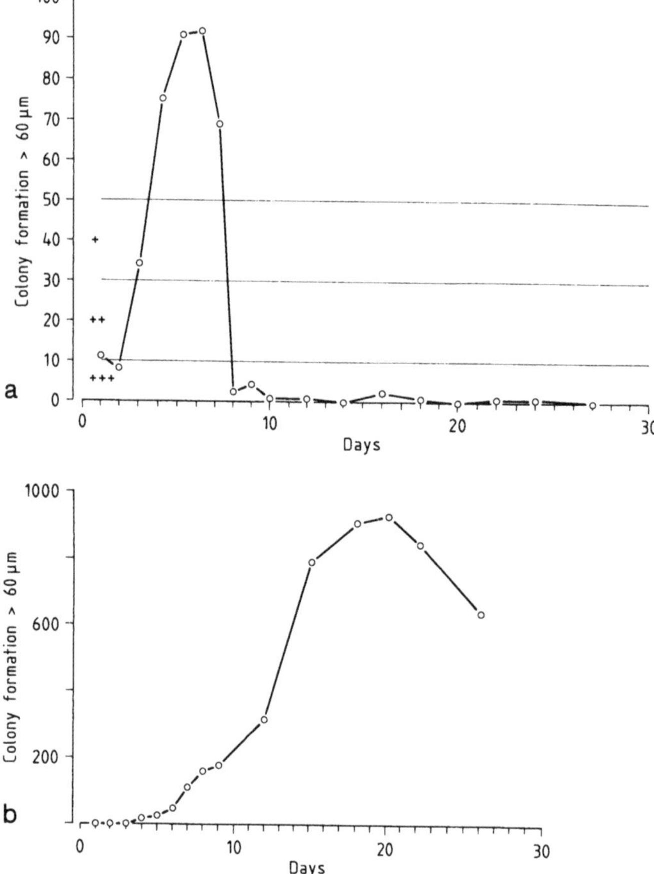

Fig. 2a, b. Colony development versus time after plating of **a** the rapidly growing thyroid cancer XF 117 and **b** the slowly growing melanoma MEXF 276. Each *point* represents the mean of three culture dishes, which were stained with tetrazolium chloride 1 day before evaluation, and frozen at $-20°$ C after decantation with glycerin until final counting

Detection of Heat Sensitivity

Clonogenic survival of heated tumors was expressed in T/C values (percent surviving colonies related to the normothermal control groups). Thermosensitivity was defined as T/C values <10 at 45° C or <30 at 43.5° C and graduated as shown in Table 2.

Results and Discussion

We examined 18 different human tumors in 25 assays. The heat response of the nine lung carcinomas tested (Table 3) was very different. Two small cell carcinomas had a low sensitivity and two a high sensitivity. One large cell carcinoma had a low sensitivity and the other one was resistant. Three adenocarcinomas of the lung were tested: one was heat resistant and two had a low sensitivity. Similar results were obtained with the other tumors examined (Table 4): one malignant melanoma was sensitive, the other one had only low sensitivity; one renal cell cancer

Table 2. Graduation of in vitro thermosensitivity

T/C value[a]	Sign	Heat sensitivity
<30 at 40.5° C[b]	+++	High sensitivity
<10 at 42.0° C		
<30 at 42.0° C	++	Sensitive
<10 at 43.5° C		
<30 at 43.5° C	+	Low sensitivity
<10 at 45.0° C		
All others	–	Resistant

[a] $T/C = \frac{\text{colonies found after hyperthermia}}{\text{colonies found in normothermal control groups}} \times 100$ (%).

[b] Heat exposure for 90 min.

Table 3. In vitro thermosensitivity of human lung carcinomas

Tumor	Histology	Thermo-sensitivity	No. of tests
LXFK 538	SCLC	+	1
LXFK 650	SCLC	+++	2
LXFK 688	SCLC	+	1
LXFK 737	SCLC	+++	1
LXFG 529	Large cell carcinoma	+	2
LXFG 625	Large cell carcinoma	–	2
LXFA 629	Adenocarcinoma	–	1
LXFA 677	Adenocarcinoma	+	2
LXFA 737	Adenocarcinoma	+	1

Table 4. In vitro thermosensitivity of other human tumors

Tumor	Histology	Thermo-sensitivity	No. of tests
MEXF 514	Malignant melanoma	+	2
MEXF 520	Malignant melanoma	++	1
PXF 698	Pleural mesothelioma	++	1
CXF 158	Colon cancer	–	1
RXF 423	Renal cell carcinoma	+++	1
RXF 631	Renal cell carcinoma	+	1
MAXF 449	Breast cancer	–	2
XF 546	Pancreatic carcinoma	+	1
SXF 627	Soft tissue sarcoma	++	2

had low sensitivity, and the other high sensitivity. These results suggest the intrinsic thermosensitivity to be a special characteristic of each tumor and not determined by its morphology. The feasibility of this test system as a predictive assay should be examined by correlation with clinical results. Combined hyperthermia and radiotherapy might be effective in tumors of low cellular heat sensitivity, since decrease in pH, malnutrition, and chronic hypoxia are thermosensitizing measures and are found in the most radioresistant parts of a tumor in vivo.

References

Alley MC, Uhl CB, Lieber MM (1982) Improved detection of drug cytotoxicity in the soft agar colony formation assay through use of a metabolizable tetrazolium salt. Life Sci 31: 3071-3078

Fiebig HH, Neumann H, Henß H, Hoch H, Kaiser D, Arnold H (1985) Development of three human small cell lung cancer models in nude mice. In: Seeber S (ed) Small cell lung cancer. Springer, Berlin Heidelberg New York, pp 77-86 (Recent results in cancer research, vol 97)

Fiebig HH, Widmer KH, Fiedler L, Wittekind C, Löhr GW (1984) Development and characterization of 51 human tumor models for large bowel, stomach and esophageal cancers. Progr Rep Dig Surg 1: 225-235

Hamburger AW, Salmon SE (1977) Primary bioassay of human tumor stem cells. Science 197: 461-463

Henss H, Fiebig HH, Meinhardt K, Löhr GW (1984) Clonal growth of human tumor xenografts: first experiences in drug testing. J Cancer Res Clin Oncol 108: 233-235

Meyer IL, van Kersen I, Hahn GM (1986) Tumor responses following multiple hyperthermia and X-ray treatments: role of thermotolerance at the cellular level. Cancer Res 46: 5691-5699

Overgaard J (1985) Rational and problems in the design of clinical studies. In: Overgaard J (ed) Hyperthermic oncology, vol 2. Taylor and Francis, London, pp 325-328

Reinhold HS, Endrich B (1986) Tumor microcirculation as a target for hyperthermia. Int J Hyperthermia 2: 111-137

Salmon SE (1984) Human tumor colony assay and chemosensitivity testing. Cancer Treat Rep 68: 117-125

Importance of Thermotolerance for Radiothermotherapy as Assessed Using Two Human Melanoma Cell Lines

D. van Beuningen and C. Streffer

Institut für Medizinische Strahlenbiologie, Universitätsklinikum Essen, Hufelandstraße 55, 4300 Essen 1, FRG

In the combined treatment of tumors by means of hyperthermia and ionizing radiation, the sequence, the interval between the two treatments, and the frequency of heat treatments are still open questions. In this discussion the development of thermotolerance plays an important role. It has frequently been observed that cells become more thermoresistant during prolonged heating at relatively low temperatures or during fractionated application of hyperthermia (review see: Henle and Dethlefsen 1978; Dewey et al. 1971; van Beuningen and Streffer 1985; Field and Law 1978; Law 1979; Law et al. 1979; Palzer and Heidelberg 1979; Law 1981; Field and Anderson 1982). The phenomenon of thermotolerance could be very important for the clinical use of hyperthermia if it also occurred in connection with radiosensitization by hyperthermia in human tumors. Up to now most studies on thermotolerance have been performed with hyperthermia alone and only a few experiments have been done with the combination of ionizing radiation and hyperthermia (Henle et al. 1979; Freeman et al. 1979; Law 1979; Nielsen and Overgaard 1979; Stewart and Denekamp 1980; van Beuningen et al. 1982; Nielsen 1984; Holohan 1982; Dewey 1984; Havemann 1983a; Streffer and van Beuningen 1983; Jorritsma et al. 1984; van Rijn et al. 1984; Jung et al. 1986; Streffer et al. 1984). The results are conflicting. Furthermore, it is very difficult to prove the existence of thermotolerance in vivo. The aim of the presented studies is to show how radiation can interact with heat treatments, especially after fractionated modalities.

Methods

Two human melanoma cell lines were used (MeWo and Be 11). The cell lines have been described previously (van Beuningen et al. 1982). Cells were treated with hyperthermia in a water bath at 42° C. At the time of treatment cells grew exponentially as a monolayer. Conditions for X-irradiation have been described previously (van Beuningen et al. 1979). Immediately after treatment cells were plated. The medium was MEM with 20% fetal calf serum and 1 mM sodium pyruvate. It was buffered with $NaHCO_3$ at pH 7.4. No feeder cells were used. Colonies with more

Recent Results in Cancer Research, Vol. 109

than 50 cells were counted 11–14 days after plating. Plating efficiency was 30%–50%. For each experiment the cells of three to four cultures were pooled and plated into four Petri dishes. Each experiment was repeated at least three times. The mean of all experiments was formed and the standard error of the mean was calculated. The terms "synergism," "supra-additive values," "more than additive values," and "radiosensitization" were used synonymously. The additive values were calculated by forming the product of survival rates after each single treatment.

Results

In Fig. 1 the survival of MeWo cells after continuous heating from 1 to 6 h at 42° C is shown. The cells show the typical survival curve after heat treatment alone. After the initial shoulder the survival decreases, but after 3 h incubation at 42° C the curve flattens. Thermotolerance occurs. When X-irradiation precedes hyperthermia (1.88 Gy and 3.76 Gy) the shoulder is reduced. The resulting cell death after combined exposures is more than additive. The expression of thermotolerance is apparently reduced under these conditions. In Fig. 2 data are presented from experiments which were done under the same treatment conditions with the other

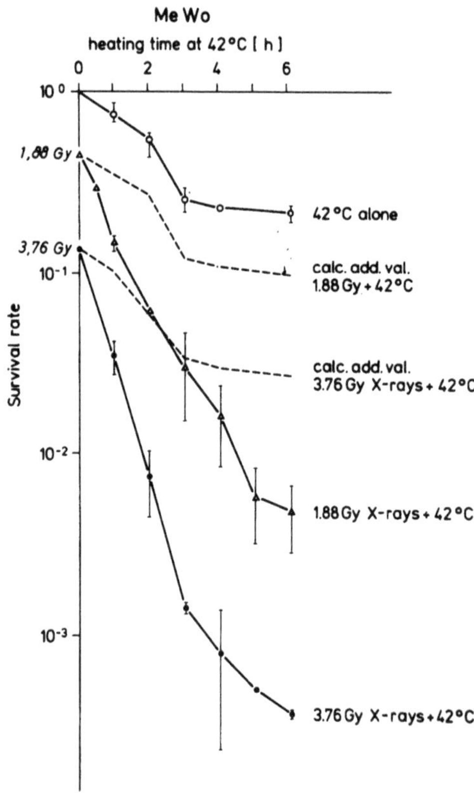

Fig. 1. Survival of MeWo cells after continuous heating at 42° C. ○—○, heating alone; △—△, 1.88 Gy X-rays followed by continuous heating; ●—●, 3.76 Gy X-rays followed by continuous heating; -----, calculated additive values

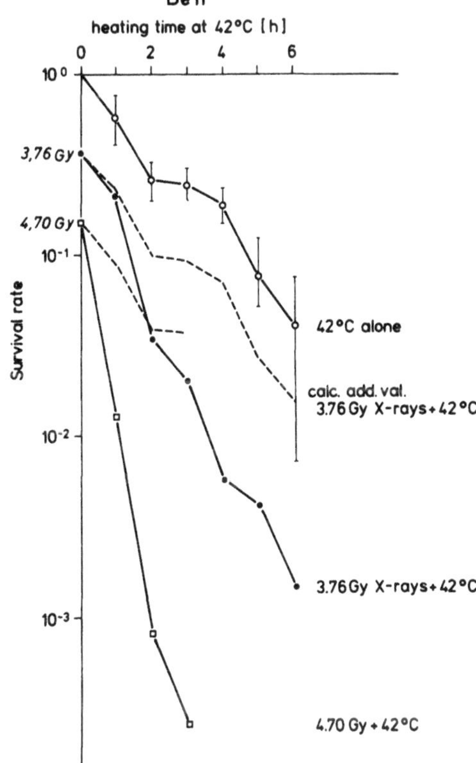

Fig. 2. Survival of Be 11 cells after continuous heating at 42° C. ○—○, heating alone; ●—●, 3.76 Gy X-rays followed by continuous heating; □—□, 4.7 Gy X-rays followed by continuous heating; -----, calculated additive values

cell line (Be 11). After heat treatment alone the shape of the survival curve is unusual. The cells develop a transient thermoresistance after about 2 h, but after heat treatment longer than 4 h the observed resistance disappears again. When irradiation precedes heating (3.76 Gy and 4.7 Gy), the Be 11 cells show a survival curve comparable to that of the MeWo cells after combined treatments with radiation doses of 1.88 and 3.76 Gy; the dose-effect curves are almost exponential under these conditions. Again, the cell death is more than additive. The above-described thermoresistance could not be observed during the 6-h heat treatment. On the basis of these experiments with continuous heating the heat treatments were split into one, two, or three fractions with an interval of 24 h and the cell survival after these treatments was compared with that after continuous heating. The same radiation dose was given (Fig. 3).

After the fractionated treatment with heat alone, the Be 11 cells showed a higher survival than after continuous heating. The same recovery was observed in the MeWo cells. When X-irradiation preceded the first fraction of heat treatment, the second and third fractions of heat alone had no further effect on the Be 11 cells. However, in the previously irradiated MeWo cells a "recall" effect was seen after the second and third heat treatments. The application of the higher X-ray dose caused a "sensitizing" effect also for the later heat treatments. No difference between the fractionated and continuous hyperthermia was observed. In the case of

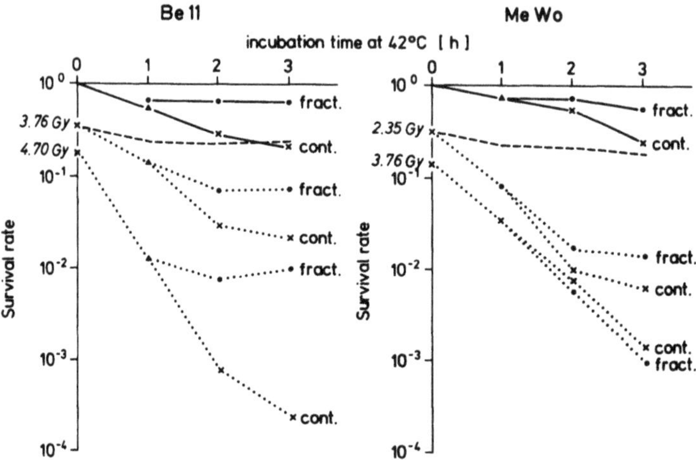

Fig. 3. Survival of MeWo cells and Be 11 cells after fractionated and continuous heating, alone and with one preceding radiation dose. ●—●, fractionated heating alone; ×—×, continuous heating alone; ●.....●, fractionated heating with one X-ray dose; ×.....×, continuous heating with one X-ray dose; -----, calculated additive value

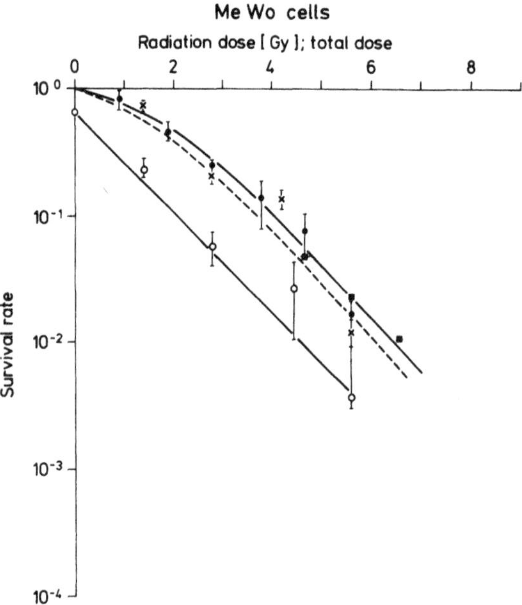

Fig. 4. Survival of MeWo cells after fractionation of X-rays and heat. ●—●, single X-ray dose; ×—×, X-rays, three doses, 24-h interval; ■—■, X-rays, two doses: first dose 3.76 Gy, 24-h interval, further X-ray doses; ○—○, X-rays followed by 1 h at 42° C, three times, 24-h interval; -----, calculated additive value

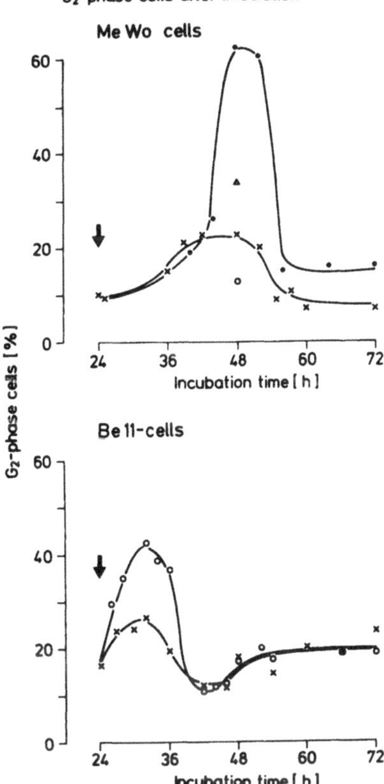

Fig. 5. G_2-block of MeWo and Be 11 cells after irradiation. *Arrow,* time of irradiation. MeWo cells: O, 1.88 Gy; ×, 3.76 Gy; Δ, 5.64 Gy; ●, 7.52 Gy. Be 11 cells: ×, 3.76 Gy; O, 5.64 Gy

Be 11 cells, too, fractionated heat treatments caused a synergistic effect with ionizing radiation. Cell death was always higher than would be expected from additive effects.

While in the foregoing experiments a heat-sensitizing effect of radiation could be shown, in the following experiments the radiosensitizing effect of heat was studied.

In Fig. 4 survival curves of MeWo cells after a single radiation dose and after two and three fractions of X-rays are shown. The interval between each fraction was 24 h. It was surprising that the MeWo cells showed no repair of sublethal radiation damage under these conditions. When in the "three fraction" experiments heat was given to each radiation dose, a strong sensitizing effect was observed. Under these conditions cell death was again more than additive.

The reason for the lack of the shoulder after fractionation of X-rays could depend on changes in the distribution of cells in the cell cycle. Flow cytometric analysis of the distribution of cells in the cell cycle showed a dose-dependent, radiation-induced G_2-block of MeWo cells which occurred just at the time when the second X-ray dose was given (Fig. 5). The Be 11 cells also showed a G_2-block, which was shorter than with the MeWo cells. Twenty-four hours after the first fraction the distribution of cells in the cell cycle was the same as in untreated cells.

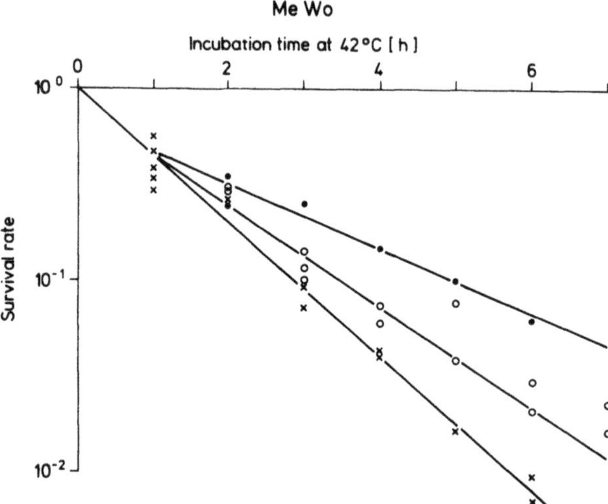

Fig. 6. Induction of thermotolerance in MeWo cells. ×—×, survival after heating at 42° C without pretreatment; ●—●, survival after heating 24 h after pretreatment for 1 h at 42° C; ○—○, survival after heating 48 h after pretreatment for 1 h at 42° C. Each *point* represents one separate experiment

Therefore, experiments were performed for the MeWo cells with a longer interval between the X-ray doses (48 h). Another question to be solved was whether cells were still thermotolerant 48 h after the first treatment. In Fig. 6 dose-effect curves after continuous heating without and with a priming dose of 1 h at 42° C are shown. Without heat pretreatment the D_0 was 76 min; with pretreatment the D_0 increased to 160 min when the cells were heated 24 h later and to 100 min when they were heated 48 h later. The cells were still thermotolerant with an interval of 48 h, but thermotolerance had started to decay at the later period.

Figure 7 shows survival of MeWo cells after fractionation experiments were performed with the 48-h interval. Under these conditions the dose-effect curves demonstrated recovery from sublethal damage after X-ray exposure alone. After the combination of X-rays followed by heat (1 h at 42° C) the survival decreased exponentially. When the first treatment was by X-rays immediately followed by heat for 1 h at 42° C and the cells were treated again with X-rays alone after an interval of 48 h, the survival curve was shifted to even lower survival values than after the single combined treatment. Although the cells were thermotolerant (Fig. 6), they could apparently "remember" the first combined treatment and were still highly sensitized.

In further experiments we investigated how long MeWo cells can preserve this "recall" effect. After 4.7 Gy (total dose) immediately followed by 1 h at 42° C the survival was 0.57 (57%) and after 5.64 Gy 0.25 (25%). In these experiments cells were plated 48 h after treatment and not immediately after treatment as in the former experiments. When the interval between radiation doses was 48 h, the survival was 0.19 and 0.04 respectively. After an interval of 120 h survival increased to 0.41 and 0.18 respectively. This means that cells show this "recall" even after 120 h, but the effect is reduced at the later period.

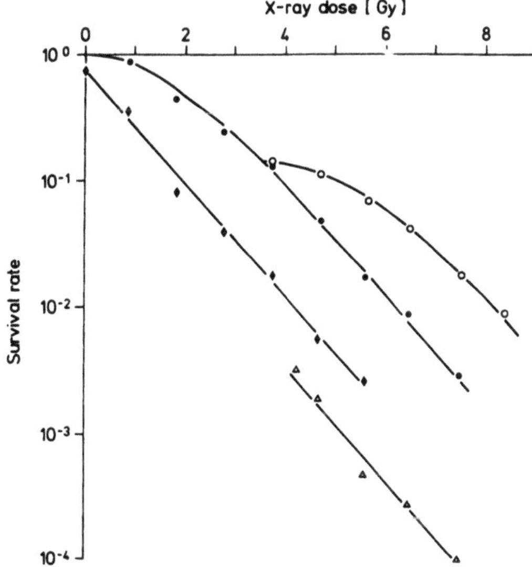

Fig. 7. Survival of MeWo cells after fractionation with X-rays and heat (48-h interval). ●—●, X-rays alone; ○—○, two X-ray doses alone; ◆—◆, X-rays followed by heat, single treatment; △—△, X-rays followed by heat, 48-h interval, X-rays alone

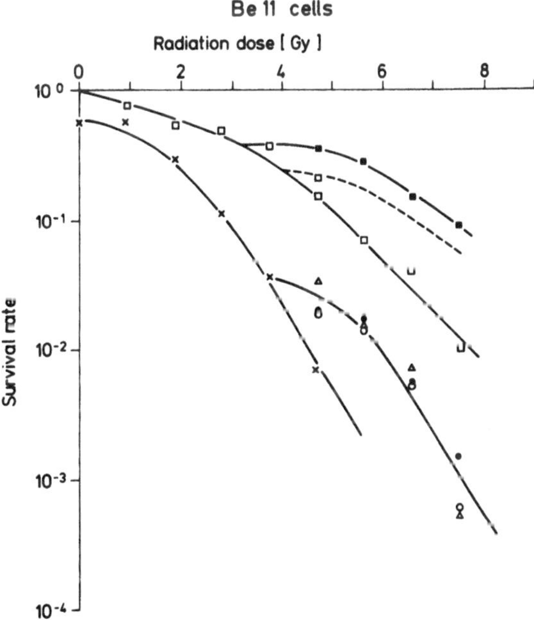

Fig. 8. Survival of Be 11 cells after fractionation with X-rays and heat (24-h interval). □—□, X-rays alone, single treatment; ■—■, X-rays alone, two fractions; ×—×, X-rays plus 1 h at 42° C, single treatment; ○—○, X-rays plus heat, 24-h interval, X-rays alone; ●—●, X-rays plus heat, 48-h interval, X-rays alone; △—△, X-rays plus heat, 72-h interval, X-rays alone; -----, calculated additive values (X-rays vs. X-rays plus heat, 24-h interval)

Similar experiments were done with the Be 11 cells. Be 11 cells were also thermotolerant 24 h after pretreatment with heat for 1 h at 42° C. However, it was not possible to describe thermotolerance by changes in D_0 because the dose-effect curve showed a strange shape (Fig. 2). Survival rates after 1 h pretreatment at 42° C were 0.52 at 2 h, 0.38 at 3 h, 0.22 at 4 h, 0.09 at 5 h, and 0.06 at 6 h; without pretreatment they were 0.26, 0.25, 0.19, 0.07, and 0.04 respectively. In Fig. 8 dose-effect curves after single and fractionated X-ray treatments are shown. The interval between the two X-ray doses was 24 h. The D_q after the split-dose experiment was 2.0 Gy, while after a single X-ray dose it was 2.6 Gy. After the combined treatment (X-rays immediately followed by hyperthermia for 1 h at 42° C) the survival curve still had a shoulder; the D_q was reduced to 1.7 Gy for the single treatment. When the first X-ray treatment was followed by heat and after an interval of 24 h X-rays only were given, the D_q was further reduced to 1.25 Gy. Thus, the Be 11 cells were also sensitized by the pretreatment (X-rays and heat), but the effect was not so pronounced as with the MeWo cells. The Be 11 cells showed the "recall" phenomenon, although they were thermotolerant or thermoresistant with respect to the strange dose-effect curve after continuous heating (Fig. 2). The decreasing D_q resulted in an enhanced cell loss, which was more than additive. Figure 8 also shows how long Be 11 cells have the "recall" effect. The interval between X-rays plus heat and the second X-ray dose without heat was prolonged to 48 and 72 h. The D_q remained the same during that time.

In another experiment we combined the fractionated heat treatments (Fig. 3) with preceding X-ray doses (Fig. 9). The interval between the three combined

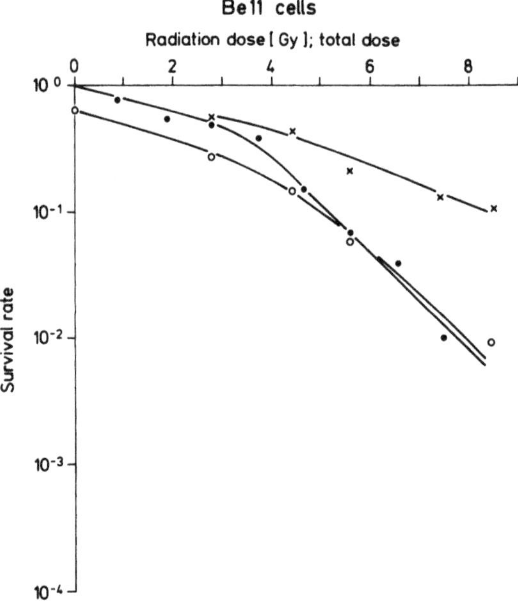

Fig. 9. Survival of Be 11 cells after three fractions of X-rays alone or X-rays plus heat, 24-h interval. ●—●, X-rays alone; ×—×, three X-ray doses alone, 24-h interval; ○—○, three doses of combined treatment (X-rays plus 1 h at 42° C), 24-h interval

treatments was 24 h. After three X-ray doses alone the survival increased as expected. After the fractionation of X-rays always followed by heat treatments for 1 h at 42° C the fractionation effect of X-rays disappeared completely. The effect was again more than additive, although the cells showed an increased resistance after fractionation of heat alone as well as after fractionation of X-rays alone (Figs. 3, 9).

Discussion

Nielsen (1984) reported that preheating reduced the sensitivity to a subsequent treatment with radiation alone as well as with simultaneous heat and radiation in L1A2 cells. He reached this conclusion from the reduction of the D_0 of the dose-effect curve. However, the TER was not influenced by the preheating treatment. The D_q of irradiated cells is reduced after prior heating as well as after simultaneous treatments. A similar phenomenon was observed in the Be 11 cells. Van Rijn et al. (1984) found with Reuber H 5 hepatoma cells that thermotolerance decreased the extent of radiosensitization. Similar data were obtained by Haveman (1983). In the latter experiments the reduction of radiosensitization by thermotolerance was even observed in the shoulder region. Streffer et al. (1984) and Jorritsma et al. (1984) reported that radiosensitization was not modified by thermotolerance. Thus, the results seem to be conflicting.

Jung et al. (1986) induced thermotolerance in R1H cells and treated these cells 16 h later with heat and X-rays. The radiosensitizing effect of heat was not influenced by thermotolerance. Data from Holohan et al. (1982, 1984) and Dewey (1984) show that thermotolerance decreased the radiosensitizing effect in the higher dose range but did not affect the shoulder region. Apparently a dose dependence existed for the radiosensitizing effect in thermotolerant cells. This phenomenon could partly explain the differing results. As in clinical use the dose per fraction is in the range of 2–3 Gy, one could assume that thermotolerance plays no role in the radiosensitizing effect under clinical conditions.

While in the above-mentioned data a priming heat dose was given to induce thermotolerance which was followed by combined radiothermotherapy, this priming heat dose was combined with a radiation dose in the results here reported. We think that this treatment design is more realistic for clinical use, because in clinical situations treatment commences with radiotherapy and heat fractions are usually added after radiation.

From our data we can assume that thermotolerance after continuous heating can be prevented by preceding irradiation (Figs. 1, 2). In each case the cell killing effect was more than additive. This means that there is synergism between heat and radiation treatment, which is important for clinical application.

After fractionation of heat both cell lines showed a fractionation effect. It is difficult or impossible to distinguish between thermotolerance and repair of heat damage after fractionation. However, if a radiation dose preceded heat fractionation, Be 11 cells still showed the fractionation effect, but the cell-killing effect was nevertheless synergistic. MeWo cells were more sensitized especially after the higher doses. They were sensitized for heat treatments by radiation. This effect is unusual and cannot be explained at present.

Further, after split-dose experiments cell cycle effects can play a role, as the experiments with the MeWo cells show, and these effects must be taken into account. Split-dose experiments clearly show that after heat alone both cell lines are thermotolerant at the time of the second dose; however, both cell lines show a "recall phenomenon" for the first combined treatment. In the MeWo cells the survival curve is shifted to lower survival rates, whereas in the Be 11 cells the shoulder is more reduced. This means that survival rates are decreased in each case in a synergistic way. Cell death is increased more than additively if the first treatment is irradiation and this is followed by heat. The same effects were observed after the split-dose experiments with the Be 11 cells.

From these data we would assume that each irradiation should be followed by one heat treatment or that heat should be given as often as possible when it is combined with X-rays. Thermotolerance has but little or no meaning.

On the other hand, when cells show the recall phenomenon it is not necessary for each radiation dose to be combined with hyperthermia. From the data reported here, one could propose that it is sufficient under these conditions when heat is given every third day during a radiation course.

References

Dewey WC (1984) Interaction of heat with radiation and chemotherapy. Cancer Res (Suppl) 44: 4714s-4720s

Dewey WC, Westra A, Miller HH, Nagasawa H (1971) Heat induced lethality and chromosomal damage in synchronized Chinese hamster cells treated with 5-bromodeoxyuridine. Int J Radiat Biol 20: 505-520

Field SB, Anderson RL (1982) Thermotolerance: A review of observations and possible mechanisms. Natl Cancer Inst Monogr 61: 193-201

Field SB, Law MP (1978) The response of skin to fractionated heat and X-rays. Br J Radiol 51: 221-222

Freeman ML, Raaphorst GP, Dewey WC (1979) The relationship of heat killing and thermal radiosensitization to the duration of heating at C. Radiat Res 78: 172-175

Haveman J (1983a) Influence of a prior heat treatment on the enhancement by hyperthermia of X-ray-induced inactivation of cultured mammalian cells. Int J Radiat Biol 43: 267-280

Haveman J (1983b) Influence of pH and thermotolerance on the enhancement of X-ray-induced inactivation of cultured mammalian cells by hyperthermia. Int J Radiat Biol 43: 281-289

Henle KJ, Dethlefsen LA (1978) Heat fractionation and thermotolerance: a review. Cancer Res 38: 1843-1851

Henle KJ, Tomasovic SP, Dethlefsen LA (1979) Fractionation of combined heat and radiation in asynchronous CHO cells. I. Effects on radiation sensitivity. Radiat Res 80: 369-377

Holohan EV, Highfield DP, Dewey WC (1982) Induction during G_1 of heat radiosensitization in Chinese hamster ovary cells following single and fractionated heat doses. Natl Cancer Inst Monogr 61: 123-125

Holohan EV, Highfield DP, Holohan PK, Dewey WC (1984) Hyperthermic cell killing and hyperthermic radiosensitization in Chinese hamster ovary cells: effects of pH and thermal tolerance. Radiat Res 97: 108-131

Jorritsma JBM, Kampinga HH, Konings ATW (1984) Role of DNA polymerase in the mechanisms of damage by heat and heat plus radiation in mammalian cells. In: Overgaard J (ed) Hyperthermic oncology. Taylor and Francis, London, pp 61-64

Jung H, Dikomey E, Zywietz F (1986) Ausmaß und Entwicklung der Thermoresistenz und deren Einfluß auf die Strahlenempfindlichkeit von soliden Transplantationstumoren. In: Streffer C, Herbst M, Schwabe H (eds) Lokale Hyperthermie. Deutscher Ärzte-Verlag, Cologne, pp 23-28

Law MP (1979) Some effects of fractionation on the response of the mouse Ear to combined heat and X-rays. Radiat Res 80: 360-368

Law MP (1981) The induction of thermal resistance in the ear of the mouse by heating at temperatures ranging from 41.5 to 45.5° C. Radiat Res 85: 126-134

Law MP, Coultas PG, Field SB (1979) Induced thermal resistance in the mouse ear. Br J Radiol 52: 308-314

Nielsen OS (1984) Fractionated hyperthermia and thermotolerance. Laege foremingeus, Arhus

Nielsen OS, Overgaard J (1979) Hyperthermic radiosensitization of thermotolerant tumour cells in vitro. Int J Radiat Biol 35: 171-176

Palzer RJ, Heidelberger C (1973) Studies on the quantitative biology of hyperthermic killing of HeLa cells. Cancer Res 33: 415-421

Stewart FA, Denekamp J (1980) Fractionation studies with combined X-rays and hyperthermia in vivo. Br J Radiol 53: 346-356

Streffer C, van Beuningen D (1983) Hyperthermia as a radiosensitizing and cytotoxic agent: cell biological and biochemical considerations. Verh Dtsch KrebsGes 4: 89-97

Streffer C, van Beuningen D, Uma Devi P (1984) Radiosensitization by hyperthermia in human melanoma cells: single and fractionated treatments. Cancer Treat Rev 11: 179-185

van Beuningen D (1983) Hyperthermie als zytotoxisches und strahlensensibilisierendes Agens: zelluläre Effekte. Strahlentherapie 159: 60-66

van Beuningen D, Streffer C (1985) Die Hyperthermie. In: Heuck F, Scherer E (eds) Strahlengefährdung und Strahlenschutz. Springer, Berlin Heidelberg New York, pp 641-681 (Handbuch der medizinischen Radiologie, vol XX)

van Beuningen D, Streffer C, Zamboglou N, Schubert B, Lindscheid K-R (1979) Effekte nach der Kombination von Hyperthermie mit ionisierenden Strahlen auf Melanomzellen. In: Wannenmacher M, Gauwerky F, Streffer C (eds) Kombinierte Strahlen- und Chemotherapie. Urban and Schwarzenberg, Baltimore, pp 75-81

van Beuningen D, Streffer C, Zamboglou N, Kersting S (1982) Proliferation of human melanoma cells after single and fractionated exposure to hyperthermia and radiation. Natl Cancer Inst Mongr 61: 137-139

van Rijn J, van den Berg J, Schamhart DHJ, van Wijk R (1984) Effect of thermotolerance on thermal radiosensitization in hepatoma cells. Radiat Res 97: 318-328

In Vitro Thermochemotherapy in Ovarian Cancer

H. M. Runge, H. A. Neumann, K. Braun, and A. Pfleiderer

Universitäts-Frauenklinik, Lehrstuhl für Gynäkologie und Geburtshilfe II,
Hugstetter Straße 55, 7800 Freiburg, FRG

Introduction

Clinical therapy for advanced ovarian cancer is largely based on radical surgery and even more so on chemotherapy. Of ovarian carcinomas 85%, are diagnosed at stages III and IV. The advanced ovarian carcinoma of stage III or IV is characterized by carcinomatosis of the peritoneum. The aim of therapy is the induction of a clinical and histopathological complete remission (Pfleiderer 1984).

The most important prognostic factors in advanced ovarian carcinomas are (Meerpohl 1985): (a) the residual tumor after surgery, (b) the age of the patient, and (c) the stage. If the residual tumor is less than 2 cm after the debulking surgery, with cis-platin chemotherapy we can expect a complete remission in 30%-50% of cases. If the residual tumor is more than 2 cm after surgery, a complete remission can be achieved only in 10%. Thus the 5-year survival ranges between 20% and 25% in stage III ovarian cancer with cis-platin containing chemotherapy. We can see that even with maximum surgical effort and highly potent chemotherapy, the prognosis of stage III and IV ovarian cancer remains poor.

Many experiments in vivo and in vitro have demonstrated that the effect of cytostatic drugs can be enhanced under hyperthermic conditions. These effects have been demonstrated mostly at temperatures of 42° C or higher. Discussing the clinical application of hyperthermia, Hahn and Shiu (1983) have pointed out that an enhancement of cell killing under whole-body hyperthermia might affect cancer cells and critical normal tissue like bone marrow cells or gastrointestinal crypt cells as well. If so, no therapeutic gain could be expected from a combination of whole-body hyperthermia and cytostatic drugs.

It was the aim of our study to test the effect of hyperthermia and cytostatic drugs on tumor colony forming cells from human ovarian carcinomas and from bone marrow progenitor cells. To have conditions that could be employed for clinical whole-body hyperthermia, we chose a hyperthermic temperature of 40.5° C for 2 h.

Recent Results in Cancer Research, Vol. 109

Material and Methods

For our in vitro experiments we cultivated 25 freshly explanted, untreated stage III and IV ovarian carcinomas. The cultivation was performed in the colony forming assay in a methylcellulose monolayer (Fig. 1). For this reason the tumor specimens were brought into single cell suspension and 2×10^5 tumor cells/dish were plated in the methylcellulose (0.9% w/v). We mainly used tissue from abdominal metastases, because we could prove a better plating efficiency for these specimens than for ascitic or primary tumor cells (Runge et al. 1986).

In 16 cases (64%) the cultivation was successful in that further chemosensitivity testing was possible. We used the methylcellulose monolayer assay for the cultivation of clonogenic tumor cells and bone marrow progenitor cells because we could prove no significant difference between the agar double layer assay, as described by Hamburger et al. (1978), and the methylcellulose monolayer (Runge et al. 1985).

The cultivation of the human bone marrow progenitor cells was performed as described by Fauser and Messner (1979). Briefly, bone marrow cells were aspirated from eight volunteers from the iliac crest. The mononuclear cells were plated in the presence of phytohemagglutinin-leukocyte-conditioned medium. The cytostatic drugs used were cis-platin, vincristine, bleomycin and its analogue peplomycin (Umezawa 1979), adriamycin, epirubicin, and melphalan. The cultures of the tumor cells and the bone marrow cells were continuously incubated with the drugs.

Hyperthermia was induced by incubation of the culture dishes at 40.5° C for 2 h. Afterwards, the culture dishes were placed in a normal 37° C incubator for the rest of the incubation period. The temperature was monitored directly in the methylcellulose with an electronic thermometer.

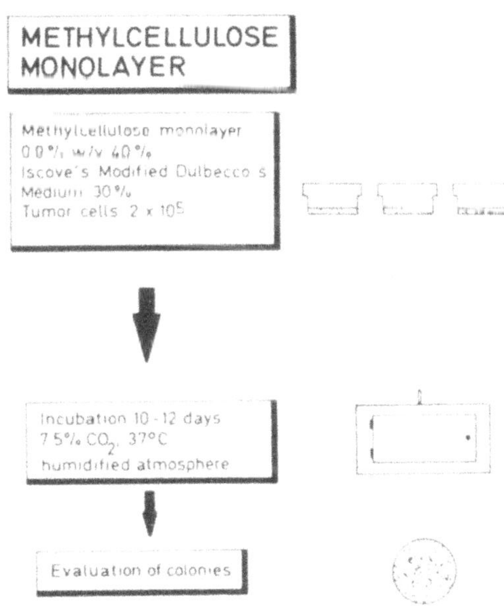

Fig. 1. The cultivation of clonogenic human ovarian carcinoma cells in the methylcellulose monolayer assay

Results

Figure 2 shows that after 30 min 40.5° C hyperthermic conditions were reached. The pH in the cultures was not altered by the 2 h of hyperthermic treatment, compared with the pH found in the normothermic cultures under the conditions used (Neumann et al. 1985).

Table 1 shows the influence of hyperthermia for 2 h on the colony formation of the tumor cells. In the colony assay an inhibition of the colony survival is measured. The supposed standard deviation for the colony formation was 10%. Thus we could find a slight inhibition in three cases and in another three cases a slight stimulatory effect. However, from what we know so far about sensitivity parame-

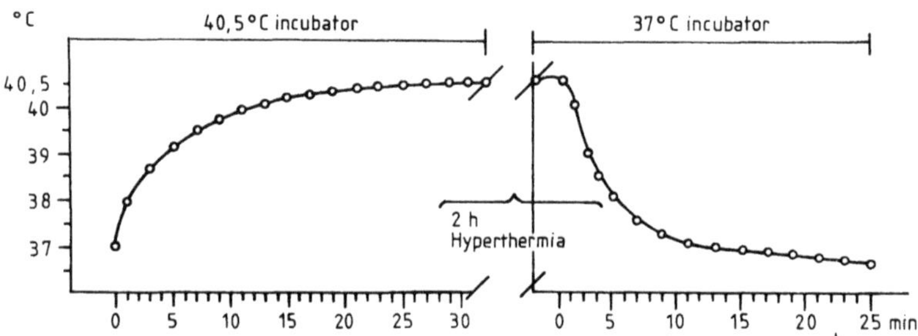

Fig. 2. Temperature profile in the methylcellulose monolayer dish under hyperthermic (40.5° C) and normothermic (31° C) conditions

Table 1. Influence of a hyperthermic incubation (40.5° C) for 2 h on the colony formation of clonogenic human ovarian cancer cells in the methylcellulose monolayer assay (%)

Patient	Colony formation at 37° C (%)	Colony formation at 2 h, 40.5° C (%)[a]
1	100	100 ± 8
2	100	116 ± 10
3	100	66 ± 6
4	100	91 ± 8
5	100	100 ± 9
6	100	78 ± 7
7	100	125 ± 8
8	100	100 ± 12
9	100	84 ± 11
10	100	109 ± 4
11	100	112 ± 5
12	100	91 ± 7
13	100	103 ± 13
14	100	100 ± 8
15	100	95 ± 6
16	100	100 ± 10%

[a] ± SD.

ters in the colony assay, we do not think that this observation has any clinical meaning. The normothermic and hyperthermic incubation of the bone marrow progenitor cells did not show a significant difference with regard to the colony formation. Figure 3 demonstrates the influence of the normothermic and hyperthermic drug incubation on the bone marrow cells. We found no significant difference between normothermic and hyperthermic incubation with our seven cytostatic drugs: in every case the incubation revealed typical and reproducible dose-response curves under normo- and hyperthermic conditions. Only the incubation of the bone marrow with vincristine (Fig. 3) did not show colony formation at 40.5° C at a drug concentration of 10^{-1} µg/ml, whereas at 37° C colony formation was still observed.

To assess therapeutic gain using hyperthermia treatment, compared with the drug effects on the bone marrow, we plotted the dose-response curves of the tumor colonies together with the dose-response curves of the bone marrow colonies (see Neumann et al., this book) (Figs 4-7). In addition, a comparison of bone marrow and tumor cell toxicity allows the assessment of the cytotoxicity of a drug independent of pharmacological doses and exposure time. Figure 4 shows an individual dose-response curve of the influence of cis-platin incubation on the bone marrow cells and on tumor colony formation. There was a marked difference in the colony formation of the tumor cells between the normothermic and hyperthermic curve below. The standard deviation of the colony formation of the tumor cells usually was less than 10%. Thus we can suggest enhanced cytotoxicity under hyperthermic conditions if the two curves differ by at least 10%-20%. In the case of patient number 1 we could prove enhanced cytotoxicity under hyperthermic conditions, with an 85% inhibition of colony formation versus 55% in the normothermic samples (at 10^{-1} µg/ml).

Figure 5 shows a vincristine case without a hyperthermic effect. The dose-response curves of the tumor colony formation under normo- and hyperthermic conditions were identical.

Figure 6 proves an enhanced hyperthermic cytotoxicity for bleomycin. The normothermic dose-response curve from the tumor colony formation revealed an inhibition of colony formation of about 55% whereas the hyperthermic dose-response curve showed a 90% inhibition. An inhibition of colony formation of more than 70% usually signalizes tumor sensitivity to the drug tested. Thus, in this case, we can conclude that the tumor, which showed only a slight sensitivity under normothermic conditions, became obviously sensitive under hyperthermic conditions.

In one case we saw a stimulation of colony formation by hyperthermic incubation with cis-platin. This phenomenon was a single observation within 57 tests we did under hyperthermic conditions. The stimulated colony formation by cis-platin (Fig. 7) could be explained by an irritated diffusion of cis-platin into the tumor cells under our hyperthermic conditions. Another single case of platin-stimulated colony formation has been reported by Neumann et al. (1985), who treated a "schwannoma" with cis-platin under hyperthermic conditions.

Table 2 summarizes our results for the seven cytostatic drugs tested.

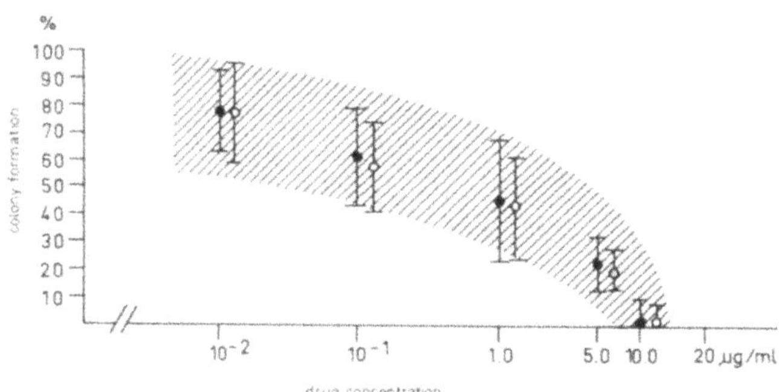
Cis-Platin
%
100
90
80
70
60
50
40
30
20
10
colony formation
10⁻²
10⁻¹
1.0
5.0
10.0
20 µg/ml
drug concentration

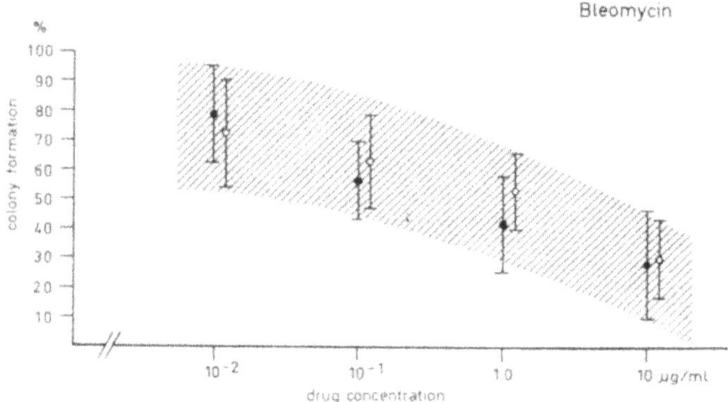
Bleomycin
%
100
90
80
70
60
50
40
30
20
10
colony formation
10⁻²
10⁻¹
1.0
10 µg/ml
drug concentration

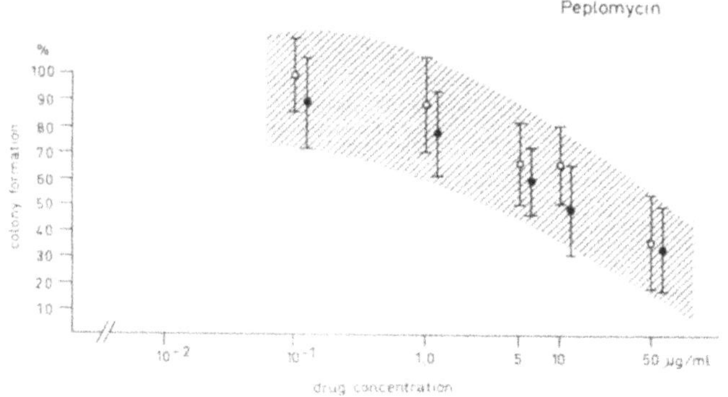
Peplomycin
%
100
90
80
70
60
50
40
30
20
10
colony formation
10⁻²
10⁻¹
1.0
5
10
50 µg/ml
drug concentration

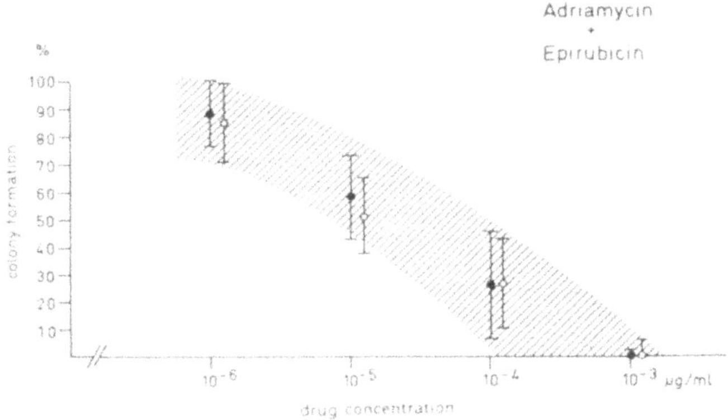

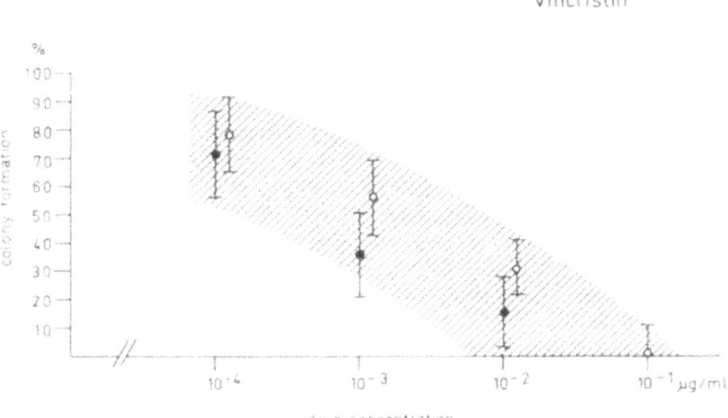

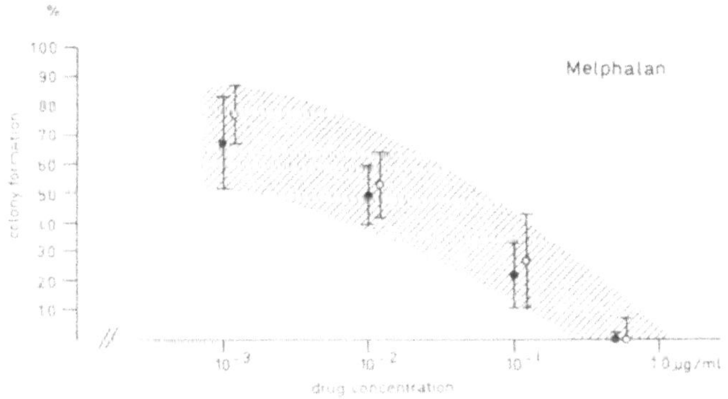

◀ **Fig. 3.** Influence of normothermic (⊢○⊣) and hyperthermic (⊢●⊣, 2 h at 40.5° C) incubation of human bone marrow progenitor cells with various cytostatic drugs in the colony assay. Values represent means of triplicate cultures of bone marrow samples from eight healthy volunteers. *Points*, % colony formation of the controls (100%)

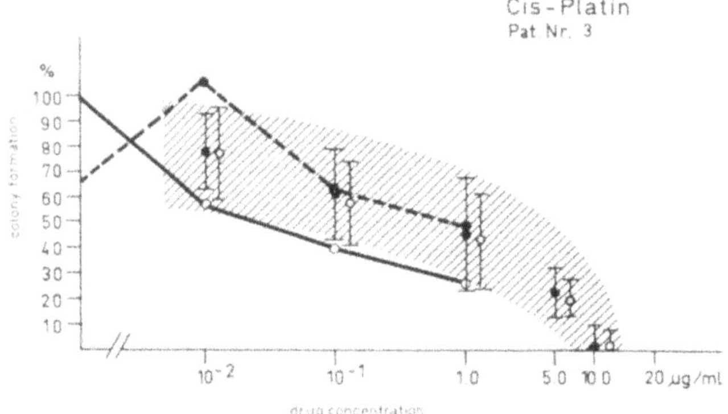

Fig. 4

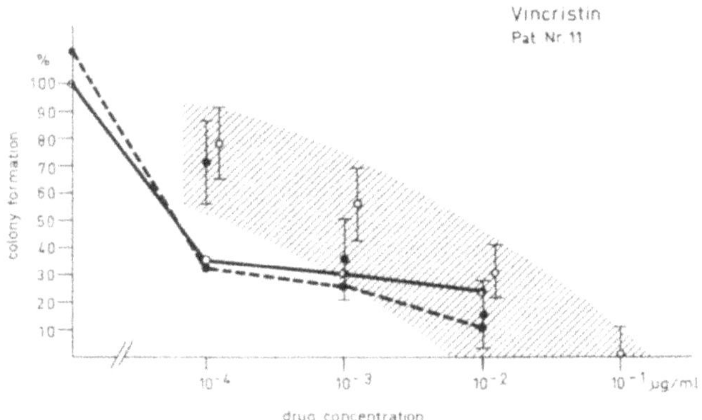

Fig. 5

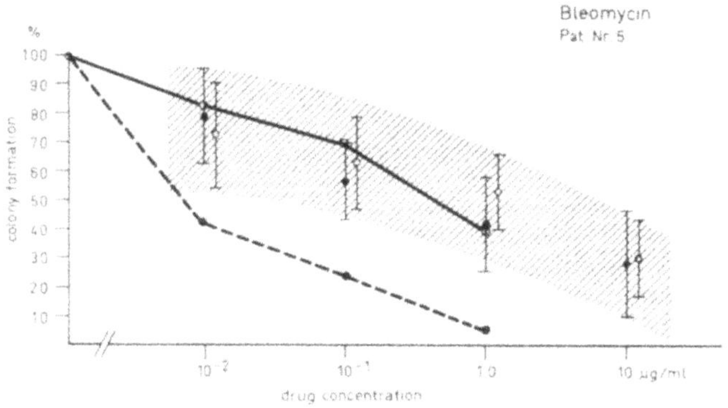

Fig. 6

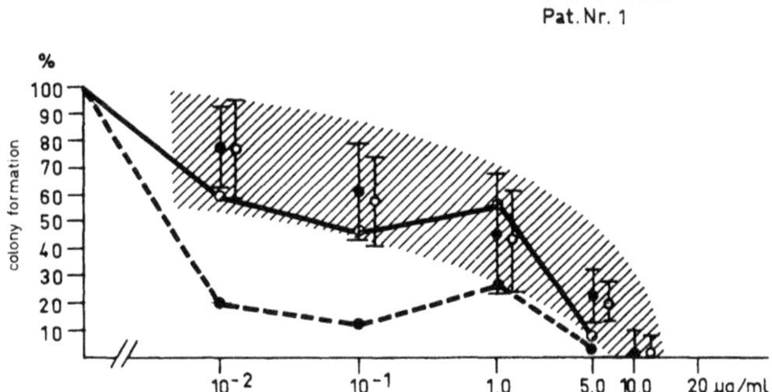

Fig. 7

Fig. 4-7 *(p. 220, 221).* Influence of continuous incubation of colony formation from various human ovarian carcinoma cells with cis-platin, bleomycin, and vincristine. The duplicate cultures of the tumor cells were incubated under normothermic (37° C, O—O) and hyperthermic (2 h at 40.5° C, ●-----●) conditions. The *shaded* area indicates the influence of the cytostatics on the colony formation of bone marrow progenitor cells under normothermic (⊢O⊣) and hyperthermic (⊢●⊣) conditions

Table 2. Hyperthermic enhancement of the tumor cytotoxicity of seven cytostatic agents under hyperthermia at 40.5° C for 2 h

Cytostatic agent	Hyperthermic enhancement	
	Cases (100%)	(%)
Cis-platin	3 (7)	43
Vincristine	3 (6)	50
Bleomycin	4 (11)	36
Peplomycin	7 (13)	53
Adriamycin	3 (8)	37
Epirubicin	0 (4)	0
Melphalan	2 (4)	50

Discussion

For cis-platin, a very commonly used drug in the treatment of ovarian cancer, we assessed an enhancement of cytotoxicity in 43%. Alberts et al. (1980) described a synergistic effect of hyperthermia and cis-platin in animals whereas the bone marrow was not affected. Probably our results in human ovarian carcinomas support these findings.

Vincristine is a phase-specific acting drug that binds to the microtubules during the mitotic phase (Lin et al. 1982). As hyperthermia affects tubular structures, one could expect an enhancement of the vincristine effect by hyperthermia. In our experiments we assessed an enhanced vincristine cytotoxicity in 50%.

Bleomycin and peplomycin are both glycopeptide antibiotics and cytotoxic drugs. Both drugs showed a good enhancement of their cytotoxic effects under hyperthermic conditions. Experiments by Braun and Hahn (1975), Hahn and Li (1982) and Hahn and Shiu (1983) described bleomycin as a cytotoxic drug whose effect can be enhanced only by temperatures above 42° C. Our experiments already showed a thermal enhancement at 40.5° C. The experiments by Hahn were done in animals, whereas our experiments were in human tumors.

Adriamycin has been described by other authors (4) as a drug whose effect is not enhanced at temperatures below 42° C. In our experiments on eight human ovarian carcinomas we found thermal enhancement of cytotoxicity in 37%.

The alkylating agent melphalan, another common drug in ovarian cancer treatment, showed an enhanced cytotoxicity of 50%. Melphalan is already widely used for the regional hyperthermic perfusion of the limbs in the treatment of malignant melanoma.

From our experiments we conclude that:

1. Hyperthermia at 40.5° C for 2 h causes no significant inhibition of the colony formation of bone marrow progenitor cells and ovarian carcinoma cells.
2. There was no significant difference between the normothermic and hyperthermic incubation of bone marrow cells with several cytostatic drugs. Therefore we conclude that hyperthermia at 40.5° C seems to be clinically achievable.
3. Hyperthermic incubation of the tumor cells with several cytostatic drugs revealed a significant enhancement of the cytotoxicity in 30%-50% of the cases.
4. A comparison of tumor and bone marrow cell toxicities in vitro might not reflect in vivo conditions, but more relevant and adequate in vitro drug concentrations seem possible.
5. The enhancement of drug cytotoxicity by hyperthermia seems to be dependent on individual properties of the tumor.
6. The classification of cytostatic drugs into drugs whose cytotoxic effects can be enhanced in a linear way and those showing a temperature threshold, as suggested by Hahn and co-workers (1982), was obtained within experimental cell lines and animal tumors. Our experiments cannot confirm these findings.
7. Our results support the idea that patients with advanced ovarian carcinoma could profit from thermochemotherapy. A moderate 40.5° C thermochemotherapy could be performed, for example, as whole-body hyperthermia. This systemic hyperthermia could be used for induction chemotherapy. On the other hand there is a strong clinical rationale for the use of intraperitoneal chemotherapy in patients with ovarian cancer. Most patients with ovarian cancer suffer from bulky abdominal disease that has already spread to peritoneal surfaces throughout the abdomen. Thus, intraperitoneal chemotherapy could be combined with hyperthermic peritoneal washings.

References

Alberts DS, Peng YM, Chen HSG, Moon TE, Cetas TC, Höschele JD (1980) Therapeutic synergism of hyperthermia and cis-platinum in a mouse tumor model. JNCI 65: 455-461

Braun J, Hahn GM (1975) Enhanced cell killing by bleomycin and 43° C hyperthermia and the inhibition of recovery from potentially lethal damage. Cancer Res 35: 2921-2927

Fauser AA, Messner HA (1978) Granuloerythropoietic colonies in human bone marrow peripheral blood and cord blood. Blood 52: 1234-1248

Hahn GM, Li GC (1982) Interactions of hyperthermia and drugs: treatment and probes. Natl Cancer Inst Monogr 61: 317-323

Hahn GM, Shiu EC (1983) Effect of pH and elevated temperature on the cytotoxicity of some chemotherapeutic agents on Chinese hamster cells in vitro. Cancer Res 43: 5789-5791

Hamburger AW, Salmon SE, Kim MB, Trent JM, Söhnlein BJ, Alberts DS, Schmidt HJ (1978) Direct cloning of human ovarian carcinoma cells in agar. Cancer Res 38: 3438-3444

Lin PS, Turi A, Kwock E, Lu RC (1982) Hyperthermic effect on microtubule organization. Natl Cancer Inst Monogr 61: 57-60

Meerpohl HG (1985) Prognosefaktoren des Ovarialkarzinoms. Onkologie 8: 296-304

Neumann HA, Fiebig HH, Löhr GW, Engelhardt R (1985) Effects of cytostatic drugs and 40.5° C hyperthermia on human clonogenic tumor cells. Eur J Cancer Clin Oncol 21 (4): 515-523

Pfleiderer A (1984) Das Ovarialkarzinom. In: Döderlein G, Wulf KH (eds) Klinik der Frauenheilkunde und Geburtshilfe. Urban and Schwarzenberg, Munich, pp 1-174

Runge HM, Neumann HA, Bauknecht T, Pfleiderer A (1986) Growth patterns and hormonal sensitivity of primary tumor, abdominal metastasis and ascitic fluid from human epithelial ovarian carcinomas in the tumor colony forming assay. Eur J Cancer Clin Oncol 22 (6): 641-646

Runge HM, Neumann HA, Bücke W, Pfleiderer A (1985) Cloning ovarian carcinoma cells in an agar double layer versus a methylcellulose monolayer system. J Cancer Res Clin Oncol 110: 51-55

Salmon SE, Hamburger AW, Söhnlein BJ, Durie BG, Alberts DS, Moon TE (1978) Quantitation of differential sensitivity of human tumor stem cells to anticancer drugs. N Engl J Med 298: 1321-1327

Umezawa H (1979) Bleomycin: discovery, chemistry and action. Cancer Res 19: 3-36

Effect of Hyperthermia at 40.5° C and Chemotherapy on Various Human Tumors in Vitro

H. A. Neumann[1], H. H. Fiebig[2], and R. Engelhardt[2]*

[1] St. Josef Hospital, Medizinische Klinik, Ruhr-Universität, Gudrunstraße 56, 4630 Bochum, FRG
[2] Medizinische Klinik, Albert-Ludwigs-Universität, Hugstetter Straße 55, 7800 Freiburg, FRG

Introduction

The possibility of enhancing the effect of cytostatic drugs on tumor cells by means of hyperthermia has been clearly shown by many in vitro and in vivo experiments (Hahn 1982, 1983). In most experiments, experimental cell lines and experimental animal tumors have been used: in only a few have data been obtained using human tumor samples (Mann et al. 1983). With the use of a tumor colony forming assay it is possible to test human tumor samples for their individual drug sensitivity and the possible influence of hyperthermia.

It was the aim of this study to test the influence of moderate hyperthermia on the cytotoxicity of drugs using cells derived from spontaneous human tumors. Most of the experiments concerning thermochemotherapy have been performed at temperatures above 42° C (Hahn 1982). These temperature ranges are of interest for local or locoregional hyperthermia. With respect to whole body hyperthermia, which might be employed for the treatment of disseminated malignancies, we have chosen hyperthermic conditions that are clinically achievable and well tolerable, i.e., a temperature of 40.5° C for 2 h.

Material and Methods

Tumors

Human tumor samples were plated in a methylcellulose monolayer. Eighteen tumors were used immediately after surgical resection. Eight tumor probes were used after growth in NMRI nude mice (laboratory of Dr. Fiebig). In this way it was possible to receive tumor material for repeated in vitro experiments. The mice were kept under laminar flow conditions and fed with the nude mice diet C 14 (Altrumin, Lage). The probes from the mice were used after the second and the sixth passages.

* The authors thank Mrs. Marlies Braun for excellent technical assistance.

Recent Results in Cancer Research, Vol. 109

Tumor Colony Assay

After surgical resection or after excision from the animals, the tumor samples were disaggregated mechanically into single cell suspension. 1×10^5 tumor cells were seeded in 30% fetal calf serum and Iscove's modified Dulbeccos medium. Methylcellulose (0.9% v/v) was used as viscous support. The final volume was 1 ml including drugs. Cultivation was performed in a moist atmosphere at 7.5% CO_2 at 37° C (Neumann et al. 1983).

Hyperthermia was performed at the initiation of the cultures in an incubator at 40.5° C for 2 h; afterwards the dishes were placed in an incubator at 37° C.

Drugs

The following drugs were tested: actinomycin D (MSD), doxorubicin (Farmitalia), vincristine (Lilly), vinblastine (Lilly), bleomycin (Mack), melphalan (Wellcome), and cis-platin (Bristol). The drugs were diluted in aqua bidest. Melphalan had to be dissolved in ethanol; further dilutions were performed with aqua bidest. The drugs remained in the cultures continuously.

Results

Cells from spontaneous human tumors were plated at 37° C and at 40.5° C for 2 h. There was no significant difference between the colony formation obtained at 37° C and that at 40.5° C. The sensitivity patterns of the human xenografts are shown in Figs. 1-9.

In order to establish a possible therapeutic gain compared with the bone marrow toxicity, the dose-response curves for the bone marrow progenitors (CFU-C) (a description of the method appears on pp. 57-59) were plotted together with the dose-response curves from the tumors when a difference was seen between normo- and hyperthermic exposure. In this way the toxicity of a drug can be evaluated in vitro independent of the exposure time or pharmacokinetics (Hug et al. 1983; Neumann et al. 1985). Analyzing the different reactions to drugs and hyperthermia, typical patterns were observed: Figure 10 shows the dose-response curves from a squamous cell carcinoma of the lung exposed to vincristine. No difference between normothermic and hyperthermic exposure was observed. The killing of the tumor cells occurs at a drug concentration far below the concentrations lethal for the bone marrow. The case of complete resistance to a drug is shown in Fig. 11. Under normothermic as well as under hyperthermic conditions no reduction in colony formation from a malignant melanoma is observed at concentrations that are lethal for the bone marrow cells.

Figure 12 shows thermal enhancement of the effect of melphalan on a malignant melanoma. At 37° C colony formation of the tumor is less affected than the bone marrow colonies, whereas after hyperthermic exposure tumor colony formation is reduced in such a way that inhibition occurs at a drug concentration that is not lethal for the bone marrow. Thermal enhancement of actinomycin D is shown

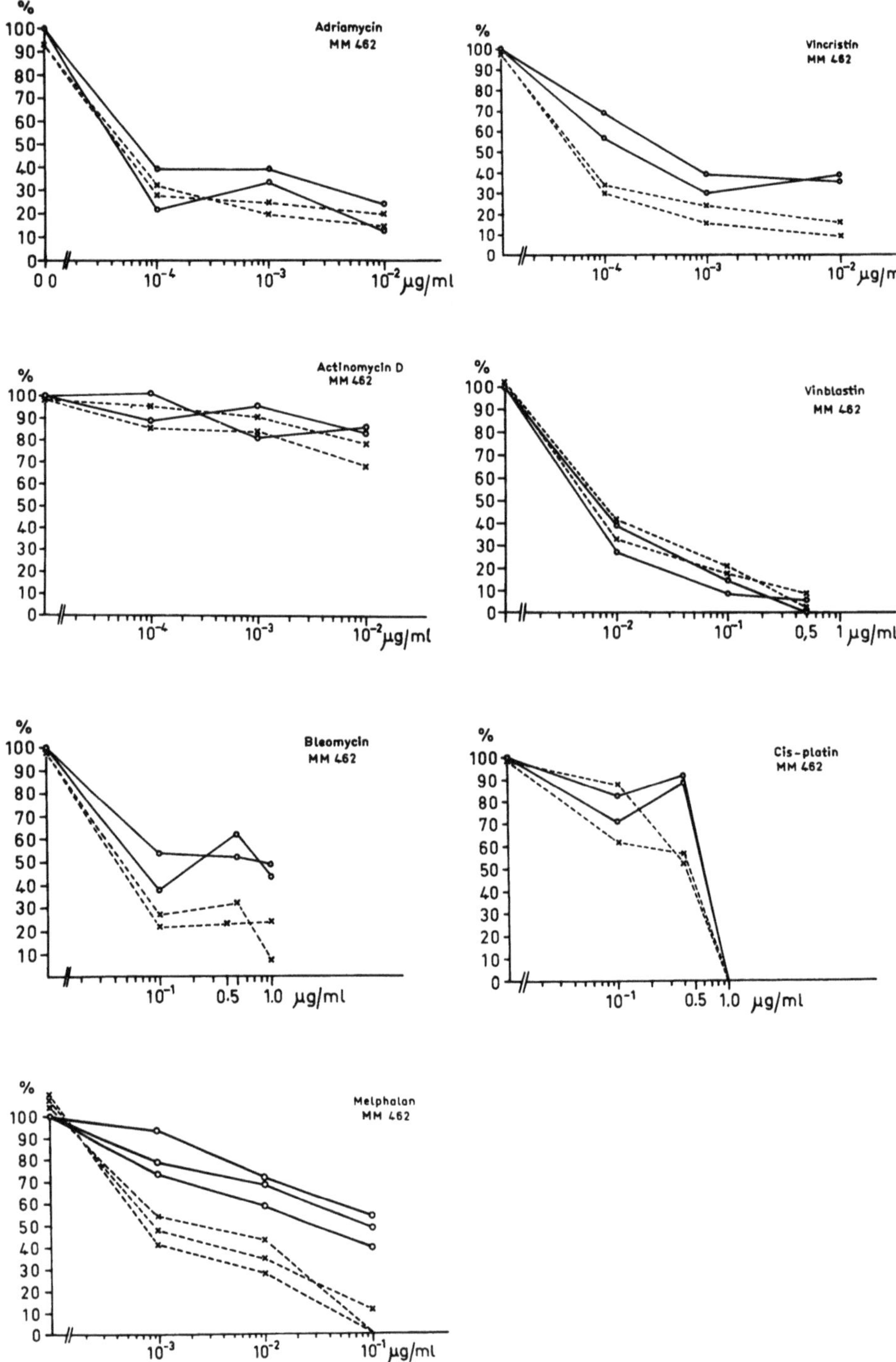

Fig. 1. MM 462: malignant melanoma

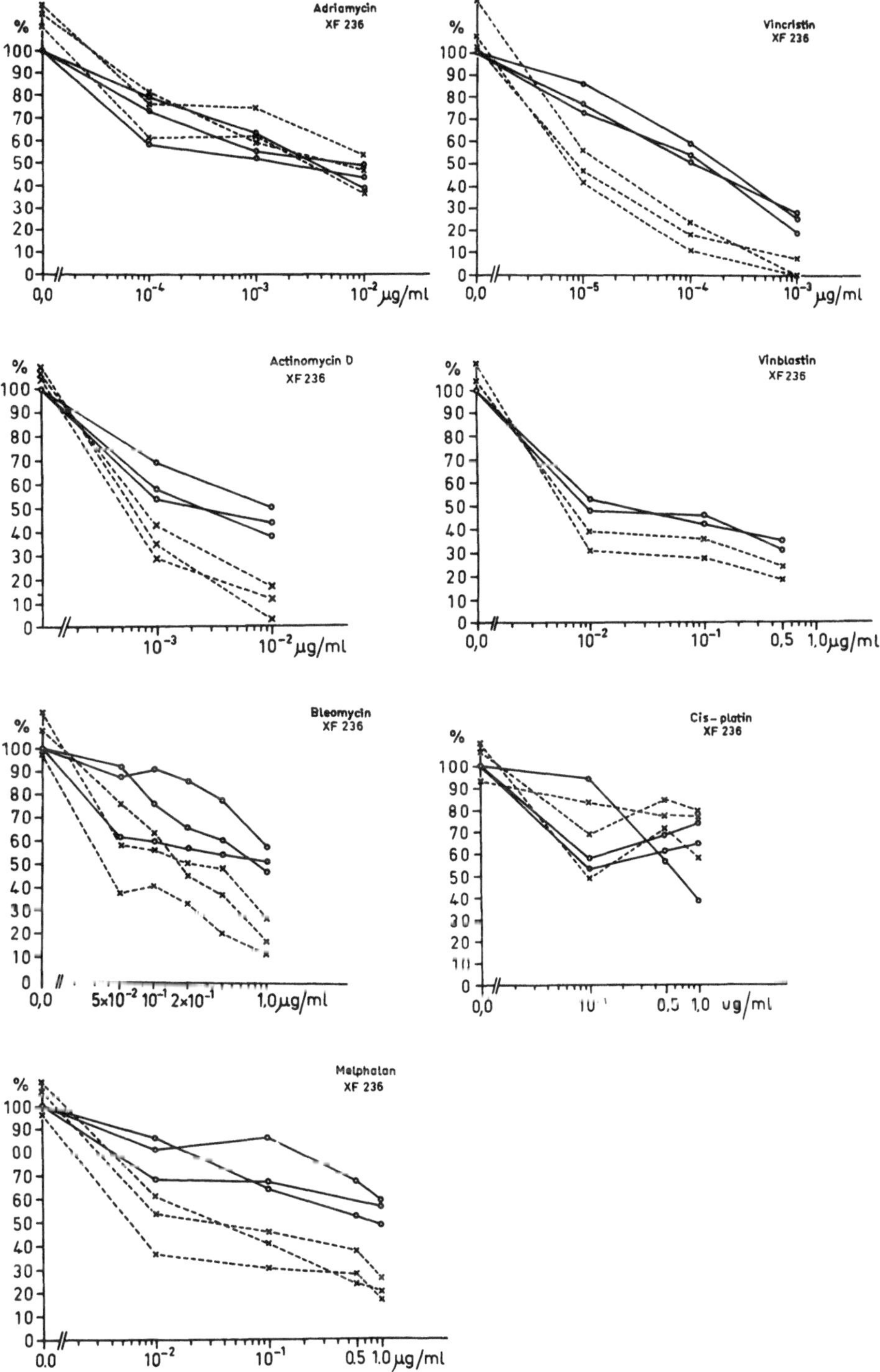

Fig. 2. XF 236: malignant melanoma

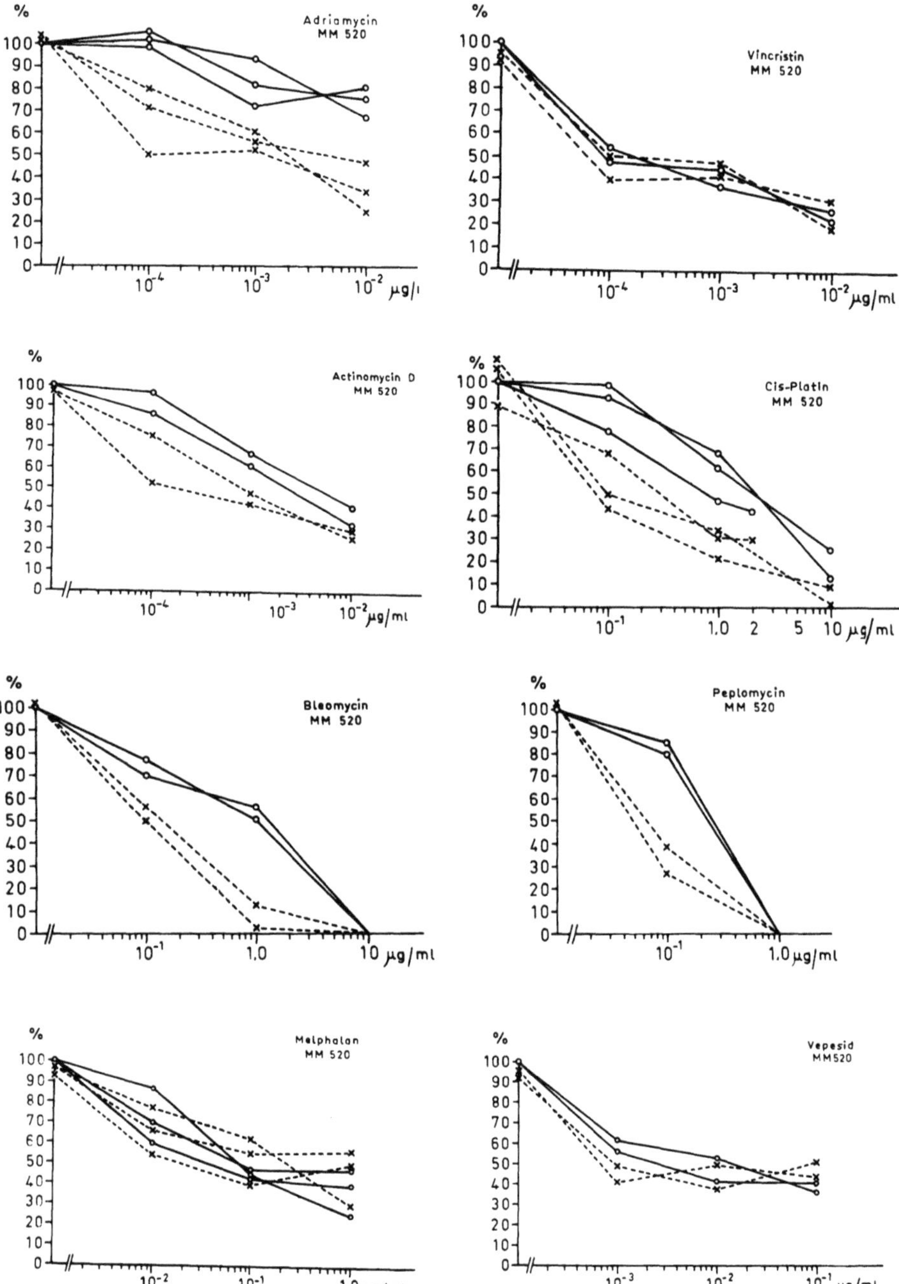

Fig. 3. MM 520: malignant melanoma

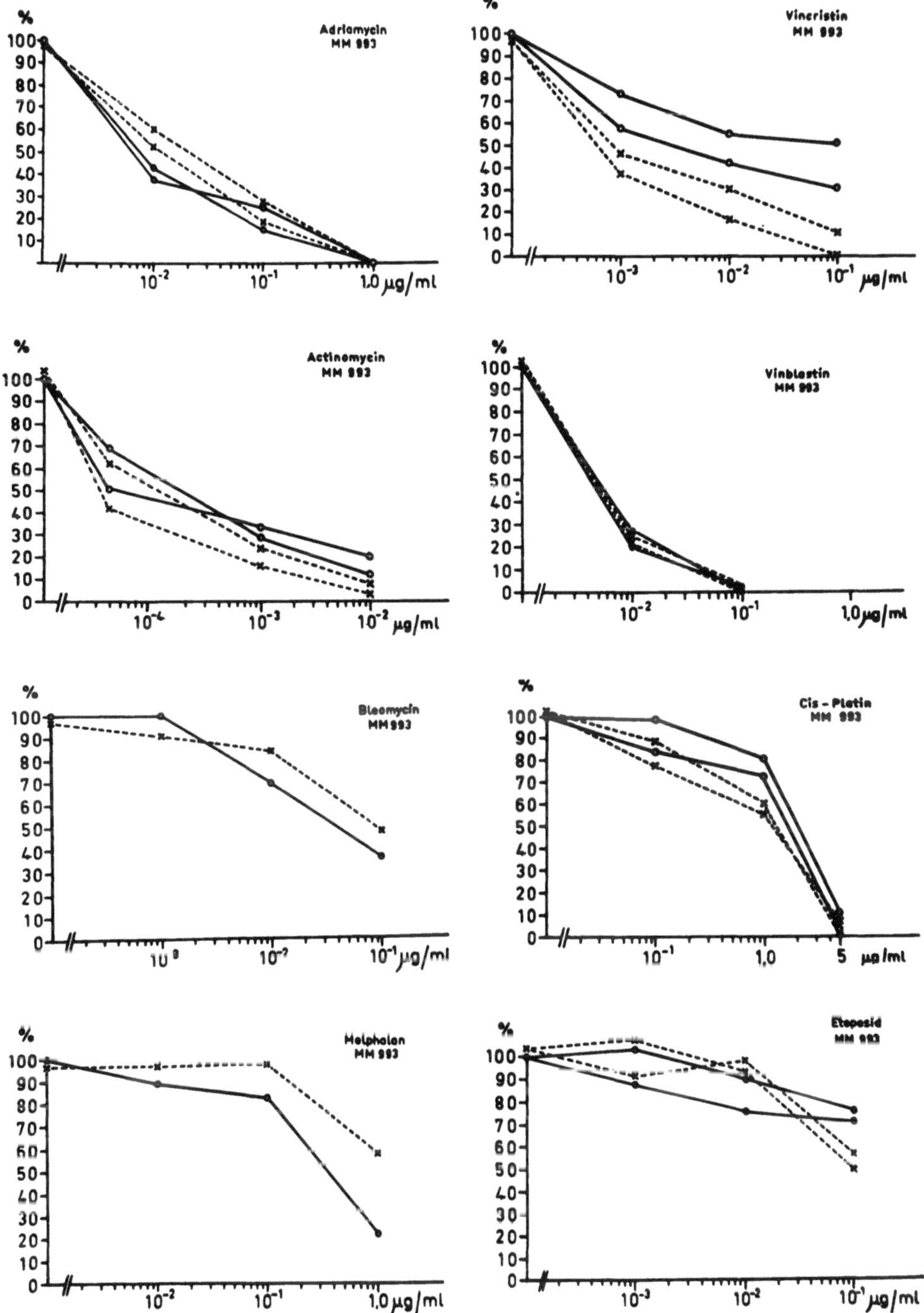

Fig. 4. MM 993: malignant melanoma

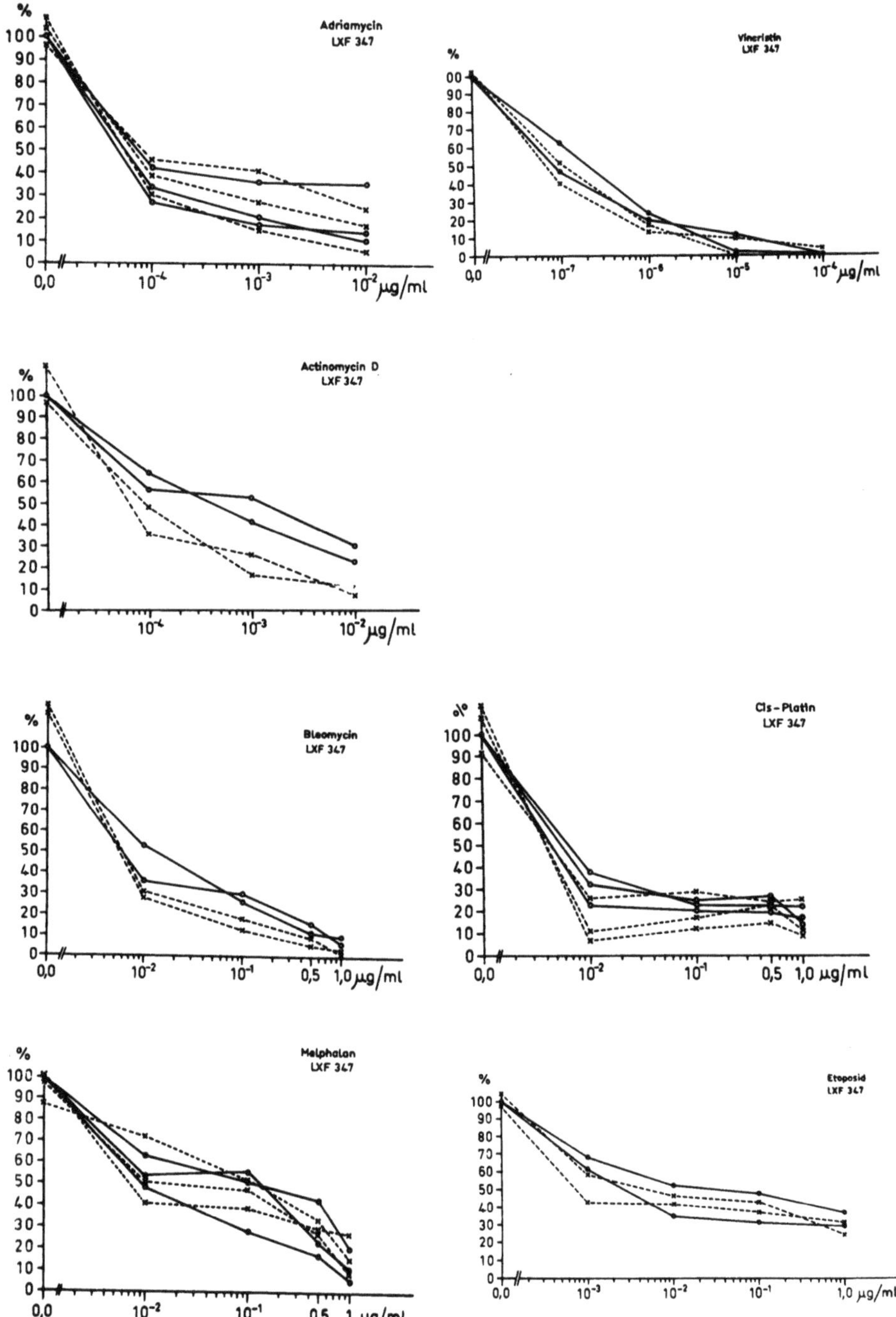

Fig. 5. LXF 347: squamous cell carcinoma of the lung

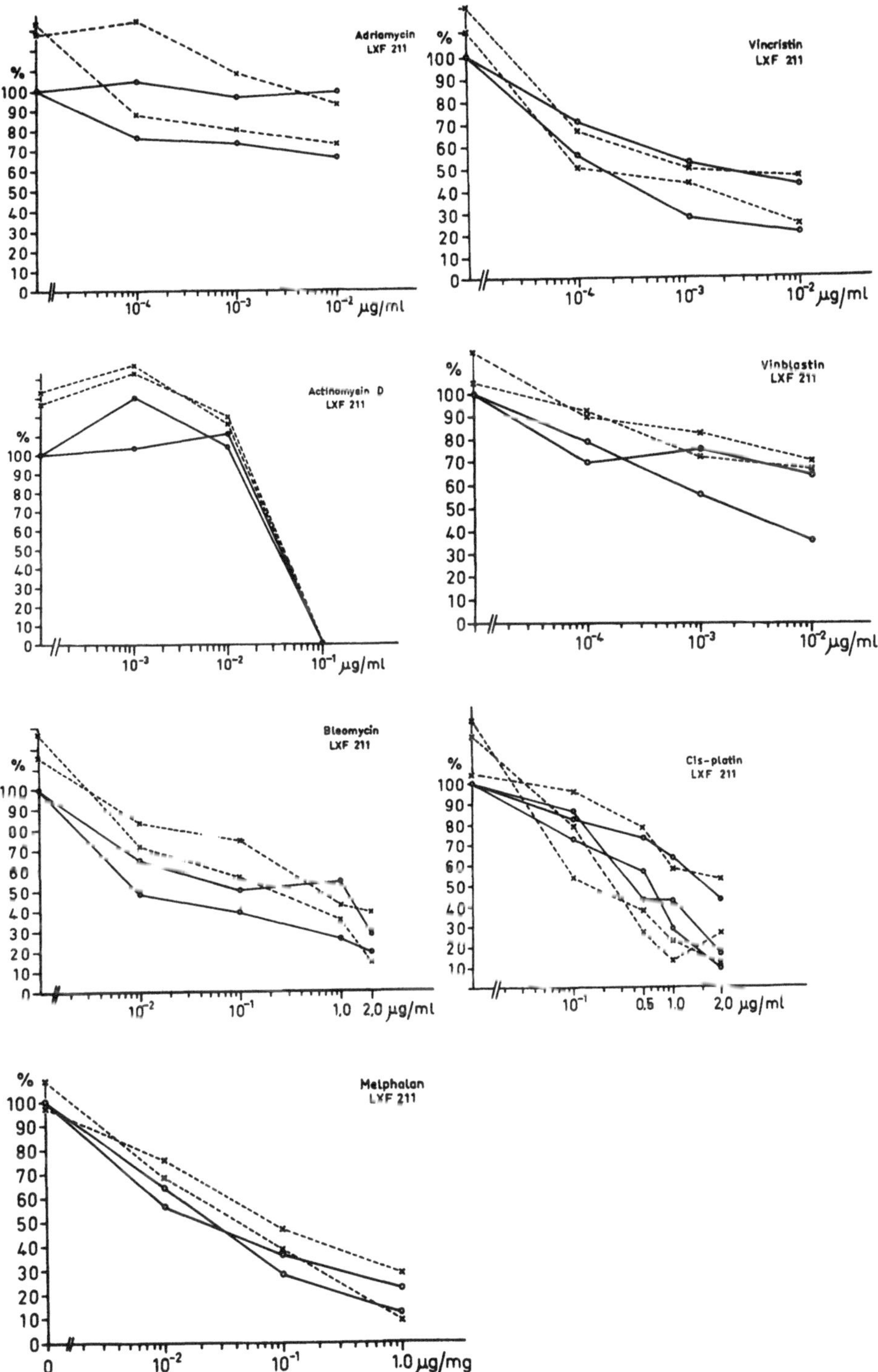

Fig. 6. LXF 211: squamous cell carcinoma of the lung

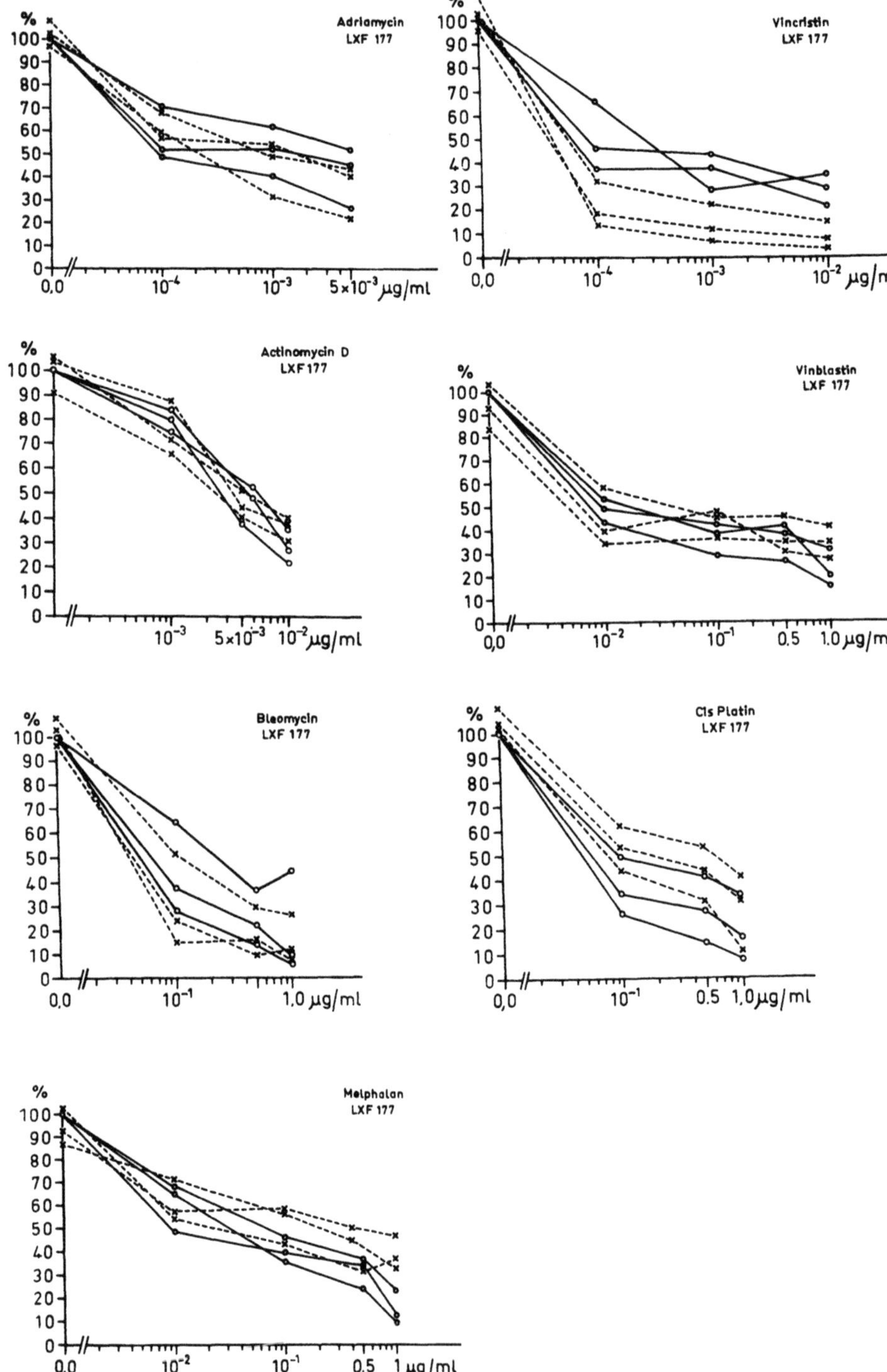

Fig. 7. LXF 177: small cell carcinoma of the lung

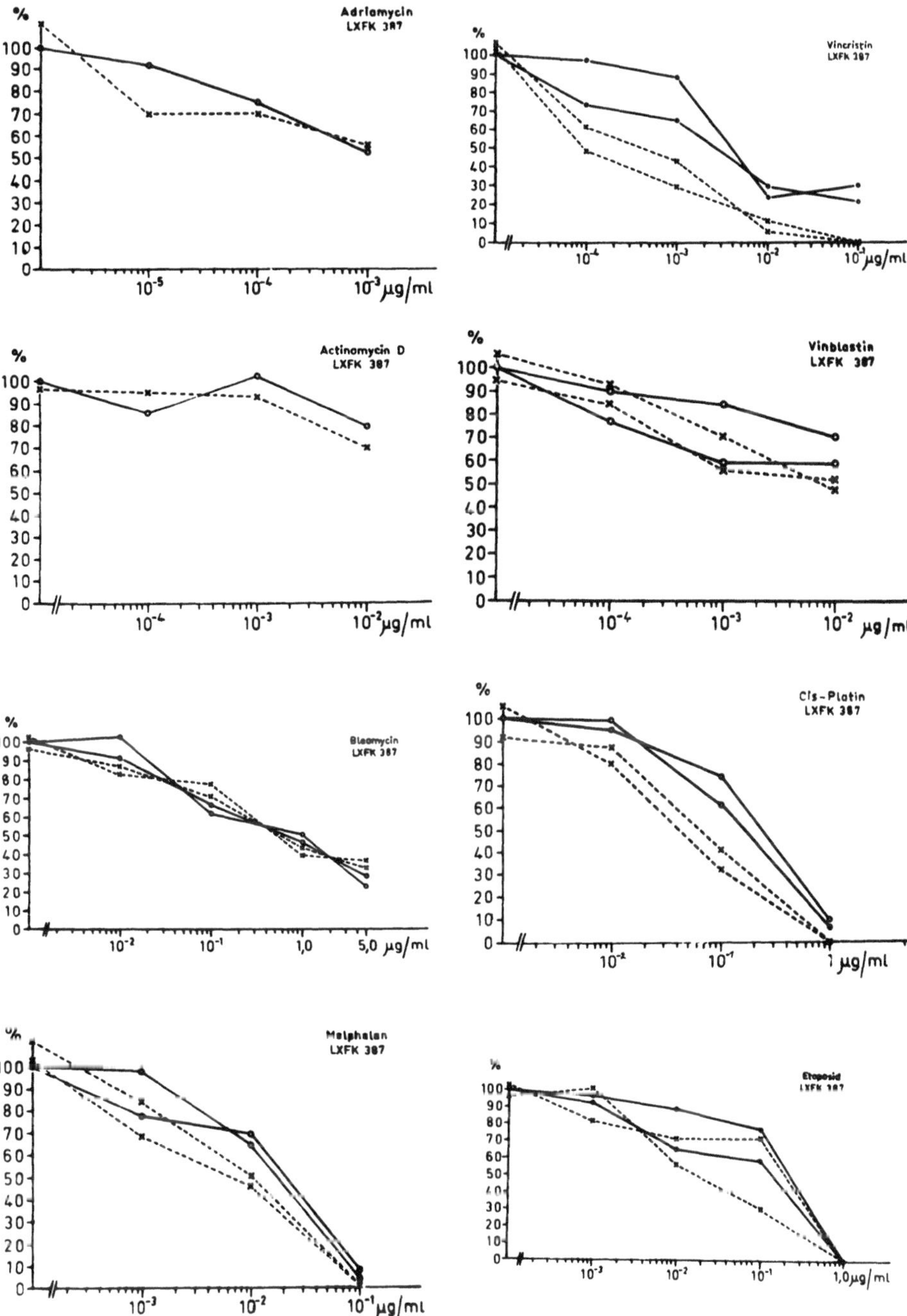

Fig. 8. LXF 387: small cell carcinoma of the lung

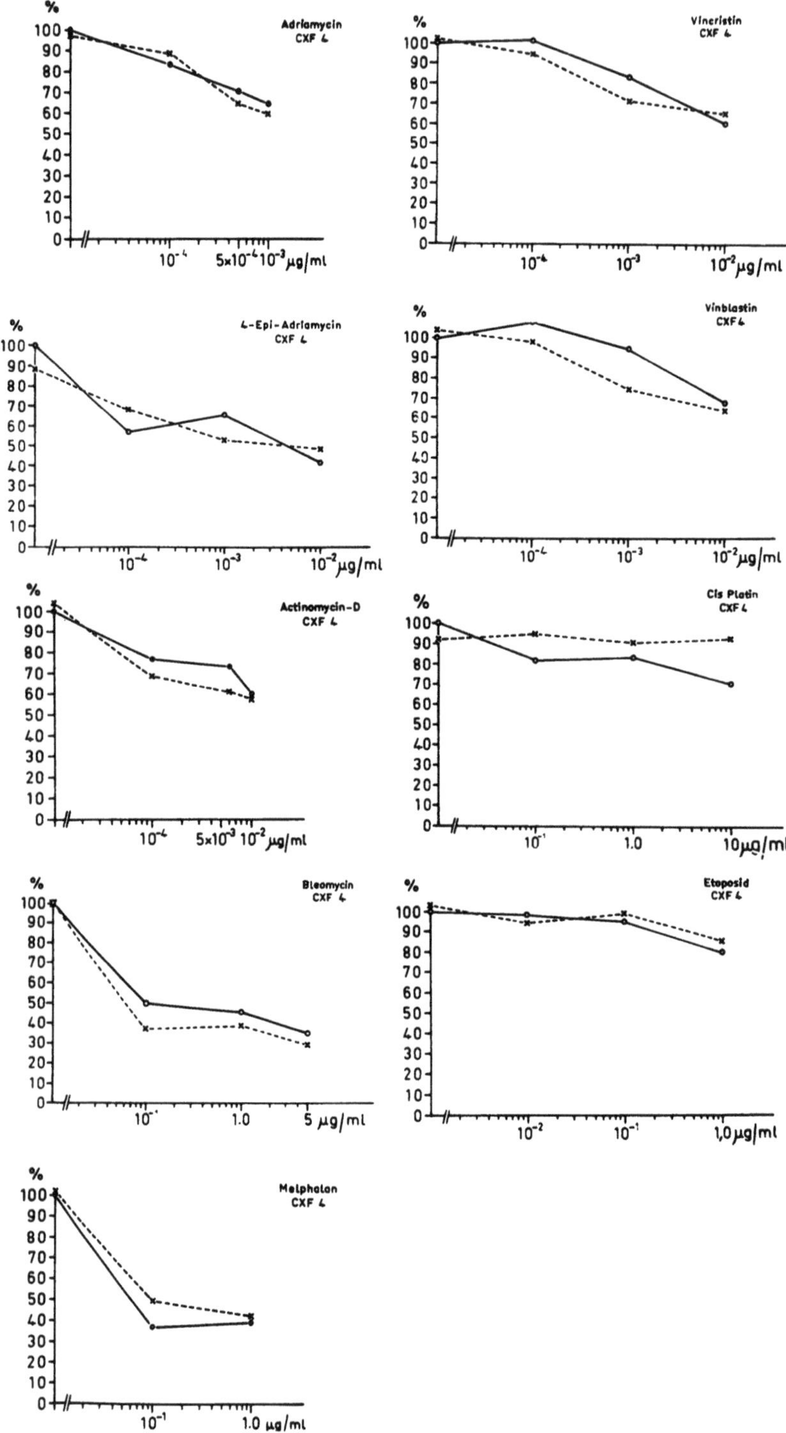

Fig. 9. CXF 4: carcinoma of the colon

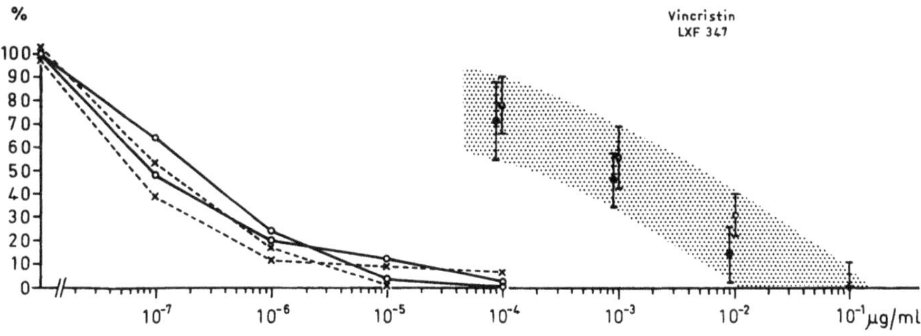

Fig. 10

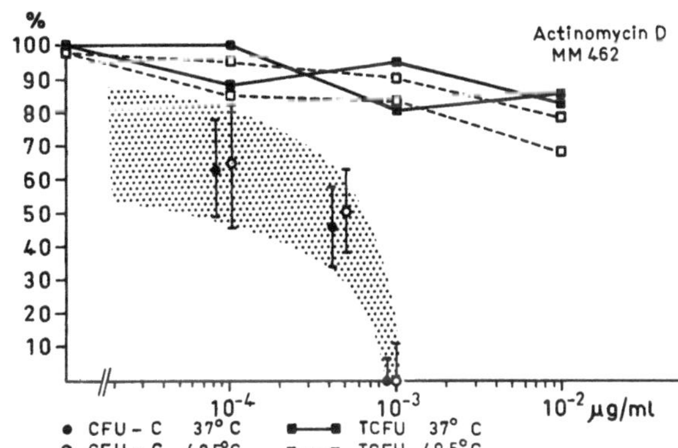

Fig. 11

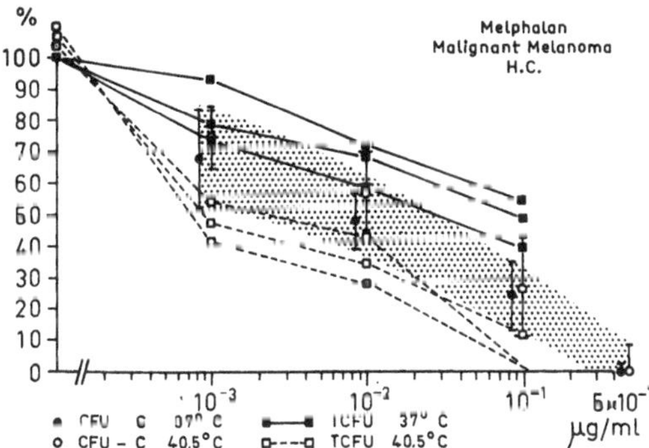

Fig. 12

◀ **Figs. 1-9** *(pp. 226-234).* Dose-response curves of human tumor xenografts with different cytostatic drugs. The drugs employed are indicated in the figures. The *solid lines* and *open circles* indicate the normothermic incubation; the *broken lines* and *crosses* indicate the dose-response curves from cultures that were incubated at 40.5° C for 2 h at the initiation of the cultures. Each *line* represents tumor samples from one nude mouse tumor sample at identical tumor passages. The dose-response curves proved to be well reproducible

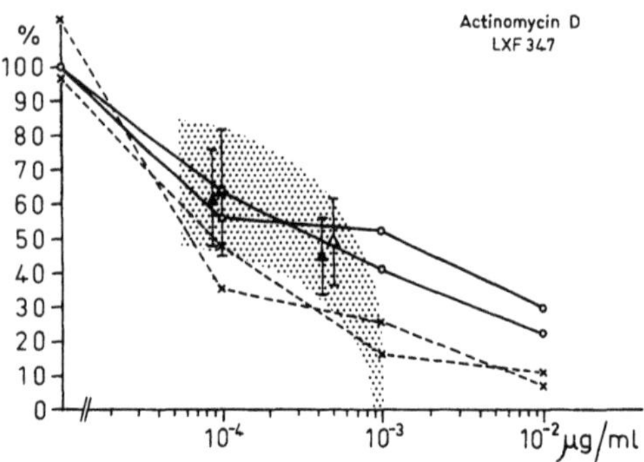

Fig. 13

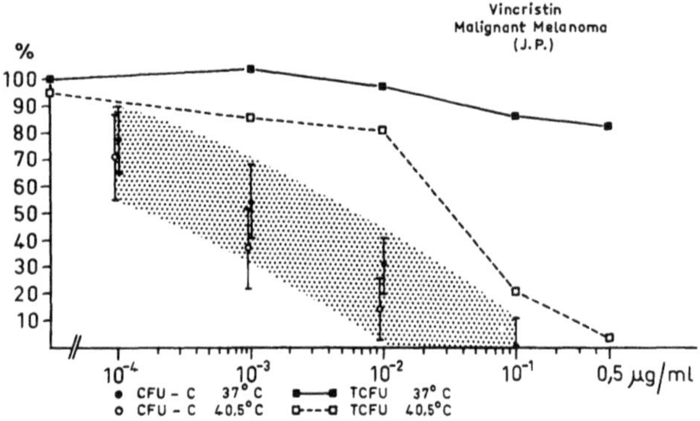

Fig. 14

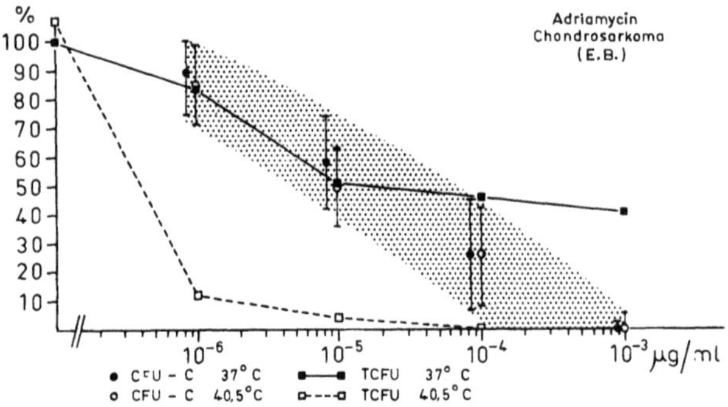

Fig. 15

Figs. 10-15 *(pp. 235, 236).* Dose-response curves from different tumors under normothermic conditions *(solid lines* and *open circles)* and after 40.5° C treatment for 2 h *(broken lines* and *crosses).* The drugs used and the tumors tested are indicated on the figures. In order to compare the cytotoxicity with the bone marrow toxicity of the drugs, dose-response curves from bone marrow cells are plotted together with the tumor dose-response curves. The bone marrow cells were obtained from healthy volunteers; for each curve at least seven or eight different bone marrow samples were used. The *bars* represent the standard deviation of colony formation; the *open circles* indicate the normothermic, the *closed circles* the hyperthermic incubation at 40.5° C for 2 h

in Fig. 13. In this case a clear enhancement of cytotoxicity is seen but at a drug concentration that is higher than that which is tolerable for the bone marrow. This situation is more pronounced in Fig. 14. The tumors proved to be completely resistant to vincristine at 37° C, whereas a dramatic reduction in colony formation is seen under hyperthermic treatment. This configuration probably does not reflect in vivo conditions because in clinical use vincristine treatment is not limited by bone marrow toxicity. To this extent the in vitro doses are probably too high for in vivo conditions.

A configuration that demonstrates a clear therapeutic benefit is seen in Fig. 15. Colony formation from a chondrosarcoma is only slightly reduced by doxorubicin at 37° C, whereas with hyperthermic incubation the dose-response curve falls rapidly even at low drug concentrations and shows complete inhibition of colony formation at a drug concentration that is not lethal for the bone marrow cells.

In 68 tumor-drug combinations with different xenografts, thermal enhancement to different extents was observed in 15 cases (Table 1): in one case with doxorubicin, in three cases with bleomycin, in two cases with actinomycin D, in one case with cis-platin, in five cases with vincristine, in two cases with melphalan, and in one case with peplomycin. In no case thermal enhancement was observed using vinblastine and etoposide. In the 18 tumor-drug combinations performed with different tumor samples plated immediately after surgical resection, thermal enhancement was seen in six cases: in three cases using vincristine (one squamous cell carcinoma of the lung, two malignant melanomas), in one case using melphalan (small cell carcinoma of the lung), in one case using cis-platin (malignant melanoma), and in one case using doxorubicin (chondrosarcoma). These results suggest that thermal enhancement is possible at a comparatively low hyperthermic treatment at 40.5° C for 2 h. The classification by Hahn (1983) which suggest that some drugs can be enhanced by hyperthermia in a linear way and some only above a temperature threshold could not be confirmed by our studies. Cis-platin,

Table 1. Tumor-drug combinations from nine different human tumor xenografts. MM 462, XF 236, MM 520, MM 993 are grown from malignant melanomas; LXF 347 and LXG 211 are derived from squamous cell carcinomas of the lung; LXF 177 and LXF 387 are from small cell carcinomas of the lung; CXF 4 is from carcinoma of the colon. +, thermal enhancement, –, no thermal enhancement, ∅, not performed

Drugs	Tumors								
	MM 462	XF 236	MM 520	MM 993	LXF 347	LXF 211	LXF 177	LXF 387	CXF 4
Doxorubicin	–	–	+	–	–	–	–	–	–
Bleomycin	+	+	+	–	–	–	–	–	–
Actinomycin D	–	+	–	–	+	–	–	–	–
Cis-platin	–	–	+	–	–	–	–	–	–
Vincristine	+	+	–	+	–	–	+	+	–
Vinblastine	–	–	∅	–	∅	–	–	–	–
Melphalan	+	+	–	–	–	–	–	–	–
Etoposide	–	∅	–	∅	–	–	∅	–	–

for example, is described as a drug which is enhanced in a linear way (Barlogie et al. 1980; Fisher and Hahn 1982; Meyn et al. 1980); however, in our studies only in one case did it show enhancement at 40.5° C whereas bleomycin and vincristine, described as threshold drugs (Hahn 1983; Hahn et al. 1975), showed thermal enhancement in three and eight cases respectively.

These individual reactions of tumors to hyperthermic treatment should be taken into account when clinical trials for whole-body hyperthermia are planned.

References

Barlogie B, Corry PM, Drewinko B (1980) In vitro thermochemotherapy of human colon cancer cells with cis-dichlorodiammineplatinum (II) and mitomycin C. Cancer Res 40: 1165-1166

Fisher GA, Hahn GM (1982) Enhancement of cis-diaminedichloroplatinum (cis-DDP) cytotoxicity by hyperthermia. Natl Cancer Inst Monogr 61: 255-257

Hahn GM (1982) Hyperthermia and cancer. Plenum, New York

Hahn GM (1983) Hyperthermia to enhance drug delivery. In: Chabner A (ed) Rational basis for chemotherapy UCLA symposia on molecular and cellular biology-new series, vol 4. UCLA symposium on the rational basis for chemotherapy, Keystone, CO, 1982. Liss, New York, pp 427-436

Hahn GM, Braun J, Har-Kedar I (1975) Thermochemotherapy: synergism between hyperthermia (42-43°) and adriamycin (or bleomycin) in mammalian cell inactivation (cancer chemotherapy/cell membranes). Proc Natl Acad Sci USA 72: 937-940

Hug V, Thames H, Spitzer G, Blumenschein G (1983) Normalization of in vitro sensitivity testing of human tumor progenitor cells. Int J Cell Cloning 1: 257

Mann BD, Storm FK, Morton DL, Bertelsen CA, Korn EL, Kaiser RL, Kern DH (1983) Predictability of response to clinical thermochemotherapy by the clonogenic assay. Cancer 52: 1389-1394

Meyn RE, Corry PM, Fletcher SE, Demetriades M (1980) Thermal enhancement of DNA damage in mammalian cells treated with cis-diamminedichloroplatinum (II). Cancer Res 40: 1136-1139

Neumann HA, Löhr GW, Fauser AA (1983) Tumor colony formation from human spontaneous tumors in a methylcellulose monolayer system. Res Exp Med 184: 137-143

Neumann HA, Fiebig HH, Löhr GW, Engelhardt R (1985) Cytostatic drug effects on human clonogenic tumor cells and human bone marrow progenitor cells (CFU-C) in vitro. Res Exp Med 185: 51-56

Predictive Assays for Tumor Response to Single and Multiple Fractions of Hyperthermia

R. L. Anderson, D. S. Kapp, S. Y. Woo, G. C. Rice, K.-J. Lee, and G. M. Hahn

Department of Therapeutic Radiology, Stanford University, Stanford, CA 94305, USA

Introduction

Local regional hyperthermia is currently being tested clinically in combination with radiation therapy or chemotherapy. The results of several clinical trials show that for superficial tumors, hyperthermia used in conjunction with radiotherapy improves the response rate over radiotherapy alone (Overgaard 1985).

One observation commonly made during these trials is the wide range of response of human tumors to hyperthermia. The source of this variation in response is not well understood but may in part be due to variations in intrinsic cell sensitivity to heat. Other factors may relate to the sensitivity of the vascular tissue, nutrient availability, variation in intratumoral pH, immune responses of the host, thermal parameters, radiation dose, and variation in hyperthermia-radiation treatment schedules. The availability of a predictive assay would permit the clinician to determine in advance whether the patient might benefit from the addition of hyperthermia to his therapy protocol.

The development of thermotolerance in a tumor is a further problem for the rational design of multifraction hyperthermia treatments. In animal models, thermotolerance has been shown to greatly influence tumor response to heat (Urano et al. 1982; Meyer et al. 1985) and to heat plus radiation (Nielsen et al. 1983; Meyer et al. 1986). It has been accepted generally that the decay of thermotolerance is rapid enough that heat treatments can be given once or even twice a week. However, recent data from Meyer et al. (1986) show that thermotolerance accumulates in a radiation-induced fibrosarcoma (RIF-1) of the mouse even when heat treatments are given at 1-week intervals. After three treatments, thermotolerance accumulates to a high level and persists for at least 15 days. The availability of an assay that can measure the level of residual thermotolerance would have obvious clinical potential.

In parallel with the clinical trials, much research has been focused on the biological effects of heat on cells and tissues. Unlike radiation, heat affects many organelles and pathways in the cell and damage to some, but not all of these may be critical for the survival of a cell. If the magnitude of a specific response within the cell indicates the heat survival of that cell or tumor, we may be able to predict the

Recent Results in Cancer Research, Vol. 109

intrinsic heat sensitivity and the level of thermotolerance present after a heat treatment.

In this paper, we present a variety of biochemical techniques that may predict intrinsic heat sensitivity or the level of thermotolerance, or both.

Results and Discussion

A clinically useful assay for predicting tumor response needs to meet three criteria: (1) it should be simple enough that it can be done in a clinical laboratory on a routine basis; (2) it should be rapid enough to be completed within 24 h, and finally, (3) it needs to be sensitive enough to be performed on the number of cells obtainable from a needle or punch biopsy - probably no more than 10^6 cells.

So far, we, and others, have identified five techniques that fulfill these three criteria and, in tissue culture, have been shown to reflect either intrinsic heat sensitivity or level of thermotolerance, or both. These techniques are: (1) inhibition of protein synthesis, (2) capping of membrane glycoproteins by Concanavalin A, (3) cyclic AMP synthesis, (4) levels of heat shock proteins and (5) uptake of dansyl lysine. The data that we have accumulated so far are summarized below.

Inhibition of Protein Synthesis

Synthesis of proteins is a heat-sensitive process. In Chinese hamster ovary (CHO) cells, the loss of protein synthesis is dependent on the severity of the heat dose, but in cells made thermotolerant by prior heating, protein synthesis is much less sensitive to heat (Hahn and Shiu 1985). The development of protection of protein synthesis by prior heating mirrors the development of thermotolerance in CHO cells, but the decay of the protection of protein synthesis is more rapid than the decay of thermotolerance as assayed by clonogenic survival (Fig. 1). A similar result was reported by Sciandra and Subjeck (1984).

The extent of inhibition of protein synthesis depends on the sensitivity of the cells to heat. In heat-resistant mutants selected from two mouse tumor lines, B16 melanoma (Anderson et al. 1984) and RIF-1 (Fig. 2), protein synthesis is more resistant to heat than in the wild type cells.

The preliminary conclusion from these studies is that inhibition of protein synthesis may be useful as an index of intrinsic heat sensitivity but not as useful as an indicator of residual thermotolerance.

Capping of Membrane Glycoproteins by Concanavalin A

Concanavalin A (Con A), a plant lectin, exhibits multivalent binding of plasma membrane glycoproteins which subsequently aggregate into patches, or caps (Edidin and Weiss 1972). In CHO cells, exposure to hyperthermia causes a dose-dependent reduction in the extent of Con A capping which correlates well with heat-induced cell killing (Stevenson et al. 1981). We have not yet attempted to

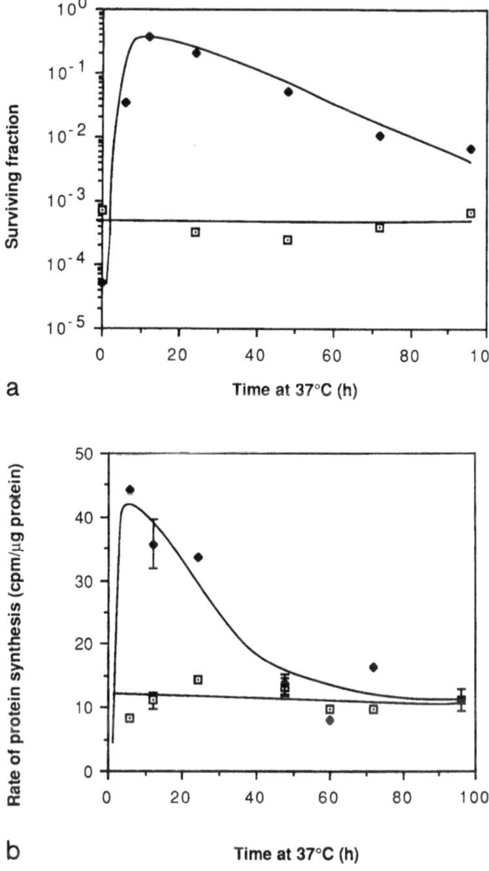

Fig. 1 a, b. The kinetics of decay of thermotolerance in CHO cells as reflected by **a** cell survival and **b** protein synthesis after a challenge dose of heat. CHO cells were grown to plateau phase over 7 days in Eagle's MEM containing 15% fetal calf serum with medium changes daily after day 2. On day 7, cells were heated for 10 min at 45° C and held at 37° C for various times before being given a challenge heat dose to measure either colony formation (80 min at 44° C) or rate of protein synthesis (10 min at 44° C). Colony formation was assayed using the method of Puck and Marcus (1956). Rate of protein synthesis was determined by the extent of incorporation of a ^3H-amino acid mix into TCA-precipitable material over a 30-min period immediately after the second heat dose (Peterson 1979). Control cells (⊡) were treated identically except that they did not receive the 10 min/45° C priming dose given to the tolerant cells (◆)

demonstrate the protection of the capping process in thermotolerant cells; however, we have demonstrated that Con A binding to the cell surface is protected during heat challenge in thermotolerant cells as compared with control cells (unpublished data), suggesting that capping may also be protected. Therefore, the determination of the extent of Con A capping following thermal exposure may provide information on intrinsic cell sensitivity and possibly on the level of residual thermotolerance in previously heated cells.

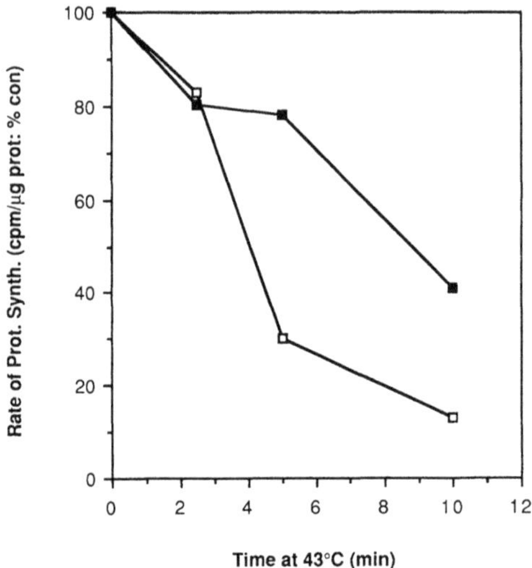

Fig. 2. Effect of 43° C heat on the rate of protein synthesis in wild type RIF (RIF-1) (□) and in a heat-resistant mutant (RIF-TR_5) (■). Exponential cells growing in RPMI plus 15% fetal calf serum were heated for varying times at 43° C followed immediately by measurement of rate of protein synthesis at 37° C. The rate was determined as described in the legend for Fig. 1, except that a 10-min incubation period in ^{3}H-amino acids was used

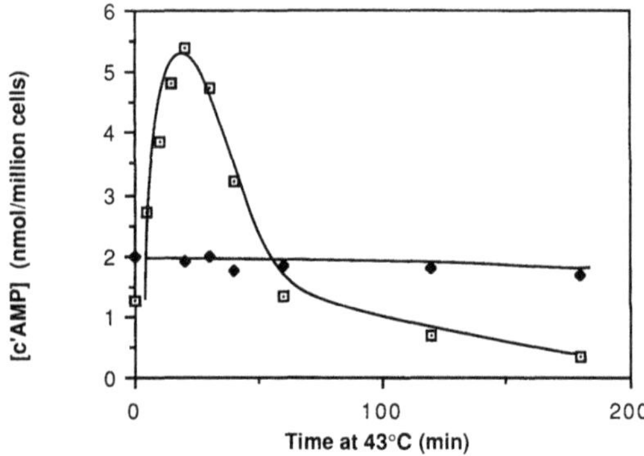

Fig. 3. Effect of 43° C heating on cyclic AMP *(c'AMP)* concentrations in control (⊡) and thermotolerant (◆) CHO cells. Thermotolerance was induced with a 10-min/45° C pretreatment 8 h prior to heating. c'AMP levels were measured immediately after heating using the competitive binding assay of Gilman (1970) on cell extracts. Redrawn from Calderwood et al. (1985)

Cyclic AMP Synthesis

Heat shock leads to a transient increase in c'AMP levels in CHO cells (Calderwood et al. 1985). The increase correlates temporally with the induction of thermotolerance in these cells. If cells are thermotolerant, they no longer respond to heat by synthesizing c'AMP (Fig. 3). This assay may therefore be useful in detect-

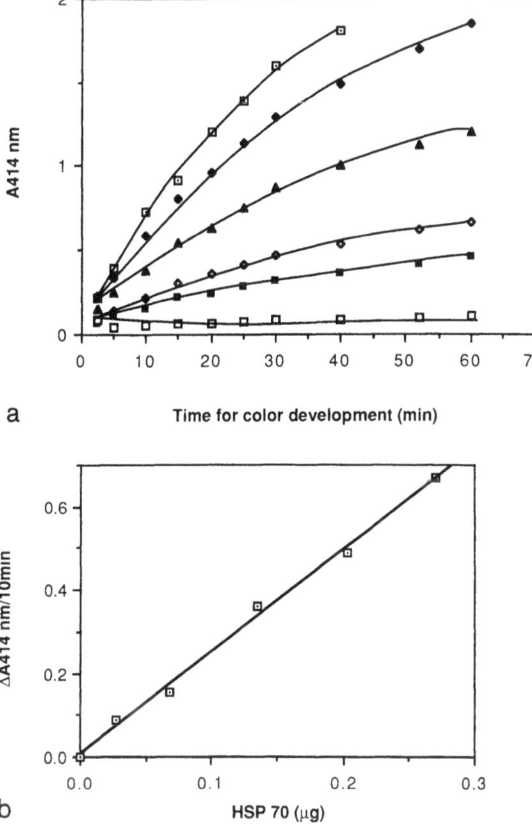

Fig. 4 a, b. Measurement of amounts of HSP 70 using an ELISA technique. Varying amounts of purified HSP 70 were placed in a 96-well polystyrene dish and left overnight at 4° C to bind to the wells. A standard ELISA technique was employed, using a mouse monoclonal antibody against HSP 70 (supplied by Dr. W. Welch, Cold Spring Harbor Laboratory) followed by addition of horseradish peroxidase linked goat anti-mouse IgG (Zymed Laboratories). The kinetics of color development due to the reaction of the peroxidase with 2,2'-azino-di-(3-ethylbenzthiazoline sulfonic acid) and hydrogen peroxide in citrate buffer, pH 4.0, were measured at 414 nm using a Titertek Multiscan photometer (Flow Laboratories). **a** The kinetics of color development for a range of amounts of HSP 70 (0 μg: □; 0.027 μg: ■; 0.068 μg: ◇; 0.135 μg: ▲: 0.203 μg: ◆; 0.27 μg: ⊡). **b** The initial velocity of enzyme reaction plotted against the amount of HSP 70 present in the well

ing the presence of thermotolerance in cells but, so far, its usefulness in measuring intrinsic heat sensitivity is unknown.

Levels of Heat Shock Proteins

It has been shown that the increase in levels of heat shock proteins (HSPs) occurs with similar kinetics to the increase in thermotolerance (Subjeck et al. 1982; Landry et al. 1982; Li et al. 1982). Li (1985) has also followed the kinetics of decay of

HSP levels during the decay of thermotolerance. Using a time intensive gel separation approach, a good correlation was found for the major HSP of mammalian cells; HSP 70. In addition, Li and Mak (1985) have characterized the kinetics of development and decay of HSPs in rodent tumor models.

In an attempt to determine more rapidly the levels of HSP, we have used an ELISA technique (enzyme linked immunosorbent assay) in tissue culture cells, normal tissues, and human tumor specimens obtained at surgical resection. The monoclonal antibodies against HSP 70 were provided by Dr. W. Welch (Cold Spring Harbor Laboratory), a collaborator on this aspect of the project. An example of the technique is shown in Fig. 4 for purified HSP 70 isolated by Dr. Welch from HeLa cells (Welch and Feramisco 1985). With increasing amounts of HSP 70 in the well, there is an increasing rate of enzyme reaction (Fig. 4a). As expected, there is a linear relationship between the rate of enzyme reaction and the amount of HSP 70 present (Fig. 4b). This technique requires very few cells. Non-heat-shocked CHO cells typically contain 6-8 μg HSP 70 per 10^6 cells or 0.03-0.04 μg/μg total cell protein. As the assay can detect satisfactorily 0.2 μg of HSP 70, less than 5×10^4 cells are required for assay.

Results similar to those obtained by others who employed a gel electrophoretic separation of HSP 70 have been obtained using the ELISA technique in CHO cells at various times after a heat shock (Fig. 5). The amount of HSP 70 increases approximately three-fold during the development of thermotolerance.

Data from a human adenocarcinoma of the colon are shown in Fig. 6. The preheated cells show elevated levels of HSP 70 compared to unheated cells. From the calibration curve obtained using purified HSP 70 (Fig. 4), we can estimate that the tolerant cells contain 0.11 μg HSP 70/μg total cell protein compared to 0.045 μg in the control cells.

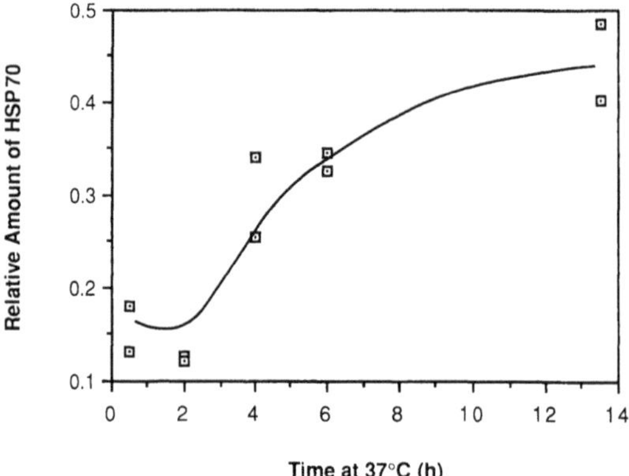

Fig. 5. Amounts of HSP 70 present in CHO cells after heat shock. Exponentially growing CHO cells were heat shocked for 10 min at 45° C and then returned to the 37° C incubator. At varying times later, cells were harvested, and the cell pellet was suspended in PBS and lysed by sonication. Aliquots of a 12000 g × 15 min supernatant solution containing known amounts of total cell protein were assayed for levels of HSP 70 as described in the legend to Fig. 4. The relative amount of HSP 70 refers to the initial velocity of enzyme reaction per μg total cell protein (see Fig. 4)

From our studies of heat-resistant mutants selected from a mouse tumor line, we conclude that the levels of HSP 70 do not indicate the level of intrinsic heat sensitivity of cells. In heat-resistant cells derived from B 16 melanoma (Anderson et al. 1986), there was no substantial increase in the level of HSP 70 detectable by gel electrophoresis or by ELISA, despite the enormous decrease in heat sensitivity. However, a 50% increase in HSP 70 has been demonstrated in heat-resistant mutants of CHO cells (Li 1985). In conclusion, the levels of HSP 70 are promising as indicators of the level of residual thermotolerance but not for the intrinsic heat sensitivity of a cell.

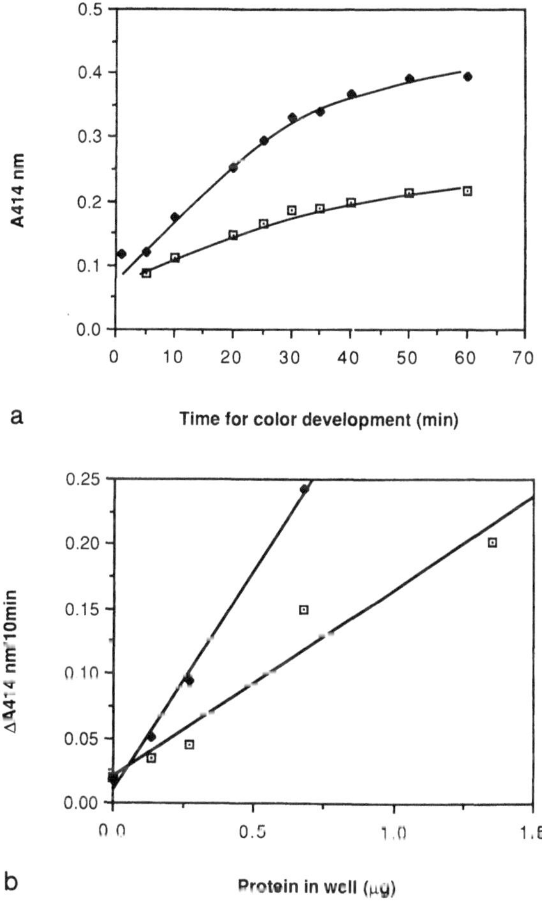

Fig. 6a, b. HSP 70 levels in a human tumor after hyperthermia. Human adenocarcinoma obtained during surgical resection was dissociated into single cells by chopping and filtration through a single layer of gauze. The ELISA assay (see legend to Fig. 4) was performed on a cell lysate of control cells (◻) and on cells made tolerant by a heat shock of 60 min at 45° C followed by 16 h at 37° C (◆). Amounts of lysate containing 0–1.5 μg total cell protein were assayed. **a** The enzyme kinetics for one of several protein concentrations used. **b** The initial velocity of enzyme reaction plotted against the amount of total cell protein in the well

Uptake of Dansyl Lysine

Dansyl lysine (DL) is a nontoxic fluorescent compound with a high partition coefficent (Rice et al. 1985) that selectively partitions into cholesterol-poor domains in binary model systems (Humphries and Lovejoy 1983). Staining is generally all-or-none in mammalian cells, with a thermal dose-dependent increase in the fraction of cells stained by DL. Fluorescence-activated cell sorting reveals that all the DL staining cells are nonviable as measured by clonogenic survival, with a concomitant enrichment of viable cells in the DL excluding fraction (unpublished). A comparison of cell survival functions measured either by colony formation or by the fraction of cells excluding DL reveals a good, but not absolute, correlation (Rice et al. 1985). The correlation can be improved by allowing a longer time (> 24 h) between the heat treatment and DL staining (Rice et al. 1985). We have gone on to show that DL can provide a rapid estimate of the kinetics and magnitude of thermotolerance in vivo in murine RIF tumors (Fisher et al. 1986) and epidermal tissue (Sekiguchi et al. 1987).

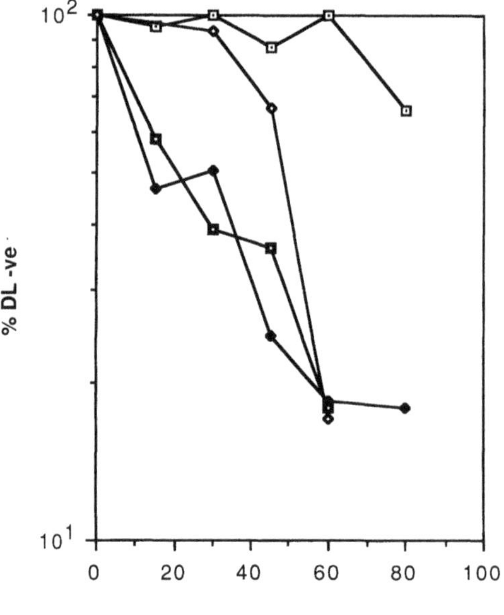

Fig. 7. Dansyl lysine *(DL)* exclusion in four different human tumors after heat challenge at 45° C. Four human tumors [colon adenocarcinoma (◇), malignant mesothelioma (■), cervical squamous cell carcinoma (⊡), and ovarian carcinoma (◆)] were obtained at surgical resection. After removal of gross blood and necrotic tissue, the tumor was separated mechanically into single cells. The cells were filtered through gauze, centrifuged at low speed, diluted to 5×10^4 cells/ml, gassed with 5% CO_2/95% air, and heated at 45° C for varying times. Following heating, the cells were held at 37° C with gentle shaking for 12–15 h before DL staining (Rice et al. 1985). The fraction of DL excluding cells was quantitated by flow cytometry with the inclusion of appropriate gates which allowed for the exclusion of most normal cell infiltrates

The technique has recently been extended to human tumor samples obtained during surgical resection. Single cells were obtained by mechanical disaggregation. The four human tumors shown in Fig. 7 exhibit variability in the heat dose dependence of DL exclusion, which may reflect differences in intrinsic sensitivity. Thermotolerance for DL staining was demonstrated in two of the tumors by preheating cells at 45° C, 16 h prior to a challenge dose of 60 min at 45° C (Fig. 8).

In conclusion, it appears that exclusion of DL may be a useful assay both for measurement of intrinsic heat sensitivity and residual thermotolerance.

A summary of the five techniques and their potential applications is shown in Table 1. The only assay that appears to be useful for both purposes is DL staining. The fluorescence can be measured rapidly on a single cell basis by flow cytometry and few cells are required. In addition, it may be possible in some tumors to distinguish between normal and tumor cells on a size basis and to look at the individual response of each cell type present in the sample. However, it is necessary for this assay, and for Con A capping, to prepare a single cell suspension of the tumor. So far, we have used mechanical disaggregation of the human tumors but certain types of tumor may require enzymic disaggregation as performed on the RIF-1 tumor (Fisher et al. 1986) and mouse skin (Sekiguchi et al. 1987). A possible

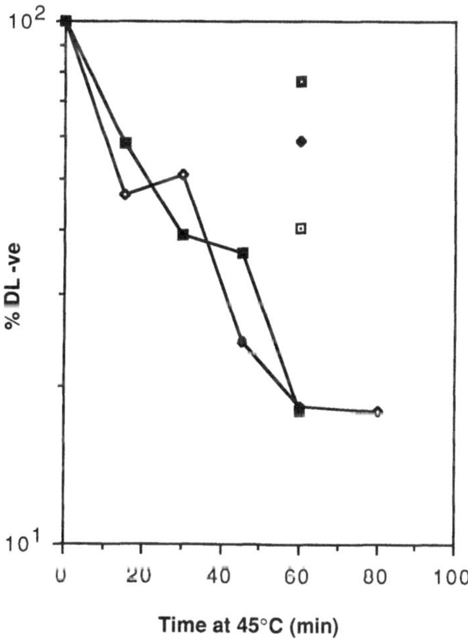

Fig. 8. Thermotolerance in human tumor cells as measured by the DL exclusion assay. For two of the tumors shown in Fig. 7, the ovarian carcinoma (◇) and the malignant mesothelioma (■), thermotolerance was induced by heating for 20 min (⊡) or 25 min (◆) in the carcinoma or 15 min (■) in the mesothelioma followed by incubation at 37° C for 16 h prior to a second heat dose of 60 min at 45° C. All other procedures are described in the legend for Fig. 7

Table 1. Summary of techniques for the determination of intrinsic heat sensitivity and level of residual thermotolerance

Technique	Intrinsic heat sensitivity	Level of thermotolerance
1. Rate of protein synthesis	Yes	No
2. Con A capping	Yes	?
3. c'AMP levels	?	Yes
4. HSP 70 level	No	Yes
5. DL staining	Yes	Yes

limitation may be the difficulty in obtaining single cell suspensions from certain human tumors, as has been found previously (Lieber 1984).

The measurement of HSP levels offers one major advantage over the other techniques. Apart from high sensitivity, there is no need to give an in vitro heat dose before measurement. However, while indicating the presence of thermotolerance, HSP levels do not appear to be a reliable indicator of intrinsic heat sensitivity.

There are potential sampling errors associated with obtaining the biopsy samples from tumors. There may be heterogeneity within the tumor due to differences in intrinsic cellular sensitivity, and local variations in environmental factors, such as blood flow, pH, and nutrient status, may also alter the level of heat damage to individual tumor cells. Nonuniform heating may result in variation in levels of thermotolerance in the tumor. Further, the DL assay is the only one able to deal with the problem of normal tissue contamination in the biopsy samples. In addition, we must be aware that all the assays described here measure a cellular heat response. If the primary response of a tumor is due to other factors, such as vascular effects, then none of the assays presented here will be useful in a predictive capacity.

We are continuing to test these assays in both animal model systems and on human tumor samples to establish further their suitability for prediction of the response of human tumor to hyperthermia and for the level of residual thermotolerance. Using the RIF-1 tumor model, we are currently testing the reproducibility of results from multiple biopsy samples taken from a single tumor after heating. Only by obtaining additional in vitro and in vivo data can we establish the usefulness of these techniques in predicting tumor response to hyperthermia and in aiding in the design of multifraction clinical trials.

References

Anderson RL, Tao TW, Hahn GM (1984) Cholesterol-phospholipid ratios decrease in heat resistant variants of B 16 melanoma cells. In: Overgaard J (ed) Hyperthermic oncology, vol 1. Taylor and Francis, London, pp 123-126

Anderson RL, Tao TW, Betten DA, Hahn GM (1986) Heat shock protein levels are not elevated in heat-resistant B 16 melanoma cells. Radiat. Res. 105: 240-246

Calderwood SK, Stevenson MA, Hahn GM (1985) Cyclic AMP and the heat shock response in Chinese hamster ovary cells. Biochem. Biophys. Res Comm 126: 912-916

Edidin M, Weiss A (1972) Antigen cap formation in cultured fibroblasts: a reflection of membrane fluidity and of cell motility. Proc Natl Acad Sci USA 69: 2456-2459

Fisher G, Rice GC, Hahn GM (1986) Dansyl lysine, a new probe for assaying heat-induced cell killing and thermotolerance in vitro and in vivo. Cancer Res 46: 5064-5067

Gilman AG (1970) A protein binding assay for adenosine 3′:5′-cyclic monophosphate. Proc Natl Acad Sci USA 67: 305-312

Hahn GM, Shiu EC (1985) Protein synthesis, thermotolerance and step down heating. Int J Radiat Oncol Biol Phys 11: 159-164

Humphries GMK, Lovejoy JP (1983) Dansyl lysine: a structure-selective fluorescent membrane stain? Biophys J 42: 307-310

Landry J, Bernier D, Chretien P, Nicole LM, Tanguay RM, Marceau N (1982) Synthesis and degradation of heat shock proteins during the development and decay of thermotolerance. Cancer Res 42: 2457-2461

Li GC (1985) Elevated levels of 70000 dalton heat shock protein in transiently thermotolerant Chinese hamster fibroblasts and in their stable heat resistant variants. Int J Radiat Oncol Biol Phys 11: 165-177

Li GC, Mak JY (1985) Induction of heat shock protein synthesis in murine tumors during the development of thermotolerance. Cancer Res 45: 3816-3824

Li GC, Peterson NS, Mitchell HK (1982) Induced thermal tolerance and heat shock protein synthesis in Chinese hamster ovary cells. Int J Radiat Oncol Biol Phys 8: 63-67

Lieber MM (1984) Technical problems with soft agar colony formation assays for in vitro chemotherapy sensitivity testing of human solid tumours: Mayo Clinic experience. In: Hofmann V, Berens ME, Martz G (eds) Predictive drug testing on human tumor cells. Springer, Berlin Heidelberg New York, pp 51-55 (Recent results in cancer res vol 94)

Meyer JL, van Kersen I, Becker B, Hahn GM (1985) The significance of thermotolerance after 41° C hyperthermia: in vivo and in vitro tumor and normal tissue investigations. Int J Radiat Oncol Biol Phys 11: 973-981

Meyer JL, van Kersen I, Hahn GM (1986) Tumor responses following multiple hyperthermia and X-ray treatments: role of thermotolerance at the cellular level. Cancer Res 46: 5691-5695

Nielsen OS, Overgaard J, Kamura T (1983) Influence of thermotolerance on the interaction between hyperthermia and radiation in a solid tumor in vivo. Br J Radiol 56: 267-273

Overgaard J (1985) Rationale and problems in the design of clinical studies. In Overgaard J (ed) Hyperthermic oncology, vol 2. Taylor and Francis, London, pp 325-328

Peterson G (1979) Review of the Folin phenol protein quantitation method of Lowry, Rosebrough, Farr and Randall. Anal Biochem 100: 201-220

Puck TT, Marcus PI (1956) The action of X-rays on mammalian cells. J Exp Med 10: 653-669

Rice GC, Fisher G, Devlin M, Humphries GMK, Mehdi SQ, Hahn GM (1985) Use of N-Σ-dansyl-L-lysine and flow cytomtery to identify heat-killed mammalian cells. Int J Hyperthermia 1: 185-191

Sciandra JJ, Subjeck JR (1984) Heat shock proteins and protection of proliferation and translation in mammalian cells. Cancer Res 44: 5188-5194

Sekiguchi R, Rice GC, Hahn GM (1987) The use of dansyl lysine to assess heat damage of normal tissues. Cancer Res (in press)

Stevenson MA, Minton KW, Hahn GM (1981) Survival and Concanavalin-A-induced capping in CHO fibroblasts after exposure to hyperthermia, ethanol and X irradiation. Radiat. Res. 86: 467-478

Subjeck JR, Sciandra JJ, Johnson RJ (1982) Heat shock proteins and thermotolerance; a comparison of induction kinetics. Br J Radiol 55: 579-584

Urano M, Rice LC, Montoya V (1982) Studies on fractionated hyperthermia in experimental animal systems 2. Response of murine tumors to two or more doses. Int J Radiat Oncol Biol Phys 8: 227-233

Welch WJ, Feramisco JR (1985) Rapid purification of mammalian 70000-dalton stress proteins: affinity of the proteins for nucleotides. Mol Cell Biol 5: 1229-1237

Predicting the Sensitivity of Human Cancers to Combined Chemotherapy and Hyperthermia

K. Yamada[1], H. A. Neumann[1], H. H. Fiebig[1], R. Engelhardt[1], and H. Tokita[2]

[1] Medizinische Klinik, Albert-Ludwigs-Universität, Hugstetter Straße 55, 7800 Freiburg, FRG
[2] Research Institute, Chiba Cancer Center, Chiba, Japan

Introduction

It has been known for quite some time the action of various kinds of antitumor drugs is enhanced when they are administered in combination with hyperthermia, be it in vitro (Hahn 1975; Gross and Parsons 1977; Mizuno et al. 1980), in animals (Marmor 1979; Twentyman et al. 1980, Yamada et al. 1985), or in humans (Stehlin et al. 1975; Arcangeli et al. 1979; Storm et al. 1984). The individual tumors, however, seem to reveal different sensitivities to hyperthermia when the latter is combined with antitumor drugs. With respect to the prediction of tumor response to chemotherapy, clonogenic assay (Salmon et al. 1978; von Hoff et al. 1981; Mann et al. 1982) and subrenal capsule assay (Bogden et al. 1981; Griffin et al. 1983; Levi et al. 1984) have already demonstrated a high probability of clinical response as in vitro and in vivo assays, respectively. These results have added considerably to the possibility that the response to thermochemotherapy for human cancers can also be predicted.

In an attempt to predict thermochemosensitivity, several in vitro assays (Mann et al. 1983; Andrysek et al. 1985; Neumann et al. 1985) have recently been reported. Expecially the results of Mann et al. (1983) have provided a good correlation with clinical responses. One goal of hyperthermic treatment is to find drugs which induce synergism in combination with hyperthermia in individual tumors. Thermochemotherapy would then yield better results in clinical practice. However, a more simplified and rapid method is required for a predictive clinical assay.

In the present study we have investigated the possibility of predicting the thermochemosensitivity of human cancers using a rapid in vitro assay based on morphological changes in nuclei, which can be done in a clinical laboratory on a regular basis.

Recent Results in Cancer Research, Vol. 109

Material and Methods

Tumors

The following tumors were used: four malignant melanomas, two lung carcinomas, one renal carcinoma, and leukemia K-562. Tumor material passaged in nude mice was taken, except for leukemia K-562. The tumor tissues were chopped into 0.5-mm squares with a razor blade on a Teflon sheet to obtain the small cell clumps. These were placed in a stainless steel strainer (0.5 mm in diameter) to remove fibrous tissues. The medium containing tumor cells was then transferred to a tube (Falcon 2070) and centrifuged at 800 r.p.m. for 30 s three times to avoid contamination by the necrotic part and fat.

Drugs

The following agents were tested: nimustine, melphalan, mitomycin C, vincristine, and vinblastine. Drug concentrations are shown in Table 1. Each drug was dissolved with 0.9% NaCl solution and diluted further with RPMI 1640 medium supplemented with 10% fetal calf serum.

Culture Assay

Tumor cells were incubated in 0.4 ml medium (RPMI 1640) supplemented with 10% fetal calf serum, containing antitumor agents as shown in Table 1. Incubation was at 37° C for 4 h for the normothermic groups, while for the hyperthermic groups it was at 43° C for 1 h and afterwards at 37° C for 3 h. After incubation, tumor cells were pumped down with a 23-gauge needle injector to obtain pure single cells. The medium containing tumor cells was centrifuged at 800 r.p.m. for 5 min and then displaced by calf serum. The calf serum containing tumor cells was centrifuged again at 800 r.p.m. for 5 min and the precipitate placed on glass slides. Subsequently, the cells were fixed in absolute methanol for 3 min and stained with Giemsa.

Data Evaluation

More than 200 tumor cells per glass slide were examined through the high-power field of a microscope. Changes noted in the nucleus, karyorrhectic changes, and

Table 1. Concentration of each drug used

Nimustine (ACNU)	2.0 μg/ml
Melphalan (MPL)	0.5 μg/ml
Mitomycin C (MMC)	0.3 μg/ml
Vincristine (VCR)	0.1 μg/ml
Vinblastine (VBL)	0.1 μg/ml

other degenerative changes with each drug were compared with the controls using statistical analysis (χ^2 test).

Results

The changes in the nucleus induced by the antitumor agents used in this study were remarkable. The karyorrhectic changes shown in Fig. 1 appeared after short-term incubation with antitumor agents. An increase in karyorrhectic changes was observed after 43° C hyperthermia for 1 h. Figure 2 shows an example (case no. 8, lung carcinoma) of an in vitro sensitivity test. In this case the frequency of karyorrhectic changes produced by 43° C was less than 10% greater than the frequency in the control group at 37° C, consequently indicating a nonthermosensitive tumor.

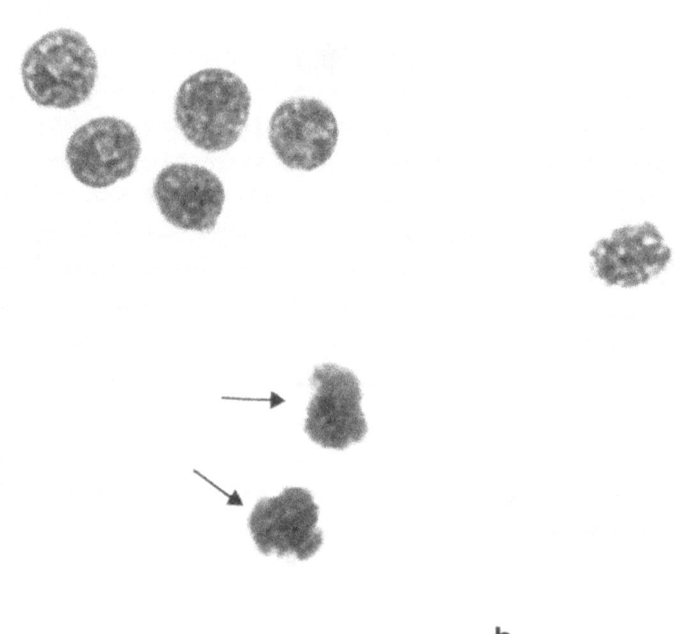

Fig. 1 a, b. Tumor cells that have developed karyorrhectic changes after incubation for 4 h with alkylating agents. **a** Karyorrhectic changes *(arrows)* caused by nimustine in case no. 5, malignant melanoma. **b** Karyorrhectic changes induced by melphalan in case no. 1, renal carcinoma. Giemsa, ×400

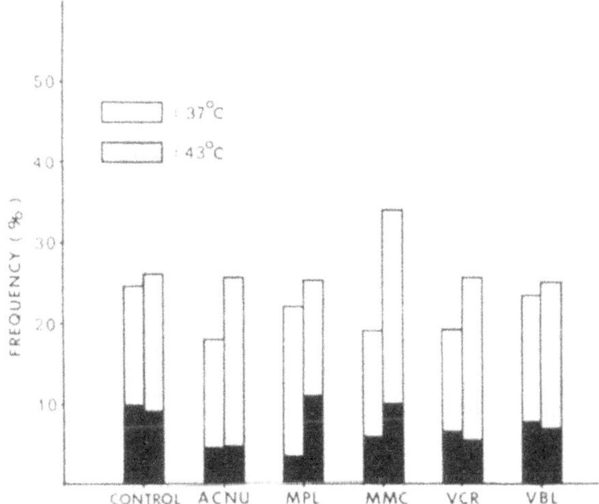

Fig. 2. The frequency of nuclear changes in case no. 8, lung carcinoma. The changes noted in the nucleus are expressed in percentages. Each *black column* shows the percentage of karyorrhectic changes, and the *white columns* indicate other degenerative changes. In this case, no significant difference was observed between 37° C and 43° C. *Abbreviations* as in Table 1

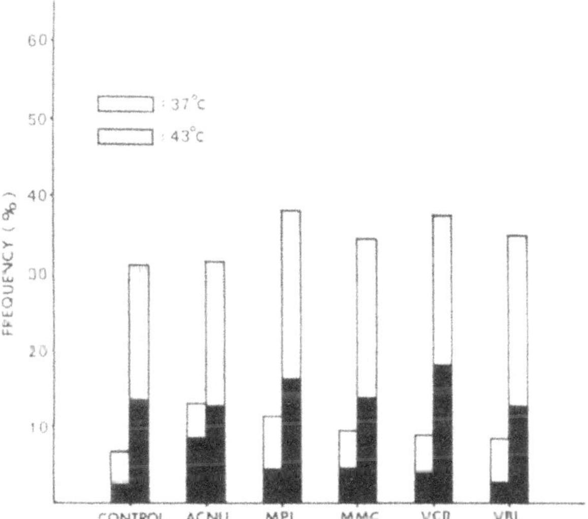

Fig. 3. The frequency of nuclear changes in case no. 1, renal carcinoma. This case reveals a high sensitivity to 43° C. The effect of melphalan and vincristine were significantly enhanced by 43° C. *Abbreviations* as in Table 1

Antitumor drugs in combination with hyperthermia at 43° C showed no significant differences as compared with hyperthermia alone. The renal carcinoma shown in Fig. 3, case no. 1, is an example of high sensitivity to hyperthermia at 43° C alone. Such hyperthermia produced karyorrhectic changes in about 14% of nuclei. However, at 37° C only 3% of nuclei developed karyorrhectic changes. The effects of melphalan and vincristine were significantly enhanced by hyperthermia at 43° C. Table 2 shows the summarized results of the in vitro sensitivity tests. Taking one example, in case no. 1, a renal carcinoma, nimustine proved effective at 37° C but there was no thermal enhancement at 43° C; on the other hand, vincristine

Table 2. Details of in vitro sensitivity tests on eight tumors. In each case the symbol on the left shows the results at 37° C, while that within parentheses indicates the results at 43° C. It was noted that in some cases drugs were significantly enhanced hyperthermia at 43° C although results were negative at 37° C

Drug	Case no.							
	1	2	3	4	5	6	7	8
ACNU	+[a] (−)	± (−)	− (−)	− (±)	− (−)	+ (−)	± (−)	− (−)
MPL	±[b] (+)	+ (−)		− (+)	− (−)	± (+)	+ (+)	− (−)
MMC	± (−)	+ (−)	+ (−)	+ (±)	− (−)	− (−)	± (−)	− (±)
VCR	− (+)	+ (−)	− (−)	+ (+)	− (−)	± (±)	± (−)	− (−)
VBL	− (±)	+ (−)	− (−)	+ (±)	− (−)	± (−)	± +)	− (−)

[a] Significantly different from controls in respect of karyorrhectic changes, $P<0.05$.
[b] Significantly different from controls in respect of the other degenerative changes, $P<0.05$.
Abbreviations as in Table 1.

Table 3. Summary of in vitro sensitivity tests. The individual tumors showed varying sensitivity to hyperthermia at 43° C, and thermal enhancement of drug cytotoxicity was also observed in some tumors

	Sensitive to heat (43° C, 1 h)	Drugs synergistically enhanced by heat (43° C, 1 h)
Case 1 (renal carcinoma)	+[a]	<u>MPL</u>,[c], <u>VCR</u>, VBL
Case 2 (leukemia K-562)	+	
Case 3 (malignant melanoma)	−	
Case 4 (malignant melanoma)	+	ACNU, <u>MPL</u>, MMC
Case 5 (malignant melanoma)	−	
Case 6 (malignant melanoma)	+	
Case 7 (lung carcinoma)	±[b]	<u>MPL</u>, <u>VBL</u>
Case 8 (lung carcinoma)	−	MMC

[a] Significantly different from control (37° C) in respect of karyorrhectic changes, $P<0.05$.
[b] Significantly different from control (37° C) in respect of the other degenerative changes, $P<0.05$.
[c] Significantly different from control (43° C) in respect of karyorrhectic changes, $P<0.05$.
Abbreviations as in Table 1. Underlined drug names are those enhanced in an overadditive manner.

showed no effect at 37° C but was significantly enhanced at 43° C. In case no. 5, a malignant melanoma, no response to the drugs used was seen either at 37° C or at 43° C.

Table 3 indicates the final results obtained from in vitro sensitivity tests. Individual tumors showed a different sensitivity to 43° C. The karyorrhectic changes in case no. 1 were significantly enhanced with melphalan as well as with vincristine at 43° C. The other degenerative changes were significantly enhanced with vinblastine. Enhancement of these drug cytotoxicities by 43° C was synergistic in nature.

In this study we observed no thermal enhancement of the drugs used at 43° C in cases 2, 3, 5, and 6. Case no. 2 was sensitive to 43° C without drugs, but thermal enhancement of drug cytotoxicity could not be proven. In case no. 6 we found the most pronounced thermal sensitivity to 43° C without drugs; however, an additive effect was induced only when we used melphalan and 43° C.

Discussion

By means of clonogenic assay using soft agar, attempts have been made to predict clinical response to chemotherapy (von Hoff et al. 1981; Mann et al. 1982). The usefulness of this clonogenic assay has, however, been limited by its low success rate and time factors (it takes 14-21 days to obtain results). Especially its low success rate seems a problem, including the fact that the assay cannot be applied to intestinal cancer contaminated with bacteria. An in vitro predictive assay that is to be performed in a clinical laboratory on a regular basis must aim at a higher success rate.

In this present study a rapid in vitro assay based on morphological changes in the nucleus was developed in order to predict the chemosensitivity of human cancers (Tokita et al. 1982, 1986a). This method has the following advantages: (a) it can be applied to any kind of tumor, including intestinal tumors contaminated with bacteria; (b) the results are obtained within 8 h; and (c) it can be done in a clinical laboratory on a regular basis. A good correlation with clinical response has already been demonstrated in osteosarcomas and ovarian carcinomas (Takamizawa et al. 1985; Tokita et al. 1986b). The ability to predict the response to thermochemotherapy using this simple method based on morphology appears to be a novelty. In the present study, five of the eight tumors tested were proven sensitive to hyperthermia at 43° C by statistical comparison with controls. In four tumors synergistic effects of antitumor agents with hyperthermia at 43° C were observed. Furthermore, it was noted that there was no thermal enhancement of drug cytotoxicity in two tumors despite sensitivity to 43° C. These results seem to suggest strongly that in the clinical application of combinations of antitumor agents and hyperthermia, predictive information is needed regarding thermal enhancement of drug cytotoxicity in individual tumors before treatment is commenced. In this study, alkylating agents were mainly tested because it seemed that morphological changes induced by other antitumor agents such as bleomycin and doxorubicin should be different from karyorrhectic changes. In fact, Tokita et al. (1982) have suggested that antitumor agents, including antimetabolic agents or antibiotic agents, cause karyopyknosis.

We will probably have to establish new criteria for the other antitumor agents in the prediction of response to thermochemotherapy. Evaluation of thermal enhancement of drug cytotoxicity using the present method is based on statistical comparison with controls ($P < 0.05$). We will also have to conduct comparative studies with other methods, e. g., clonogenic assay, to confirm that the parameters used here reliably reflect the response to thermochemotherapy.

Summary

In order to estimate its ability to predict the thermochemosensitivity of human cancers, a rapid in vitro assay based on morphological changes in the nucleus was performed on eight different human tumors (four malignant melanomas, two lung tumors, one renal carcinoma, and leukemia K-562). Nude mice, implanted with tumors, supplied the tumor material, with the exception of leukemia. Nimustine, melphalan, mitomycin C, vincristine and vinblastine were tested.

Tumor cells developed karyorrhectic changes after incubation for 4 h with each of the aforementioned five drugs. An increase in the karyorrhectic changes was observed with hyperthermia at 43° C. The individual tumors showed different sensitivities to 43° C. Five of the eight tumors were significantly sensitive to 43° C. However, in two thermosensitive tumors no drug enhancement was recognized at 43° C. In four tumors several drugs were synergistically enhanced by hyperthermia at 43° C. This study suggests that this simple method may be of clinical use in predicting response to thermochemotherapy.

References

Andrysek O, Bláhová E, Gregora V, Rezný Z (1985) An experimental model for predicting the synergism of hyperthermia with cytostatics. Neoplasma 32: 93-101

Arcangeli G, Cividalli A, Mauro F, Nervi C, Pavin G (1979) Enhanced effectiveness of adriamycin and bleomycin combined with local hyperthermia in neck node metastases from head and neck cancers. Tumori 65: 481-486

Bogden AE, Cobb WR, Lepage DJ, Haskell PM, Gulkin TA, Ward A, Kelton DE, Esber HJ (1981) Chemotherapy responsiveness of human tumors as first transplant generation xenografts in the normal mouse: six day subrenal capsule assay. Cancer 48: 10-20

Griffin TW, Bogden AE, Reich SD, Antonelli D, Hunter RE, Ward A, Yu DT, Greene HL, Costanza ME (1983) Initial clinical trial of the subrenal capsule assay as a predictor of tumor response to chemotherapy. Cancer 52: 2185-2192

Gross P, Parsons PG (1977) The effect of hyperthermia and melphalan on survival of human fibroblast strains and melanoma cell lines. Cancer Res 37: 152-156

Hahn GM (1975) Thermochemotherapy: synergism between hyperthermia (42°-43° C) and adriamycin (or bleomycin) in mammalian cell inactivation. Proc Natl Acad Sci USA 72: 937-940

Levi FA, Blum JP, Lemaigre G, Bourut C, Reinberg A, Mathe G (1984) A four-day subrenal capsule assay for testing the effectiveness of anticancer drugs against human tumors. Cancer Res 44: 2660-2667

Mann BD, Kern DH, Giuliano AE, Burk MW, Campbell MA, Morton DL (1982) Clinical correlation with drug sensitivity in the clonogenic assay. Retrospective pilot study. Arch Surg 117: 33-36

Mann BD, Storm FK, Morton DL, Bertelsen CA, Korn EL, Kaise LR, Kern DH (1983) Predictability of response to clinical thermochemotherapy by the clonogenic assay. Cancer 52: 1389-1394

Marmor JB (1979) Interaction of hyperthermia and chemotherapy in animals. Cancer Res 39: 2269-2276

Mizuno S, Amagi M, Ishida A (1980) Synergistic cell killing by antitumor agents and hyperthermia in culture cells. Gann 71: 471-478

Neumann HA, Fiebig HH, Löhr GW, Engelhardt R (1985) Effect of cytostatic drugs and 40.5° C hyperthermia on human clonogenic tumor cells. Eur J Cancer Clin Oncol 21: 515-523

Salmon SE, Hamburger AW, Soehlnen B, Durie BG, Albert D, Moon TE (1978) Quantitation of differential sensitivity of human tumor stem cells to antitumor drugs. N Engl J Med 298: 1321-1327

Stehlin JS, Giovanella BC, Ipolyi PD (1975) Results of hyperthermia perfusion for melanoma of the extremities. Surg Gynecol Obstet 149: 17-21

Storm FK, Silberman AW, Ramming KR, Kaise LR, Harrison WH, Elliot RS, Haskel CM, Sarna G, Morton DL (1984) Clinical thermochemotherapy: a control trial in advanced cancer patients. Cancer 53: 863-868

Takamizawa H, Sekiya S, Iwasawa H, Ishige H, Tokita H, Tanaka N (1985) A new in vitro chemosensitivity test: individualized chemotherapy against ovarian cancer and its clinical effect. Gan To Kagaku Ryoho 12: 2293-2297

Tokita H, Tanaka N, Ueno T (1982) Morphological changes of tumor cells by antitumor drugs - comparison of in vivo and in vitro. Proceedings of the 41st Japanese Cancer Congress, p 263

Tokita H, Tanaka N, Fugimoto S, Nakao K (1986a) The in vitro cytotoxic test for predicting human colon and rectum cancer chemosensitivity. Med Biol 112: 171-175

Tokita H, Tanaka N, Ueno T, Fujimoto S, Nakao K, Takada N, Takamizawa H (1986b) In vitro cytotoxic test for predicting human cancer chemosensitivity. The 14th International Cancer Congress, No 3883 PP 1009 (abstr) Budapest, Hungary

Twentyman PR, Morgan JE, Donaldson J (1980) Enhancement by hyperthemia of the effect of BCNU against the EMT 6 mouse tumor. Cancer Treat Rep 64: 439-443

von Hoff DD, Casper J, Bradley E, Sandbach J, Jones D, Makuch R (1981) Association between human tumor colony-forming assays results and response of an individual patient's tumor to chemotherapy. Am J Med 70: 1027-1032

Yamada K, Someya T, Shimada S, Nakagawa H, Kukita A, Tokita H, Tanaka N (1985) Thermochemotherapy for malignant melanoma: overcoming heterogeneity in drug sensitivity. J Invest Dermatol 85; 43-64

Subject Index

Recent Results in Cancer Research

Volume 100: Therapeutic Strategies in Primary and Metastatic Liver Cancer
Edited by Ch. Herfarth, P. Schlag, P. Hohenberger
1986. 163 figures, 104 tables. ISBN 3-540-16011-6

Volume 101: Locoregional High-Frequency Hyperthermia and Temperature Measurement
Edited by G. Bruggmoser, W. Hinkelbein, R. Engelhardt, M. Wannenmacher
1986. 96 figures, 8 tables. IX, 143. ISBN 3-540-15501-5

Volume 102: Epidemiology of Malignant Melanoma
Edited by R. P. Gallagher
1986. 15 figures, 70 tables. IX, 169. ISBN 3-540-16020-5

Volume 103: Preoperative (Neoadjuvant) Chemotherapy
Edited by J. Ragaz, P. R. Band, J. H. Goldie
1986. 58 figures, 49 tables. IX, 162. ISBN 3-540-16129-5

Volume 104: Hyperthermia and the Therapy of Malignant Tumors
Edited by C. Streffer
1987. 52 figures, 63 tables. IX, 207. ISBN 3-540-17250-5

Volume 105: Breast Cancer
Edited by S. Brünner and B. Langfeldt
1987. 59 figures, 43 tables. IX, 132. ISBN 3-540-17301-3

Volume 106: Minimal Neoplasia
Edited by E. Grundmann and L. Beck
1988. 82 figures, 61 tables. IX, 194. ISBN 3-540-18455-4

Volume 107: Application of Hyperthermia in the Treatment of Cancer
Edited by R. D. Issels and W. Wilmanns
1988. 118 figures, 56 tables. XII, 277. ISBN 3-540-18486-4

Volume 108: Supportive Care in Cancer Patients
Edited by H.-J. Senn and L. Schmid
1988. 60 figures, 97 tables. XII, 342. ISBN 3-540-17150-9

GPSR Compliance
The European Union's (EU) General Product Safety Regulation (GPSR) is a set of rules that requires consumer products to be safe and our obligations to ensure this.

If you have any concerns about our products, you can contact us on

ProductSafety@springernature.com

In case Publisher is established outside the EU, the EU authorized representative is:

Springer Nature Customer Service Center GmbH
Europaplatz 3
69115 Heidelberg, Germany

www.ingramcontent.com/pod-product-compliance
Ingram Content Group UK Ltd.
Pitfield, Milton Keynes, MK11 3LW, UK
UKHW061656190726
13853UKWH00008B/2235
9783642832642